T0255725

POCKET GUIDE
to
INTERVENTION
in Occupational Therapy

❂❂❂

Second Edition

POCKET GUIDE

to

INTERVENTION

in Occupational Therapy

◐◉◑

Second Edition

Franklin Stein, PhD, OTR/L, FAOTA
Professor Emeritus, Department of Occupational Therapy
University of South Dakota
Vermillion, South Dakota
Editor, Annals of International Occupational Therapy

Kristine Haertl, PhD, OTR/L, FAOTA
Professor, Department of Occupational Therapy
St. Catherine University
St. Paul, Minnesota

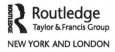

Routledge
Taylor & Francis Group

NEW YORK AND LONDON

First published in 2019 by SLACK Incorporated

Published 2024 by Routledge
605 Third Avenue, New York, NY 10158

and by Routledge
4 Park Square, Milton Park, Abingdon, Oxon OX14 4RN

Routledge is an imprint of the Taylor & Francis Group, an informa business

© 2019 by Taylor & Francis Group

Dr. Franklin Stein and *Dr. Kristine Haertl* have no financial or proprietary interest in the materials presented herein.

Trademark notice: Product or corporate names may be trademarks or registered trademarks, and are used only for identification and explanation without intent to infringe.

Cover Artist: Justin Dalton

Library of Congress Cataloging-in-Publication Data

Names: Stein, Franklin, author. | Haertl, Kristine, author.
Title: Pocket guide to intervention in occupational therapy / Franklin Stein, Kristine Haertl.
Other titles: Pocketguide to treatment in occupational therapy
Description: Second edition. | Thorofare, NJ : Slack Incorporated, 2019. | Preceded by Pocketguide to treatment in occupational therapy / Franklin Stein, Becky Roose. c2000. | Includes bibliographical references and index.
Identifiers: LCCN 2019010044 (print) | ISBN 9781630915681 (paperback : alk. paper)
Subjects: | MESH: Occupational Therapy | Handbook
Classification: LCC RM735.3 (print) | NLM WB 39 | DDC 615.8/515--dc23
LC record available at https://lccn.loc.gov/2019010044

ISBN: 9781630915681 (pbk)
ISBN: 9781003525783 (ebk)

DOI: 10.4324/9781003525783

Dedication

The book is dedicated to my wife Jennie, and my adult children David, Jessie, and Barbara, who have provided the love and support to my life career.
—FS

I dedicate the book to my dear friends Charles Christiansen, Liz Townsend, Frank Stein, Judith Reisman, Rhoda Erhardt, and in memory of Joy Huss. You each have mentored so many and have paved the way for occupational therapy. I also dedicate this book to my current and former students—you are the future of occupational therapy!
—KH

Contents

Major Terms and Interventions

Acknowledgments

Special thanks to content reviewers Barbara Plato, James McPherson, Brenda Frie, Traci Kruse, Kyle Miklik, and Paula Rabaey.

Special thanks to contributing authors Brenda Frie and Rhoda Erhardt to the current book and to Becky Roose for contributing to the previous edition of this book.

About the Authors

Franklin Stein, PhD, OTR/L, FAOTA is currently Professor Emeritus of Occupational Therapy at the University of South Dakota in Vermillion, founding editor of *Annals of International Occupational Therapy*, and life member of the American Psychological Association. Previously, he was the Director of the School of Medical Rehabilitation at the University of Manitoba in Winnipeg, Canada, Director of the Occupational Therapy Program at the University of Wisconsin, Milwaukee, and Associate Professor, Graduate Division at Sargent College, Boston, Massachusetts. He is the first author of the textbook *Clinical Research in Occupational Therapy, Fifth Edition* (2013) with Martin Rice and Susan Cutler; *Occupational Therapy and Ergonomics* (2006) with Ingrid Soderback, Susan Cutler, and Barbara Larson; *Psychosocial Occupational Therapy: A Holistic Approach, Second Edition* (2002) with Susan Cutler; *Pocket Guide to Treatment in Occupational Therapy* (2000) with Becky Roose; and *Stress Management Questionnaire* (2003), plus over 50 publications in journals and books related to rehabilitation and psychosocial research. He has also presented more than 100 seminars, workshops, institutes, short courses, and research papers at national and international conferences.

Kristine Haertl, PhD, OTR/L, FAOTA is a professor in the Department of Occupational Therapy at St. Catherine University in St. Paul, Minnesota. She is an academician and practitioner in the areas of developmental disabilities, psychiatric practice, and occupational science. Dr. Haertl has been active in mental health research related to peer-supported mental health housing models and exploration of the nature and efficacy of services at a freestanding psychiatric occupational therapy clinic. Her research has led to legislative changes regarding evidenced-based mental health practice in Minnesota and has helped secure funding for the development of Fairweather housing units in Pennsylvania. In addition to full-time faculty work, Dr. Haertl has served as the chairperson of a large mental health board in Minnesota and maintains a private practice, serving persons with psychiatric disorders and developmental disabilities. She has over 50 academic publications including her book, *Adults With Intellectual and Developmental Disabilities: Strategies for Occupational Therapy* (2014), and over 100 presentations nationally and internationally. She has received a number of awards in areas related to fitness, occupational therapy, and mental health service.

Preface

The second edition of the *Pocket Guide* builds upon the strengths of the first edition as a useful quick reference to occupational therapy terms and interventions regarding specific diagnoses and conditions. It is geared for students, occupational therapy clinicians, and occupational therapists returning to work.

In this revised edition, we have changed the title of the book from *Pocket Guide to Treatment in Occupational Therapy* to *Pocket Guide to Intervention in Occupational Therapy*. The occupational therapy profession has undergone enormous changes in the last two decades. Occupational therapy has become an evidence-based health care profession that uses scientifically based research to justify clinical practice. Interventions in hospitals, clinics, and community and school settings are continually evolving based on scientific evidence. The reason we chose the word *intervention* rather than *treatment* is that intervention is a more general term than treatment and it encompasses nonmedical techniques such as client health education or counseling, instruction in activities of daily living, modifying of the environment such as in ergonomics, teaching and demonstrating arts and crafts as therapeutic activities, and providing sensory enriching activities, especially for children. These interventions are intended to prevent injury and maintain or improve client function. On the other hand, treatment in occupational therapy is more limited in scope to the management and care of a patient with a disease or disorder.

The term *intervention* is also consistent with the *Occupational Therapy Practice Framework: Domain and Process, Third Edition* (American Occupational Therapy Association, 2014), which identifies the intervention process as a skilled service provided by occupational therapists in collaboration with clients for the purposes of facilitating engagement in "occupation related to health, well-being, and participation" (p. S14). Within the intervention process, a plan is developed, implemented, reviewed, and revised as needed.

Intervention approaches identified by the *Framework* include the following: 1) *Create/Promote* is an approach that may be used with all populations, regardless of whether or not there is a disability; 2) *Establish/Restore* is an approach designed to fix or treat the underlying issue, such as working with a person in acute stages of brain injury under the assumption that the brain is plastic and can heal; 3) *Maintain* is an approach used to continue existing function and prevent a decrease in function; 4) *Modify* is an approach that uses compensation and adaptation to facilitate occupational performance; and 5) *Prevent* is an approach that seeks to prevent disability and often is used for at-risk populations. Therapists use clinical reasoning to determine the best intervention approach, utilizing client-centered care and a collaborative approach.

We perceive the occupational therapist to assume a variety of roles, such as a healer, who may work with an individual with clinical depression or post-traumatic stress disorder; a teacher, such as when the occupational therapist teaches a mother on how to help her child with cerebral palsy become independent in activities of daily living; or an ergonomist, who helps introduce adaptive equipment such as grab bars in the bathroom for an individual who has had a stroke and kitchen aids for people with cognitive disorders.

New terms and interventions have been added to the *Pocket Guide* to reflect current practice. Practicing occupational therapists working in acute care settings, home health environments, schools, and outpatient clinics have been helpful in reviewing and updating the book's contents.

With this in mind, we want to maintain the recognized qualities of the *Pocket Guide* as a practical resource in selecting occupational therapy interventions for specific diagnoses and its pocket size so it is readily available for use in field work and in a clinical setting and as resource in planning and designing interventions.

The main purpose of this *Pocket Guide*, as originally stated, is to enable students and clinicians to have a quick reference for planning intervention strategies. The interventions suggested are pragmatic and are meant to be user friendly. They can serve as an initial step in planning an intervention strategy. However, good treatment is evidence-based, supported by clinical research. The interventions suggested are based on the authors' experiences as university professors, as occupational therapy practitioners, in carrying out clinical research, and through extensive reading in occupational therapy and medical research studies. In using this *Pocket Guide*, it is important that the reader understand what a good intervention strategy is:

1. It is individually planned to meet the needs and interests of the client. This implies that the therapist in conjunction with the client plan a strategy that is client-centered, collaborative, and in sync with the treatment team.

2. Interventions should be holistic, taking into consideration the biopsychosocial factors that affect function. For example, the hand therapist also considers the psychological and social aspects of a client's disability, and the psychosocial occupational therapist considers the client's physical functions.

3. The client is assessed before and after intervention. This implies that the therapist will establish a baseline of function, implement the intervention strategy, and then reassess function.

4. The intervention method should be operationally defined so that the strategies can be easily identified and replicated by other therapists. Intervention protocols can be established by the therapist and individualized to meet the needs of the client. Interventions should not be a cookbook formula, yet there should be structure and guidelines.

5. The effects of the interventions should be continuously reevaluated by the therapist, client, family, teacher, and interested others to determine whether they should be continued, changed, or discontinued.

6. Interventions should be theory- and evidenced-based, yet may also be eclectic, meaning that the frames of reference or theories generating treatment are selected to meet the functional goals of the client. For example, client-centered, biomechanical, psychosocial, cognitive behavioral, occupational performance, and developmental frames of reference can all be applied to the same client.

7. Interventions should be evidence-based and supported by research findings. Good treatment can be substantiated by explaining to the client how and why the intervention works.

8. It is acknowledged that in the 21st century, prevention and health and wellness are the cornerstones of good health care. Occupational therapists promote these concepts in everyday practice.

How the Pocket Guide *Is Organized*

The *Pocket Guide* is organized around the major conditions that occupational therapists encounter in their everyday practice. These include physical, psychosocial, cognitive, geriatric, and pediatric diagnoses. Intervention guidelines are outlined for the major disabilities. In addition, there are brief descriptions of the intervention techniques that therapists use and definitions of terms that are relevant to interventions, such as **abduction** in relation to anatomical position and movement, and **positive symptoms** in schizophrenia.

Each main entry is printed in bold. Each cross-referenced entry is underlined. Each main entry disorder is listed alphabetically, with subcategories of a given disorder described under the main entry.

Specific techniques, most applicable across disorders, also are alphabetized and described at their main alphabet entry. When appropriate, the reader is also referred to the conditions for which the technique is appropriate.

The appendices include an outline of essential skills for occupational therapists, general developmental guidelines, an overview of muscles and movements, orthotic devices, tables of muscles, average range of motion measurements, prime movers for upper and selected lower extremity motions, and substitutions for muscle contractions.

A

Abduction. To move a body part away from the midline. See <u>Anatomical position</u>.

Abstract Thought Process. The ability to conceptualize thoughts based on situations that are not currently present. Such thinking enables an individual to generalize from one situation to a similar situation; for instance, an individual with the ability to transfer cooking skills from a gas to an electric stove. Persons with developmental conditions such as <u>Autism</u>, certain psychiatric conditions such as <u>Schizophrenia</u>, and those with brain injuries may have difficulty with abstraction.

Acquired Brain Injury. Brain injury that results in events post-birth as opposed to genetically or in utero. Generally, it does not include brain insult from neurological conditions, but may include injuries from brain tumors, stroke, brain bleeds, and substance abuse. See <u>Traumatic brain injury</u>.

Active Assistive Range of Motion (A/AROM). The therapist gently assists the client in moving a joint. See <u>Range of motion (ROM)</u>.

Active Range of Motion (AROM). A client moves a joint without assistance. See <u>Range of motion (ROM)</u>.

Activities of Daily Living (ADLs). Everyday activities that are essential for self-care. The *Framework* (American Occupational Therapy Association, 2014) lists specific ADLs to include bathing, showering, toileting, dressing, eating, feeding, functional mobility, personal device care, hygiene and grooming, and sexual activity. See <u>Assistive technology</u>, <u>Self-care</u>, and specific diagnoses/conditions for further discussion and treatment.

Activity Analysis. The systematic process of determining the typical steps, components, and demands of an activity. The process involves consideration of body structures, functions, performance skills, and performance patterns required of the task (American Occupational

Stein, F., & Haertl, K.
Pocket Guide to Intervention in Occupational Therapy, Second Edition (pp 1-34).
© 2019 Taylor & Francis Group.

Therapy Association, 2014). When a client works toward goals, appropriate therapeutic activities are used to improve the individual's functions. Activities are chosen to address multiple performance demands while the client completes the task (e.g., a client who is completing wood sanding on an incline can increase <u>Active range of motion (AROM)</u>, muscle strength, and kinesthetic awareness). The activity can also be used to address visual field cuts/neglect, coordination, position in space, and proprioception. The analysis of an activity not only assists the therapist in choosing activities based on goals, but also helps avoid activities that may be contraindicated or adapt preferential activities that the client enjoys. The activity analysis should look at all areas of function, including sensorimotor, physical, cognitive, social, and psychosocial factors. The significance and meaning of a task to an individual are considered, along with the sequential steps necessary to complete the task. The task should be amendable to adaptation and grading so that it may be modified according to the client's progress toward goals.

Activity Group Therapy. Originally developed by Samuel Slavson (1943) to treat children with behavioral disorders and later expanded on in occupational therapy by Ann Cronin Mosey (1973), activities therapy is aimed at helping the client develop functional skills and inner controls. Mosey identified types of groups to include evaluation groups, task-oriented groups, developmental groups, thematic groups, topical groups, and instrumental groups. Tasks and creative media are often used, including clay, art media, blocks, and skill building tasks.

Acupuncture. An ancient Chinese treatment based on the concept that vital energy (ch'i) is a life force that circulates through meridians, similar to blood vessels or neuronal pathways. Practitioners insert needles into identified meridians for health benefits and pain relief. Recent research demonstrates positive benefits. Practitioners of acupuncture need to be trained in the practice; many states and countries have specific guidelines for licensure or certification. See Taylor, Pezzullo, Grant, and Bensoussan (2014) on cost-effectiveness for chronic <u>Low back pain (LBP)</u>.

Adaptation. The adjustment of a person to his or her environment as a reaction to a stressor or environmental demand. Such adaptation may be at the person level or environmental level. An individual may have to adapt to a new routine or disabling condition through psychological as well as physical adaptation. Therapists may help this process by providing adaptive equipment (e.g., a sock aid or built-up spoon), or may guide environmental adaptation such as use of ramps or <u>Assistive technology</u> in order to increase function in areas such as <u>Activities of daily living (ADLs)</u>, <u>Instrumental activities of daily living (IADLs)</u>, <u>Work</u>, and <u>Leisure</u>.

Adaptive Equipment. Devices that have been adapted to help a client complete a Self-care, Work, Leisure, Activities of daily living (ADLs), Instrumental activities of daily living (IADLs), or educational activity with increased independence and occupational performance. See Assistive technology and Self-care for further application during occupational therapy intervention.

Adaptive Skills. Practical life skills and behaviors necessary for everyday living. Such skills are required in daily life and when an individual acquires a condition or injury, such as when an individual with a brain injury uses mnemonic devices to remember people's names or a journal and calendar to remember daily obligations.

Addiction. A chronic disease of the brain resulting in compulsive use, most often of a harmful habit-forming substance. According to the American Society of Addiction Medicine (2017), genetic factors account for about one-half of all addicting behaviors, and other biopsychosocial factors contribute to the rest. Various psychosocial interventions such as Cognitive behavioral therapy and other individual and group therapies have been shown effective for addictions, including opioid addictions (Dugosh et al., 2016). In addition to cognitive behavioral techniques, therapists often use approaches using the Model of Human Occupation (MOHO) and consideration of life balance and time use, expressive techniques, and motivational interviewing techniques exploring readiness for change.

Adduction. To move a body part toward the midline. See Anatomical position.

Adhesions. Fibrous bands that connect body structures or tissues that are not normally connected. Therapists may use the term *adhesions* to refer to scar tissue that forms in collagen "clumps" and may adhere to structures such as tendons, bones, or skin. Adhesions may restrict movement and cause pain. See Hand injuries for further discussion.

Specific Interventions

- Special types of soft tissue massage, including Myofascial release
- Rehabilitation after operative surgery for adhesions
- Topical scar pads and treatments to reduce the effect of adhesions
- Stretching and prescribed exercise aimed at reducing adhesions
- Functional tasks to return to meaningful daily occupations

ADLs. Popular acronym for Activities of daily living.

Adult Day Care. Nonresidential setting that provides supervised social, recreational, nutritional, and health-related services for clients with cognitive, emotional, and physical conditions. Individuals with <u>Alzheimer's disease</u> and other neurocognitive conditions may benefit from adult day care. The service also provides respite for caregivers.

Aerobic Exercise. Repetitive movement/exercise that pumps oxygenated blood to the heart and vascular system. The heart and breathing rate are sustained such that exercise may occur for an extended period, such as what occurs in walking, running, biking, dancing, and swimming. Aerobic exercise is necessary for overall health and has been shown to benefit a number of conditions such as <u>Depression</u>, <u>Anxiety</u>, and heart conditions. Recent research also demonstrates the benefits of exercise for those with cognitive conditions. Health professionals recommend a minimum of 30 minutes of moderate exercise per day.

Affect. The observable mood of an individual such as happy, sad, depressed, angry, anxious, etc. Disorders of affect include <u>Depression</u>, <u>Bipolar disorder</u>, and those experiencing mania. Some individuals with psychiatric conditions, such as persons with <u>Schizophrenia</u>, may display a *flat affect* that is devoid of emotion. Intervention for mood disorders that result in an altered affect may include creative expression, skill training, <u>Stress management</u>, <u>Coping skills</u>, <u>Relaxation therapy</u>, <u>Biofeedback</u>, and expressive art-based modalities.

After-Care Clinic. A state or locally funded agency that is often the extension of hospital services in order to provide transition to the community. Services may include case management, supervision of medication, counseling/psychotherapy, vocational placement, occupational therapy, and other rehabilitative services. Clients with cognitive issues, as well as those with chronic mental health conditions and substance abuse, may benefit from this service.

Agnosia. Inability to interpret sensory information. See <u>Cognitive-perceptual deficits</u> for intervention ideas.

Agonist. Muscle(s) that serves as the prime mover for a motion. For instance, in elbow flexion, the agonists are the biceps (along with the brachialis and the brachioradialis). See also <u>Prime mover</u>.

Agraphesthesia. The inability to identify letters, numbers, or symbols that are traced on the skin while vision is occluded. See <u>Cognitive-perceptual deficits</u> for treatment of perceptual deficits.

Agraphia. The inability to write.

Airplane Orthosis. A padded splint (orthosis) designed to prevent limitation in shoulder abduction range of motion (ROM). The client's upper extremity is usually positioned near 90 degrees of shoulder and horizontal abduction. Clients who have had burns and skin grafts of the upper extremity may benefit from this splint. See <u>Splints/orthoses</u> for additional examples of types of splints and conditions treated.

Akinesia. Difficulty with the initiation of voluntary movement. Akinesia may be caused by a number of factors, including coma, brain injury, basal ganglia lesions, and paralysis. Clients with Parkinson's disease often have accompanying akinesia. See <u>Parkinson's disease</u> for further discussion.

Alexander Technique. A technique developed by Australian actor Frederick Matthias Alexander in order to reduce tension in the body and correct postural alignment of the head, neck, and spine through the way we move. The technique is designed to facilitate conscious movements, reduce tension, and minimize fatigue. Therapists are certified in this technique to help clients improve movement patterns through hands-on guidance. Following observation of breathing and movement patterns, recommendations are made to develop healthy movement patterns into everyday activities. Anecdotal evidence claims that it is effective in relieving tension headaches, neck and back pain, and muscle spasms. The technique may be useful for individuals with backache, stiff neck, <u>Repetitive strain injury</u>, and certain neurological conditions.

Alexia. The inability to read.

Alternative Medicine (also referred to as *Complementary and Alternative Medicine*). Techniques and interventions that are not usually taught in medical schools and are used in place of conventional medicine. Examples are <u>Acupuncture</u>, <u>Ayurveda</u> (Indian medicine), traditional Chinese medicine, and <u>Naturopathy</u>.

Alzheimer's Disease. A chronic, progressive disorder that most often occurs in people over 65 years of age. Within the DSM-5 (American Psychiatric Association, 2013) Alzheimer's disease is characterized as a neurocognitive disorder marked by decline of learning, memory, and cognition with no evidence of other causes such as <u>Cerebrovascular accident (CVA)</u> or neurological disease. It is accompanied by a degeneration of the cerebral cortex and other areas of the brain, which results in impairment of cognitive functions. The cause is unknown. It is characterized by memory loss, personality deterioration, confusion, disorganization, language distortions, sleep and eating disturbances, and difficulties with <u>Self-care</u> functions. A systematic review by Rao, Chou, Bursley, Smulofsky, and Jezequel (2014) found that occupational therapy that includes aerobic and strength training may help improve performance in <u>Activities of daily living (ADLs)</u>. Individuals with Alzheimer's disease can benefit from occupation-based interventions such as music programs, sensory stimulation, outdoor walking, arts and crafts, and <u>Pet therapy</u> in addition to occupation-focused programs to maximize current function and adapt for cognitive and functional loss. Environmental modification, family psychoeducation, and work with caregivers are often included.

Specific Interventions

- Maintain mobility through exercise and environmental adaptation.
- Utilize gross motor activities for exercise and leisure when fine motor activities become difficult.
- Fabricate orthoses to prevent contractures or deformity if weak antagonist muscles are unable to oppose strong agonist muscles.
- Maintain balance through reaching activities.
- Teach compensation techniques for memory loss such as a daily written schedule, notebook, calendar, list, use of familiar electronic devices, or map.
- Utilize cognitive techniques aimed to capitalize on existing cognitive function.
- Give simple directions (without talking down to the individual) for tasks to increase the client's ability to follow verbal commands.
- Provide orientation to person, place, time, and situation with a written orientation board, daily reminders, and other means.
- Increase or maintain the client's self-esteem through the performance of <u>Self-care</u> and <u>Leisure</u> activities.
- Implement the use of routines, schedules, and organized environments to increase the client's independence with activities and reduce <u>Anxiety</u>/fear.
- Complete community outings or involve the client in group therapy/support groups for socialization.
- Educate caregivers on strategies to maintain personal health while offering assistance to the individual with Alzheimer's disease.
- Adapt the home environment to preserve safety and function.

Contraindications/Precautions

- The client is at risk for becoming lost, even in a familiar environment such as the nursing home or neighborhood.
- Work with the team to give the individual realistic expectations regarding the prognosis of the disease and the goals of treatments.

- Avoid environments that may be overstimulating; organize treatment areas to reduce distractions.
- Monitor the client's safety judgment when responding to dangerous situations such as a hot stove or a smoke alarm.
- If a splint has been fabricated, monitor for skin breakdown or decreased circulation.
- Avoid the use of sharp objects if the client is in the final stage of Alzheimer's disease.
- Avoid "talking down" to the individual.

Americans with Disabilities Act (ADA) of 1990 (CPB-101-336). Refers to the civil rights of individuals with disabilities. It is organized into five titles. Title I, Employment, ensures that an individual with a disability who can perform a job with or without reasonable accommodation cannot be discriminated against. Title II, Government nondiscrimination, ensures that individuals with disabilities will have the necessary transportation and access to federal, state, and local public services. Title III, Private business, refers to public accommodations and services operated in the private sector. Title IV, Telecommunication, ensures that individuals with speech and hearing impairments have reasonable accommodation from telephone companies to facilitate communication. Title V refers to complaint procedures and miscellaneous items such as access to federal wilderness areas.

Amputation. Removal of all or part of an extremity that can occur spontaneously through trauma or surgically in order to remove a diseased part of the body (e.g., a client who has diabetes may have sores that will not heal and contain infection; amputation may be required to prevent the spread of infection). Amputation may also be indicated for a client who has peripheral vascular disease. Amputation is completed at a level on the extremity where the physician feels good wound healing and proper fit for prosthetics can occur.

Specific Interventions

- Use an interdisciplinary approach to facilitate client adaptation to amputation and use of prescribed prosthetics.
- Following surgery, educate the client regarding care of the amputated part, hygiene, maintenance of skin integrity, and how to don and doff the prosthesis.
- Allow the client to use the prosthesis functionally during activities; if upper extremity amputation has occurred, intervention

should begin with the prosthetic extremity assisting the unaffected extremity and progress to use of the extremity in one-handed activities.

- Instruct the client to use the unaffected limb to compensate for motor or sensory loss in the affected limb (e.g., the client should learn to test the temperature of bath water with the left hand, even though the client may have always used the right hand for this activity in the past).
- Teach the client proper care and maintenance of the prosthesis, as well as ensure skin integrity of the amputated body part.
- Desensitize the stump of the affected extremity if the client is hypersensitive and has difficulty wearing the prosthesis.
- Address the emotional adjustment to the loss of the extremity.
- Consider use of a support group, and provide opportunities for socialization.
- Train specific skills required for return to work or leisure activities as needed.
- Explore new interests and aptitudes if the client is unable to return to the previous work or leisure activities.
- Educate the client on assistive devices that can help with Self-care or transfer activities.
- Complete a home evaluation and recommend adaptations to the environment as needed for the client's safety and mobility after returning home.

Contraindications/Precautions

- Teach the client to inspect the skin of the stump to check for breakdown from use of the prosthesis.
- Monitor the prosthesis to ensure that it works correctly.

Amyotrophic Lateral Sclerosis (ALS). A nervous system disorder that affects the upper and lower motor neurons and various tracts of the spinal cord. This disease results in weakness and atrophy of all voluntary muscles except those that control the eye and sphincters. Upper motor neuron involvement results in spasticity and decreased strength, while lower motor neuron involvement results in flaccidity and muscle atrophy. Onset is frequently between 35 and 65 years of age. The cause is unknown. Symptoms often begin distally and asymmetrically, with many clients first noticing weakness in the hands. Upper motor neuron involvement and spasticity occur later in the disease process. Other symptoms include muscle fasciculations, especially in the extremities and tongue; <u>Dysphagia</u>; <u>Dysarthria</u>; hyperactive <u>Deep tendon reflexes</u>; and difficulty with breathing. Death usually occurs from respiratory failure 2 to 5 years after onset of the disease.

Specific Interventions

- Fabricate splints to maintain functional positions in the presence of weak muscles.
- Recommend assistive devices as needed to continue the completion of functional activities.
- As speech diminishes and dysarthria hinders language production, work with the client to find a new form of communication, such as a communication board.
- Adjust the client's diet as needed to reduce chewing or improve swallowing.
- Position the client appropriately, especially during meals for safety in swallowing.
- Complete upper extremity exercises to maintain endurance and range of motion; <u>Aquatic therapy</u> may be particularly useful in this situation.
- Teach <u>Pain management</u> techniques.
- Educate the client on <u>Stress management</u> and <u>Relaxation therapy</u>.
- Train the client to complete activities while using energy conservation and work simplification principles.
- Instruct the client on safe and easy transfer methods.
- Assist the client with emotional adjustment to the disease.
- Explore new leisure activities that are able to be completed as the disease progresses.
- Encourage the client and family members to join a support group.
- Educate the client on assistive devices that can make <u>Self-care</u>, home management, or transfer activities easier.
- If the client is able to continue working, provide recommendations and/or assist with adaptations to the work environment.
- Maintain meaningful occupational engagement throughout the disease progression.
- Address both physical and psychological effects of ALS.

Contraindications/Precautions

- Do not have the client complete resistive exercise, as the course of the disease eventually results in weakness, regardless of strengthening activities; instead, focus on exercise to maintain endurance and range of motion.
- Watch for signs of decreased respiration.
- Avoid fatigue.
- Monitor the purchase of expensive equipment to keep costs down if possible.

Anarithmetria. Difficulty with mathematical problems that is not due to other reading, writing, or spatial deficits. A client with this deficit may have had training and demonstrated sufficient academic mathematical skills in the past.

Anatomical Position. Anatomical position is used as the basis for describing body parts in relation to one another. Anatomical charts include various stances—the most familiar is with the person facing forward, body upright and feet forward toward the observer with arms supinated and hands open. The following are specific anatomical descriptions:

- **Planes.** Four imaginary planes that pass through the body while it is in anatomical position are used to help with relating body parts to one another.
    - **Median Plane.** An imaginary plane that divides the body (or a body part such as the hand or foot) into right and left halves by passing vertically through the body (or body part) from the front to the back.
    - **Sagittal Plane.** An imaginary plane that is parallel to the median plane but does not divide the body into equal halves.
    - **Coronal Plane.** An imaginary plane that divides the body into front and back portions by passing vertically through the body from one side to the other. This plane may also be referred to as the *frontal plane*.
    - **Horizontal Plane.** An imaginary plane that divides the body into upper and lower portions by passing horizontally through the body from one side to the other.

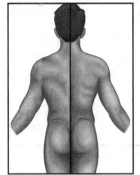
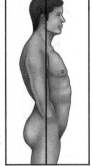
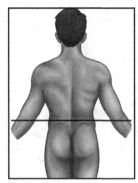

Medial plane.   Coronal plane.   Horizontal plane.

- **Positional Adjectives.** The use of common adjectives helps describe the relationship of body parts to one another.
  - **Superior.** Closer to the person's head. The term *cranial* or *cephalic* may also be used.
  - **Inferior.** Closer to the person's feet. The term *caudal* may also be used.
  - **Anterior.** Closer to the front of the body. The term *ventral* may also be used.
  - **Posterior.** Closer to the back of the body. The term *dorsal* may also be used.
  - **Medial.** Closer to the median plane of the body.
  - **Lateral.** Farther from the median plane of the body.
  - **Proximal.** Closer to the person's trunk or the body part's point of origin.
  - **Distal.** Farther from the person's trunk or the body part's point of origin.
  - **Superficial.** Closer to the surface of the skin.
  - **Deep.** Farther from the surface of the skin.
  - **External.** Closer to the exterior surface of a body part.
  - **Internal.** Closer to the interior surface of a body part.
  - **Central.** Closer to the center of the body or body part.
  - **Peripheral.** Farther from the center of the body or body part.

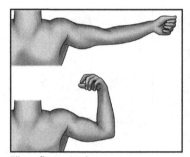

Elbow flexion and extension.

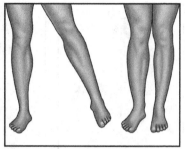

Hip abduction and adduction.

- **Movement Terms.** These terms help describe the movement of a body part at a joint. See <u>Appendices E and F</u> for specific motions and the normal ranges of those motions.
  - ○ **Flexion.** Most often refers to motion at a joint that bends a body part (such as a limb).
  - ○ **Extension.** Most often refers to a motion at a joint that straightens a body part.
  - ○ **Abduction.** A joint motion that moves a body part away from the midline of the body in the coronal plane, except when referring to fingers, toes, or the thumb. When the fingers or toes abduct, they move away from the midline of the hand or foot. The thumb abducts when it moves away from the palm of the hand.
  - ○ **Adduction.** A joint motion that moves a body part toward the midline of the body in the coronal plane, except when referring to fingers, toes, or the thumb. The fingers and toes adduct when they move toward the midline of the hand or foot. When the thumb adducts, it moves toward the palm of the hand.
  - ○ **Horizontal Abduction.** A joint motion at the shoulder that occurs when the shoulder is flexed and results in the arm being pulled away from the midline in the transverse plane.
  - ○ **Horizontal Adduction.** A joint motion at the shoulder that occurs when the shoulder is flexed and results in the arm being pulled toward the midline in the transverse plane.
  - ○ **Internal Rotation.** Also referred to as *medial rotation*. A joint motion that turns the anterior surface of a body part medially, or toward the midline of the body, in the transverse plane.

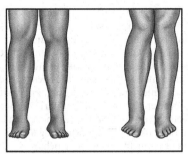

Inversion and eversion.

- ○ **External Rotation.** Also referred to as *lateral rotation*. A joint motion that turns the anterior surface of a body part laterally, or away from the midline of the body, in the transverse plane.

- ○ **Supination.** Rotation of the forearm or foot medially in the coronal plane so that the palm of the hand or the sole of the foot is facing upward/inward.

- ○ **Pronation.** Rotation of the forearm or foot laterally in the coronal plane so that the palm of the hand or the sole of the foot is facing downward/outward.

- ○ **Inversion.** A motion of the foot that combines supination with adduction of the front of the foot.

- ○ **Eversion.** A motion of the foot that combines pronation with abduction of the front of the foot.

- ○ **Circumduction.** A joint motion that moves a body part in a circular motion that results from a combination of flexion, extension, abduction, adduction, and rotation.

Ankylosis. A fixated or stiffened joint often caused by an abnormal bony or fibrous union resulting from disease or injury.

Anomia. A type of aphasia that causes difficulty with recalling the names of everyday items. See also <u>Aphasia</u>.

Anomic Aphasia. See <u>Aphasia</u>.

Anorexia Nervosa. Sometimes referred to only as *anorexia*, this is an eating disorder most prevalent in females in their teens and early twenties. Anorexia has the highest mortality rate of all psychiatric disorders, often due to the unstable medical condition caused by severe deprivation of food intake. The disorder is characterized by distorted body image and fear of becoming overweight or obese. Often, the condition begins with dieting that later becomes excessive and regimented. The disorder results in emaciation, amenorrhea, poor body disturbance, and, in extreme form, may cause organ failure. Anorexia often has comorbid conditions such as Anxiety, Depression, and substance abuse or Addiction. Initial intervention approaches are aimed at stabilizing the client's medical condition. In conjunction with the interventions listed later, in a systematic review and meta-analysis, Couturier, Kimber, and Szatmari (2013) found family-based treatment was as effective as individual treatment for adolescents with eating disorders and had positive effects extending 6 to 12 months post-therapy. Interventions often include Cognitive behavioral therapy, Dialectical behavioral therapy (DBT), Prescriptive exercise (or controlled exercise so as not to encourage addictive exercise), Creative arts, expressive therapy, Music therapy, Psychoeducational groups, and Stress management.

Anosognosia. Inability to know one is ill (e.g., difficulty knowing one has hemiplegia following a lesion). Additional information can be found in Cognitive-perceptual deficits.

Anoxia. The lack of oxygen to a part of the body, which may be caused by asphyxia, disease, or in utero. Often, anoxia results in lightheadedness and dizziness and, if serious, may cause permanent damage, particularly to the brain.

Antagonist. A muscle that completes the motion opposite to the desired motion (e.g., if the desired motion is elbow flexion, then the antagonist to elbow flexion is the triceps, which completes active extension).

Anterior. Anatomical position toward the front of the body. See Anatomical position.

Antisocial Personality Disorder. A personality disorder identified in the DSM-5 (American Psychiatric Association, 2013) as characterized by a disregard for and violation of the rights of others occurring since 15 years of age. Behaviors may include lying, stealing, aggressiveness, substance abuse, criminal activity, and disregard for authority and discipline. The individual lacks moral and ethical standards, lacks empathy toward others, and is unable (or has diminished capacity) to feel guilt. Synonymous terms historically used are *sociopathic* and *psychopathic personality*. According to the National Collaborating Centre for Mental Health (2010), there is a paucity of evidence related to effective intervention in antisocial personality disorder. According to the National Collaborating Centre, the focus for offenders is often on reducing risk of reoffense and developing therapeutic communities. Use of cognitive reasoning and behavioral approaches appear to vary from client to client.

Specific Interventions

- Intervention is aimed at helping the individual to develop inner controls and empathy toward others; response to intervention is highly individual.
- Group treatment has been effective when consensual validation is used to give feedback to the individual.
- Behavior modification and therapeutic communities have had some success in changing individuals with severe acting out.
- There is evidence to suggest some individuals may respond affirmatively to <u>Cognitive behavioral therapy</u>, particularly if there is capacity for insight and empathy.

Anxiety. A feeling of worry, apprehension, uneasiness, and fear of the future or dread. Physiological symptoms such as rapid or disturbed breathing, increased heart rate, increased sweating, hand tremors, dizziness, and possibly confusion may accompany anxiety. Interventions may include <u>Behavior rehearsal</u>, <u>Systematic desensitization</u>, <u>Paradoxical intention</u>, expressive therapy, <u>Creative arts</u>, <u>Music therapy</u>, <u>Cognitive behavioral therapy</u>, <u>Dialectical behavioral therapy (DBT)</u>, and <u>Stress management</u>.

Anxiety Disorders. Exaggerated fears and anxiety that prevent or limit an individual from performing normal activities or behavior. They include <u>Panic disorders</u>, phobias, and stress disorders. While <u>Obsessive compulsive disorder</u> and <u>Post-traumatic stress disorder (PTSD)</u> were categorized as anxiety disorders in the DSM-IV-TR, they are separated out in the DSM-5 (American Psychiatric Association, 2013). Physical symptoms often occur with anxiety disorders such as heart palpitations, sweating, hand tremors, chest pain, shortness of breath, dizziness, and nausea. There is extensive evidence for the use of <u>Cognitive behavioral therapy</u> for anxiety disorders (Kaczkurkin & Foa, 2015). Occupational therapists often pair cognitive behavioral therapy with occupation-based approaches for persons with anxiety disorder.

Specific Interventions

- Cognitive behavioral therapy paired with occupation-based approaches
- <u>Behavioral rehearsal</u>
- <u>Systematic desensitization</u>
- <u>Paradoxical intention</u>
- <u>Creative arts</u>
- <u>Music therapy</u>

- Stress management
- Relaxation therapy
- Biofeedback

Aphasia. A language disorder that causes difficulty understanding or generating language Causes include neurological damage and are manifested in persons with conditions such as Cerebrovascular accident (CVA) or Traumatic brain injury. Some individuals are profoundly affected such that they are unable to express or comprehend language. Intervention for aphasia includes use of communication devices, communication boards, and cognitive retraining programs.

Types of Aphasia

- **Global Aphasia.** Loss of all language skills, including receptive and expressive abilities.
- **Broca's Aphasia.** An expressive aphasia in which an individual is unable to express oneself to others. The individual may understand verbal and written communication but find difficulty in word generation, name recall, writing, and response to complex questions.
- **Wernicke's Aphasia.** A type of receptive aphasia marked by the inability to understand language, particularly auditory communication. The individual is able to express thoughts; however, speech is often rapid and meaningless. The individual may understand single words but have difficulty with complex sentences and reading.
- **Anomia.** Difficulty with word finding that often occurs in aphasia. If this is the only deficit demonstrated by a client, the client is diagnosed with anomic aphasia.
- **Anomic Aphasia.** A condition characterized by the inability to find words for conversation; however, the client does not demonstrate any other symptoms of aphasia.

Aphonia. The inability to produce sound from the larynx.

Approximation. A compression of joint surfaces that facilitates joint receptors and promotes stability, usually during weightbearing, within the framework of proprioceptive neuromuscular facilitation. See Motor control problems and Proprioceptive neuromuscular facilitation (PNF) for more techniques.

Apraxia. A perceptual deficit that hinders clients from completing functional or purposeful movement. The client may have normal sensory, motor, and coordination skills or may suffer apraxia as a result of brain damage. See Cognitive-perceptual deficits for further discussion and treatment.

Types of Apraxia

- **Limb Apraxia.** The inability to execute purposeful movements with the limbs, even though the motor and sensory functions of the limb are intact. Limb apraxia can be further subdivided into ideomotor apraxia and ideational apraxia.
  - ○ **Ideational Apraxia.** The inability to complete purposeful movement during functional activities, usually resulting from difficulty with sequencing.
  - ○ **Ideomotor Apraxia.** The inability to complete purposeful movement on verbal command. A client may be able to complete that same activity spontaneously but is unable to perform under a testing situation.
- **Constructional Apraxia.** The inability to design or construct pictures, images, or three-dimensional objects. It affects the individual's ability to complete purposeful movements that must occur within a specific spatial relationship or design, specifically writing or constructing dimensional objects.
- **Dressing Apraxia.** The inability to perform movements that are necessary to complete dressing, even though motor and sensory functions are intact.

Aptitude. The inherent, natural ability of an individual and the underlying capacity to learn or perform in a specific area. Aptitude tests are a measure of abilities in various areas such as mechanical, musical, or artistic capacities. Occupational therapists may also use aptitude tests in <u>Vocational rehabilitation</u> programs.

Aquatic Therapy. The therapeutic use of water, hot or cold, fresh or mineral, for the treatment of physical or psychological disorders. An equivalent term is <u>Hydrotherapy</u>. The properties of water that contribute to the effectiveness include buoyancy, which decreases a body's weight; surface tension; relative density; viscosity; temperature; and hydrostatic pressure, which increases lung capacity and venous circulation. Therapy with water can be used for decreasing pain, cleansing effects, increasing range of motion and muscle strength, increasing cardiac function, increasing respiratory output, as a diuretic, and to create a relaxing or stimulating psychological effect. Aquatic therapy has also been used successfully in increasing self-esteem and social interactions between the parent and the child. Some of the most common disorders treated with aquatic therapy include orthopedic problems, <u>Cerebral palsy (CP)</u>, arthritis, multiple sclerosis, <u>Traumatic brain injury</u>, and stroke. There are also definite implications for use with clients experiencing psychosocial disorders.

AROM. Acronym for <u>Active range of motion</u>.

Aroma Therapy. The use of natural oils in plants to enhance overall health or appearance. Evidence is increasing in this area related to various benefits of specific oils.

Arousal. The physiological state of readiness or stimulation of an individual to act, as in Selye's theory of stress (1993), or in the ability to attend to a task.

Art Therapy. The use of art as a therapeutic tool to provide the opportunity for nonverbal expression, communication, and growth. Art therapy historically was influenced by the psychoanalytic movement. One of the important goals of art therapy is to help the client express feelings. Art therapy may be used for a variety of conditions, including <u>Depression</u>, <u>Anxiety</u>, eating disorders, and phobia and for those who have difficulty with expressing feelings verbally. Art therapy may also be used with children to encourage self-esteem, use of fine motor skills, and feelings expression.

Arthroplasty. The surgical replacement of any or all parts of a joint with manufactured hinges or pieces of bone.

Types of Arthroplasty

Total Hip Arthroplasty

Many surgical approaches may be used; therefore, the therapist must communicate with the physician to know the approach used and the necessary precautions. This will ensure that all soft tissue has healed before motions are completed, which could displace the manufactured pieces of the joint. Individuals who have arthroplasty may have had an injury or have degenerative joint disease or <u>Rheumatoid arthritis</u>. The client generally must follow precautions for 6 to 8 weeks following surgery; however, the physician should be consulted to make sure healing is complete before removing the client's precautions. The client may be limited to no full weightbearing on the hip for several weeks, although the prognosis is individualized based on client factors and the procedure done.

Specific Interventions

- Increase the client's upper extremity strength to improve the client's ability to use assistive devices for ambulation.
- Complete activities to increase endurance, since any length of hospitalization results in a decrease of activity, which may affect endurance.

- Teach <u>Pain management</u> or <u>Relaxation therapy</u> if needed.
- Instruct the client regarding safe transfer methods when transferring into a low chair, bed, toilet, or tub.
- Work with the rehabilitation department to educate on the use of a walker or cane during daily activities.
- Educate the client on relevant hip precautions, depending on the approach used during surgery.
- Train the client to use energy conservation and work simplification techniques during activities.
- Complete a home evaluation as needed, and recommend appropriate equipment to ensure that the client returns to a safe environment.
- Instruct the client on assistive devices that can be used to increase the independence with dressing while observing applicable precautions; devices may include a reacher, dressing stick, sock aid, long-handled shoehorn, elastic shoelaces, or shoe buttons.
- Educate the client on equipment that may be used to complete bathroom activities independently, including grab bars, bath bench, safety frame, and toilet riser.
- Help reorganize the home to prevent the client from bending, kneeling, or reaching above the head.
- Recommend that heavy tasks, such as cleaning and laundry, be completed by others until the client demonstrates safe ambulation.
- Follow standard rehabilitation recommendations for hip recovery and strengthening.

Contraindications/Precautions

- Instruct the client to see the physician if infection occurs anywhere in the body since the site of the hip replacement is at high risk for spread of infection.
- Watch for and manage edema.
- Initial precautions for separate surgical approaches are as follows. (Note: Please follow the surgeon's advice, as individual circumstances and recovery may differ.)
  - Posterior surgical approach:
    - No hip flexion past 80 to 90 degrees
    - No hip adduction past midline

- No internal rotation of the hip; do not pivot on the affected leg
- An abductor pillow should always be placed between the knees when the client is side-lying

○ Anterior surgical approach:
- No external rotation of the hip; do not cross the legs
- No hip adduction past midline
- An abductor pillow should always be placed between the knees when the client is side-lying

○ Transtrochanteric surgical approach:
- No hip flexion past 80 to 90 degrees
- No hip adduction past midline
- An abductor pillow should always be placed between the knees when the client is side-lying
- No full weightbearing on the affected leg
- No internal rotation of the hip
- No active hip abduction

○ Direct lateral surgical approach:
- No hip adduction past midline
- An abductor pillow should always be placed between the knees when the client is side-lying
- No full weightbearing on the affected leg
- No active hip abduction

- Communicate closely with the physician regarding movement and weightbearing precautions as a wrong movement can result in displacement of the joint.

Metacarpophalangeal Joints

Clients who have rheumatoid arthritis may require this intervention. Referenced information in this section comes from Lubahn, Wolfe, and Feldscher (2011).

Arthroplasty Care

- Specific protocols for splinting, range of motion, and strengthening vary with the type of joint implant. Postoperative care protocols are coordinated with the treating physician.
- Postoperative treatment includes wound care, edema control, and scar control.

- Treatment includes joint protection and joint stabilization exercises.
- Care is taken to maintain uninvolved joints and prevent undue stress to the uninvolved extremity to prevent secondary complications.
- General goals for arthroplasty are to increase the functional arc of movement, reduce pain, and reduce joint deformity. During rehabilitation, care must be taken to maintain joint stability and alignment.

Wrist Arthroplasty

- **Splinting.** Treatment typically includes a volar wrist resting splint that positions the wrist in 10 to 20 degrees of extension for 4 to 6 weeks.
- **Range of Motion.** Gentle protected <u>Active range of motion (AROM)</u> is initiated 4 weeks postoperatively. AROM programing is guided with the goal of obtaining approximately 40 degrees active wrist flexion and 60 degrees wrist extension.
- **Functional Use.** Light functional use without resistance is initiated in a brace, progressing to light use out of the brace 4 weeks post-surgery. Light strengthening and resistive use are initiated 8 to 10 weeks postoperatively. Postoperatively, heavy lifting is restricted; protective bracing is recommended for moderate to heavy tasks.

Arthroplasty Metacarpophalangeal Joints

- **Splinting.** Treatment typically includes a night resting metacarpophalangeal (MCP) extension splint and a day dynamic <u>Dorsal splint</u> that is applied 1 to 2 weeks postoperatively. The dynamic splint is fabricated with an extension outrigger that holds MCP joints in neutral position. Care is taken in fabrication of the splint and during exercise to maintain proper joint alignment and prevent lateral stress on the implant. The dynamic splint is maintained until 6 to 8 weeks postsurgery. The night resting MCP extension splint is continued 6 to 12 months postsurgery.
- **Range of Motion.** Gentle protected AROM is initiated postoperatively within the dynamic splint. Hourly AROM is guided within the splint to promote index and middle finger stability (index finger MCP 0/45 degrees flexion, middle finger MCP 0/60) and ring and small finger mobility (ring and small finger MCP 0/70 degrees flexion). To prevent joint stiffness, treatment focuses on isolation of movement flexing the MCP joints, followed by interphalangeal

joint flexion. Care is taken to maintain the full length of intrinsic hand muscles, promote soft tissue mobility, and maintain radial deviation.

- **Functional Use.** The client may begin to use the affected hand for light functional use at 2 to 3 weeks after surgery with the splint on. Light functional use is initiated out of the brace at 6 to 8 weeks postsurgery. The client is educated in joint protection, including prevention of deforming ulnar force during pinch. At 8 weeks postsurgery, graded isometric strengthening is added to the home program.

Arthroplasty Proximal Interphalangeal Joints

Proximal interphalangeal (PIP) arthroplasty may be completed to correct a <u>Boutonniere</u> or <u>Swan neck deformity</u> from arthritis or joint trauma.

- **Splinting.** Treatment typically includes a night resting extension splint and a day dynamic PIP extension splint (or template guided exercise) within 1 week postoperatively. A night resting splint is fabricated with the wrist in 15 degrees extension, MCP at 20 degrees flexion, and IP joints in extension. Care is taken to maintain digital extension and to prevent rotational deformation and lateral stress. The dynamic splint is maintained for 6 to 8 weeks or until the PIP joint is stable enough for light functional use. Nighttime PIP extension splinting is continued on an as-needed basis.
- **Range of Motion.** Guided AROM is typically started, allowing PIP joint range from 0 to 30 degrees flexion within a dynamic splint (or guided template). The splint or template is adjusted weekly to allow a 10-degree increase in active PIP flexion. The goal is functional pain-free pinch and grip with PIP motion 0/75 degrees. The client is monitored closely to make sure full PIP joint extension and joint alignment are maintained.
- **Functional Use.** At 6 to 8 weeks, tendon gliding and graded isometric strengthening is begun. The client is educated in joint protection to avoid hyperextension, rotation, and lateral deforming forces during light functional tasks.

Assertiveness Training. A technique used in skill training, <u>Behavior therapy</u>, and some forms of <u>Cognitive behavioral therapy</u> to assist individuals to become more assertive in their interpersonal relationships and to understand the differences between passive, assertive, and aggressive actions. <u>Role playing</u> and <u>Behavior rehearsal</u> are used in the technique.

Assistive Technology (includes adaptive techniques). A device or system to assist a person with <u>Self-care</u>, work, leisure, and everyday activities. According to Cook and Polgar (2008), technology ranges on a continuum of no technology to high technology. For instance, a picture board would be considered a low-technology device to help with communication, while a Dynavox communication device would be considered high technology. Selection of assistive technology includes consideration of client factors (e.g., physical, psychological, and cognitive factors) along with lifestyle, resources, and daily needs. If possible, a client should try the equipment on a trial basis before purchasing it; this helps ensure that the individual is able to use the assistive technology successfully. In some instances, the client may need to try various types of technology and strategies before the best tool is found to promote maximal occupational performance. The following are practical suggestions for assistive technology. Adaptive techniques are also included in the list because some devices require special techniques or placement of items.

Self-Care Activities

- **Dressing**
    - Types of clothing should be chosen to fit the client's needs, with attention paid to fashion and taste. Specific garments can be used such as pullover or button-down shirts, sweatpants, elasticized pants, or clothes that are a size larger than usual while maintaining clothing style preference.
    - Brassieres with front closures or sports bras that pull over the head may be purchased. The client may also be taught to hook a back-fastening bra in the front and then turn the bra around to the back.
    - A dressing stick, which has a small hook on one end and a larger double hook on the other, helps push and pull clothing off and on the extremities.
    - A reacher can be used to help with dressing, as well as picking items up from the floor if a client who has a hip replacement is unable to bend past 90 degrees.
    - Buttons can be replaced with larger buttons.
    - <u>Buttonhooks</u> can assist a client in buttoning a shirt with one hand.
    - Complex fasteners can be replaced with easier fasteners or with Velcro.
    - Zipper pulls can be attached to enlarge the pull tab of zippers.

- ○ Elastic shoelaces, shoe buttons, or other shoe devices can allow lace-up shoes to be slipped on or tied with one hand.
- ○ Velcro or slip-on shoes may be purchased to eliminate the need for tying shoes.
- ○ Sock aids can be used with or without garter attachments to help don socks or thromboembolic deterrent (TED) hose. To increase the effectiveness of the sock aid, powder may be used on the client's foot to promote sliding of the aid on the foot.
- ○ A long-handled or regular-length shoehorn will help the client pull shoes on.

- **Grooming and Hygiene**
  - ○ A bath chair or bench allows the client to transfer into the tub safely by sitting on the edge of the chair first and then swinging the lower extremities into the tub.
  - ○ A handheld shower will convert a tub only into a shower and prevent a client from using stairs to use an upstairs or downstairs shower. This also assists the client with washing the body and hair.
  - ○ A long-handled bath sponge or brush will assist the individual in reaching the lower extremities or back when bathing if the client has bending precautions or limited range of motion (ROM).
  - ○ A wash mitt aids with weak grasp while bathing.
  - ○ Rubber strips can be placed on the bottom of the tub to prevent slipping.
  - ○ Grab bars, which are installed on the wall (in a stud) or fastened to the edge of the tub, increase the client's ability to stand from the toilet or bath chair.
  - ○ An elevated toilet seat prevents a client with hip precautions from bending past 90 degrees and may help individuals with weak lower extremities. This device also can assist an individual with standing since it will be easier to stand from a taller device than a short toilet seat.
  - ○ A safety frame around the toilet assists the client with standing and also helps prevent falls.
  - ○ A special device can be used to hold toilet paper and help a client with toilet hygiene.
  - ○ Grooming devices can be adapted with extended or built-up handles to increase independence of a client with limited ROM or weak grasp.

- String can be attached to devices to prevent them from falling all the way to the floor if a client has a tendency to drop items.
- Soap with a string attached assists the client who has decreased grasp.
- An electric razor is easier to use, and it also increases the client's safety. If a client is on medication that thins the blood, a regular razor should not be used.
- Spray deodorant is easier for a client with hemiplegia to apply to the noninvolved arm while using the noninvolved hand/arm.
- A brush that attaches to the side of the sink with suction cups can be used for cleaning dentures or to assist a client who has hemiplegia with washing the noninvolved hand.
- Electric toothbrushes may be helpful for those with oral sensitivity. In addition, the use of a toothpaste pump rather than a tube may be more accessible.
- Grooming checklists may help those with cognitive deficits complete the daily hygiene tasks.
- Suction cups may be used to secure fingernail brushes and grooming aids.
- A long-handled skin inspection mirror will be necessary for a client who has paraplegia or quadriplegia to help the client prevent pressure sores.

- **Feeding**
  - Built-up handles can increase the client's ability to hold utensils.
  - Utensils that are curved or bent can be purchased to enable the client to bring the utensil to the mouth if the client demonstrates impaired ROM.
  - Swivel spoons can help the client keep the spoon tipped appropriately to keep food on it if the client has limitations with supination or motor planning.
  - Weighted utensils may help decrease slight to moderate tremors enough to allow the client to feed him- or herself; otherwise, a weight can be placed on the client's arm to slow tremors, but the weight should not be heavy enough to cause fatigue early during the meal.
  - Universal cuffs allow a client with weak grasp to hold utensils.

- ○ A mobile arm support or deltoid aid can be positioned to assist the client with feeding if the client has impaired ROM and/or weakness. The client needs to actively extend the shoulder to lower the device to the plate, but then these devices mechanically assist with shoulder flexion and help remove the effects of gravity on movement.
- ○ Straws can increase the client's independence with drinking if the client is unable to lift or hold a cup.
- ○ Cups with a section cut out will allow the client to tip the cup and drink all the contents if the client is unable to extend the neck and tip the head back. The cut-out area allows clearance of the client's nose while tipping the cup.
- ○ Cups can also have one or two handles if the client demonstrates weakness, and lids can be placed on some cups to prevent spilling if the client has tremors or weakness.
- ○ Scoop dishes, divided dishes, or plate guards provide a rim for the client to scoop food against when attempting to get food on the utensil.
- ○ A nonslip mat or damp dish towel can be used to prevent a plate from sliding away from the client during feeding.

- **Home Management**
  - ○ Built-up grips can be placed on pens and pencils to make writing easier. Other devices that slip on the client's finger(s) can assist a client in holding a pen.
  - ○ Writing aids can be used for those with poor <u>Fine motor coordination</u> or weakness.
  - ○ Paperweights help stabilize writing paper.
  - ○ Computers and communication devices may be used to address both communication difficulties and coordination difficulties with writing.
  - ○ Bookholders allow a client to continue reading if he or she is unable to hold a book.
  - ○ A mouth stick or electric page turner can assist in turning pages for a client who has quadriplegia.
  - ○ Extended levers can be applied to doorknobs.
  - ○ Specialized holders can be attached to telephone receivers, or a voice-activated phone can be installed.
  - ○ Faucets can have extensions mounted to make turning easier.

- When organizing the kitchen cabinets, items that are used most frequently should be placed on the lowest shelves or toward the front of the shelves for easy access. Shelves can also be built to pull out from the cabinet, or lazy Susans can be installed to make the items in the back more accessible. Cabinet doors may also be removed to allow better mobility and function for a client in a wheelchair.
- A high stool can be placed in the kitchen to allow a client who has decreased endurance to sit while washing dishes or preparing a meal.
- A utility cart with wheels can assist a client in transporting items.
- Reachers can aid a client in removing light items from high shelves. Specialized reachers are able to lift heavier items such as large cans safely; refer to an assistive device catalog.
- Special nonslip mats can be placed under a cutting board or bowl while the client works.
- A specialized cutting board with two stainless steel nails through its center can assist in holding a vegetable while chopping.
- Countertops can be adapted to achieve the proper work height.
- Light kitchen utensils may be purchased and built-up handles can be added if a client demonstrates weakness. On the other hand, heavy utensils may also be used if the client demonstrates tremors or incoordination.
- Electric appliances can be used when possible to decrease the client's amount of work.
- Oven mitts that extend farther proximally on the client's arm provide more safety when removing items from the oven.
- Pots and pans with two handles can be used by a client who demonstrates weakness.
- A specialized pan holder with suction cups helps stabilize a pan on the stovetop.
- A steamer basket can be placed in a pot with boiling vegetables. This allows the client to remove the basket to strain the vegetables, which erases the need to carry and tip a hot pan.
- A stove with front controls will assist a client who is in a wheelchair.

- o Special loop scissors remain open and require very little force to close in order to cut.
- o Special knives, such as a right-angle knife or rocker knife, can be used to make cutting easier.
- o Lightweight and easy-to-open containers should be used for food storage. Groceries, such as milk, may need to be purchased in smaller amounts to allow a client to lift the items independently. Jar openers can assist a client with decreased grasp.
- o Prepared foods that can be heated in the microwave are simple for a client to make at meal time.
- o Cleaning tools such as mops or brooms with flexible handles can be used to prevent bending.
- o An adjustable ironing board can allow the client to sit while working.
- o Lightweight vacuums or self-propelled vacuums can allow a client with decreased strength to continue cleaning. Heavier vacuums assist a client with tremors or incoordination while cleaning.
- o A front-loading washer and dryer permit a client to retrieve all the clothes from the appliance.

Devices for Work, education, and Leisure activities can be located in many catalogs from assistive technology companies. Many devices can be used for specialized tasks; however, these are applicable to clients on a very individualized basis, as jobs and leisure activities vary from one person to another. This guide seeks to provide general knowledge, so a therapist seeking this specialized information should complete research independently.

Associated Reactions. Involuntary movement of a body part in reaction to movement of another body part. These are often seen in children or those with neurological or developmental conditions. See Reflexes and reactions.

Astereognosis. Inability to identify objects placed in the hand. See Cognitive-perceptual deficits.

Asymmetrical Tonic Neck Reflex (ATNR). A primitive reflex sometimes referred to as the *fencing reflex* as the infant's arm bends near the head and the opposite arm straightens in the direction the face is pointed. See Reflexes and reactions.

Ataxia. Lack of coordinated motor movement often characterized by a wide-based, unsteady gait. The client's steps may be uneven in length or timing, and the client may have a tendency to walk toward the side that has the lesion site. The client may also demonstrate little to no arm swing. This specific type of gait occurs following a cerebellar lesion. Intervention should focus on compensatory techniques to allow the client to complete necessary functional activities.

Athetosis. Involuntary movement that occurs in slow, wormlike, twisting movements and is usually arrhythmic. The extremities, face, and neck usually demonstrate this deficit; however, the client does not display athetosis while sleeping. A lesion in the basal ganglia may result in athetosis. See <u>Cerebral palsy (CP)</u> for intervention.

Attachment Disorder. Failure to develop healthy attachments to caregivers, often due to neglect or unhealthy caregiving early in life. For specifics on intervention, see <u>Reactive attachment disorder (RAD)</u>.

Attention. The ability to focus on a task, person, or object without being distracted by other stimuli. See <u>Cognitive-perceptual deficits</u> for further discussion and intervention.

Attention Deficit Disorder (ADD)/Attention Deficit Hyperactivity Disorder (ADHD). A condition in which children (often with normal or above-normal intelligence) develop hyperactivity and/or inattention. This condition affects boys more often than girls and often causes a functional deficit due to inattentive behaviors. In addition to pharmaceutical treatment that may be prescribed by a physician, there are a number of interdisciplinary and occupational therapy approaches to intervention. A meta-analysis of interventions suggested that medications should not be the only course of intervention and that positive effects are seen in combination approaches that include behavioral training, particularly when reinforced across settings such as the home, school, and community (Snead, 2005). Thus, it is important for therapists to work in conjunction with the team on approaching ADD/ADHD.

Specific Interventions

- The client may have comorbid <u>Sensory integration (SI)</u> problems and <u>Sensory processing</u> disorder, and thus specific interventions to address sensory needs are tailored to the client. Note: All sensory motor interventions should be planned after a thorough evaluation of the client's needs.

- Complete activities that require <u>Bilateral integration</u>/coordination and motor planning to address any sensory, development, and coordination needs.

- Utilize activities that increase trunk control and balance through the treatment of antigravity extension, joint stability and/or co-contraction of muscles, and righting and <u>Equilibrium reactions</u>.
- Calming activities may be used in conjunction with sensory approaches such as slow rocking, joint compression, deep pressure or massage, <u>Neutral warmth</u>, and low-frequency/low-intensity <u>Vibration</u>.
- Increase tactile stimulation to assist with sensory organization/tactile discrimination, which can increase the client's level of alertness; recommended areas of the body include the face, hands, mouth, and soles of the feet.
- Teach the client new ways to complete tasks.
- Use "tagging" strategies such as a soft reminder bell every few minutes to remind the client to return to homework or the task at hand.
- Improve problem solving by using questioning techniques.
- Educate parents on home programs (e.g., educational and sensory programs).
- Establish a behavior modification program, using rewards instead of punishment.
- Assist the client in establishing a system of reminders to improve memory.
- Help organize the environment to reduce distractions.
- Teach relaxation techniques.
- Clients with sufficient cognition may benefit from approaches such as <u>Biofeedback</u> and <u>Cognitive behavioral therapy</u>.

Contraindications/Precautions

- Observe changes in behavior while being cognizant of all the client's medications; monitor side effects.
- Follow restrictions that have been set if the client is using diet therapy.
- Monitor the behavior reward program and discontinue use if it is not effective.

Attention Span. The length of time an individual can focus on a task. A good attention span is marked by the cognitive ability to focus on a task over an extended period. It is impaired in individuals with <u>Attention deficit hyperactivity disorder (ADHD)</u> and others with impulsivity. <u>Relaxation therapy</u> can be used to help individuals self-regulate hyperactive behavior that interferes with attention span.

Auditory Defensiveness. An excessive reaction or overreaction to sound. Often, auditory defensiveness is caused by difficulty in <u>Auditory perception</u> or <u>Sensory processing</u>. See <u>Sensory deficits</u> and <u>Sensory integration (SI)/sensory processing therapy</u>.

Auditory Perception. Ability to interpret information coming into the ears. The individual has to identify, understand, and attach meaning to the sound. Individuals with learning disabilities or <u>Sensory processing</u> difficulties may have poor auditory perception.

Auditory Sensation. Receiving, discriminating, localizing, and interpreting sounds through the ears. Examples of damage to auditory sensation are otosclerosis (chronic progressive deafness of low tones), cerebral deafness (caused by brain lesion), and perceptive deafness (caused by damage to sensory receptors of the cochlea).

Augmentative Communication. Communication devices and instruments used to facilitate the ability to speak or write for those with communication disorders. Examples of devices include communication boards and electronic communication devices.

Autism. Autism is a neurodevelopmental disorder characterized by social communication deficits along with restrictive/repetitive behaviors. The DSM-5 now includes the previous Asperger's diagnosis under autism as well (American Psychiatric Association, 2013). Individuals may display extreme withdrawal, inability to establish relationships with parents or peers, difficulty in communication with others, difficulty using language, an inward turning toward self in fantasy, and highly repetitive actions. Specific behaviors may also include lack of awareness of others, absence of social play, lack of eye contact, and marked distress over minor changes in the environment. Intervention depends on client factors, communication capabilities, and intelligence. An individualized approach with consideration of the client's developmental level, skills, needs, and strengths is important for intervention planning for clients with autism spectrum disorder (Case-Smith & Arbesman, 2008). Areas of intervention include the use of <u>Augmentative communication</u>, sign language, <u>Behavior therapy</u>, <u>Gross motor coordination</u>, computer games, occupation-based approaches, <u>Sensory integration (SI)/sensory processing therapy</u>, <u>Music therapy</u>, and <u>Creative arts</u>.

Specific Interventions

- Use both remedial and adaptive strategies to address the client's needs.
- Use picture schedules and picture exchange communication systems for those who learn best visually.

- Complete gross motor coordination activities to improve gross motor skills.
- Address <u>Sensory processing</u> issues through a client-specific intervention plan.
- Reduce stress if the client engages in self-abusive or self-stimulating behaviors through adaptation of the environment for fewer distractions.
- Use catered programs such as How Does Your Engine Run/Alert Program (Williams & Shellenberger, 1996), Zones of Regulation (Kuypers, 2011), the Incredible 5-Point Scale (Buron & Curtis, 2003), and other programs for <u>Sensory modulation</u> and self-regulation.
- Address <u>Sensory defensiveness</u> issues.
- Utilize behavioral techniques and social skills training.
- Use video cameras with role play to develop social skills and assertiveness techniques.
- Develop strategies for transitions.
- Teach <u>Stress management</u> or <u>Relaxation therapy</u>.
- Use predictable routines, yet gently introduce new experiences and novel items.
- Encourage socialization through community outings, group therapy, or support groups.
- Assist the client with language and communication through the use of a communication board or other device.
- Complete <u>Self-care</u> activities to increase self-esteem and independence.
- Encourage parallel or cooperative play versus solitary play.
- Explore <u>Leisure</u> activities.
- Address employment, particularly socialization and following rules.
- Use family-based therapy and caregiver education to ensure approaches are consistent between home, school/work, and community.
- Incorporate <u>Assistive technology</u>, communication strategies, and computers per client needs.

Contraindications/Precautions

- If using a behavior modification program, understand that the child has difficulty generalizing consequences from one situation to another.
- Observe safety precautions when using sensory devices such as the hammock or scooterboard.

Autogenic Training. A system of self-regulation of the autonomic nervous system in which the client uses visualization, deep diaphragmatic breathing, and "mind-quieting phrases," such as "my hands are heavy and warm" to reach a relaxed state in treatment of <u>Anxiety</u> and stress disorders. <u>Biofeedback</u> can be combined with autogenic training.

Automatic Stepping. See <u>Reflexes and reactions</u>.

Autonomic Dysreflexia. A sympathetic reflex of the nervous system that can result in uncontrolled hypertension in a client with spinal cord injury; generally, those who have a lesion above the level of T6. The source of the reflex may include any of the following: distended bladder, impacted bowel, pressure sores, ingrown toenails, enemas, catheters, skin irritation, or certain types of muscle facilitation techniques (see <u>Motor control</u> problems). Symptoms may include hypertension, flushing, sweating, pupil constriction, headache, goosebumps, or nasal constriction.

When a client demonstrates symptoms of dysreflexia, the client's head should be elevated, possibly lower the legs, and if the cause is known, address the situation (e.g., if there is a triggering event). Dysreflexia should be treated immediately and the client's blood pressure monitored, as the condition can be fatal.

Aversion Therapy. A form of <u>Behavior therapy</u> in which punishment or unpleasant stimuli, such as creating nausea, are used to extinguish maladaptive behavior such as alcoholism, drug abuse, sexual deviance, and self-mutilation.

Avoidant Personality Disorder. Characterized by low self-esteem, feelings of inadequacy, social avoidance, lack of friends, inhibition of feelings, and <u>Hypersensitivity</u> to criticism. The individual may be a loner and avoid social groups or friendships. Intervention includes individual and <u>Group therapy</u> where the individual has the opportunity to role play and learn social skills.

Awareness. The ability to understand and be aware of one's surroundings and conditions affecting the self. In illness, the client with awareness can understand personal symptoms that limit performance in the affected areas (e.g., the client who has hemiplegia and lacks awareness that his or her left side is paralyzed is at increased risk of falls). The client may attempt to transfer while unattended since he or she does not recognize that help is required to compensate for the hemiplegia. See <u>Cognitive-perceptual deficits</u> for further discussion and treatment.

Ayurveda. An ancient Hindu medical practice that strives to improve health by harmonizing mind, body, and spirit. Its name is derived from the

Sanskrit meaning life and knowledge. It utilizes prescribed diet, herbal remedies, massage therapy, Yoga, and pulse diagnosis. The treatment prescribed is individualized to put the client in harmony, which helps to prevent illness. Ayurvedic practitioners recommend a daily routine that consists of early rising, prescribed exercises, sensitivity and response to bodily needs such as defecation and sleep, cleaning of body and use of oil massage, and maintaining good mental health and ethical standards.

B

Babinski Reflex. Primitive reflex in which the infant's sole is stroked and the big toe rises up toward the top of the foot. See Reflexes and reactions.

Balance. Our sense of body in space monitored through the inner ear and at the brainstem level. Proprioceptors and sensors in the skin, joints, and tendons along with the eyes help facilitate balance. Occupational therapy intervention for persons with balance disorders may include sensory processing/sensory integrative treatment, vestibular retraining, and compensatory techniques to maximize function.

Balanced Forearm Orthosis. An assistive device that facilitates function for individuals with upper extremity weakness. It is also referred to as a *mobile arm support*. See Assistive technology and Mobile arm support for more information.

Bathing. An Activity of daily living (ADL) that is essential to an individual's self-care. See Self-care for specific adaptive techniques, Assistive technology for adaptive equipment, and specific diagnoses/conditions for further discussion and intervention ideas.

Bed Positioning. While in bed, the client should be positioned to prevent contractures and abnormal tone, maintain skin integrity, decrease pain, and reduce reflexive postures. See Positioning for specifics on intervention.

Behavior Rehearsal. Opportunity for clients to practice different social roles to develop the skill of empathy, understanding, or compassion. The use of Role playing is a prominent method in behavioral rehearsal (e.g., the client can take the role of a parent, child, significant other, or therapist).

Behavior Therapy. The application intervention techniques based on the principles of learning theories that include Aversion therapy, Contingency management, and Systematic desensitization. The main purpose is to

Stein, F., & Haertl, K.
Pocket Guide to Intervention in Occupational Therapy, Second Edition (pp 35-44).
© 2019 Taylor & Francis Group.

change maladaptive behavior through positive reinforcement, <u>Modeling behavior</u>, and conditioning. This type of therapy often uses punishments, reinforcements, and a <u>Token economy</u>.

Bibliotherapy. A therapeutic technique in which the therapist recommends books to the client based on the content of the book and its specific relevance to the client in working out problems. Reading groups can be incorporated with group therapy.

Bilateral Clasped Activities. A treatment technique by Bobath (1990) to help the client relearn normal movement with the affected arm by allowing the nonaffected arm to assist the affected arm through movement patterns. The nonaffected arm also provides sensory input and increases the client's awareness of the affected arm. See <u>Motor control</u> problems and <u>Neurodevelopmental treatment (NDT)</u>.

Bilateral Integration. The ability to coordinate both sides of the body such as both hands or both feet while engaging in an activity. It is an important concept in <u>Sensory integration (SI)/sensory processing therapy</u>. Examples include skating, biking, driving a car with a manual transmission, and assembling parts with two tools simultaneously.

Biofeedback. A treatment method in which the client is taught to become aware of internal processes such as heart rate, blood pressure, finger temperature, or muscle tension as a means to control function. The client learns by using monitoring devices that sound a tone or show a visual display when changes in pulse, blood pressure, brain waves, or muscle contractions occur. Biofeedback is usually combined with <u>Relaxation therapy</u> so that the client can produce beneficial changes in his or her physiology. The client can apply the information learned from biofeedback to reduce stress. A training program is designed to develop the ability to control the autonomic (involuntary) nervous system. After learning the technique, the client may be able to control heart rate, blood pressure, or skin temperature or to relax certain muscles. Biofeedback has been used successfully in conjunction with relaxation therapies for clients who experience tension headaches, insomnia, hypertension, <u>Anxiety</u>, chronic pain, <u>Depression</u>, <u>Schizophrenia</u>, and <u>Attention deficit disorder (ADD)</u>. It has also been used to increase muscle control and for incontinence.

Biopsychosocial Approach. An approach that assumes human health and well-being have biological, psychological, and sociological determinants such as genetic, developmental, and environmental factors. Biopsychosocial interventions imply a holistic, multimodal treatment approach encompassing occupation, medication, psychological counseling, exercise, nutrition, <u>Stress management</u>, cultural considerations, and client factors.

Bipolar Disorder. An affective illness characterized by episodes of mania and <u>Depression</u>. Within the DSM-5, Bipolar I is distinguished by its manic and mixed episodes with some depression. Bipolar II is marked by depression with at least one hypomanic episode (American Psychiatric Association, 2013). Typically, the mania is more pronounced in Bipolar I than Bipolar II. Symptoms of the disorder fluctuate from extreme euphoria, <u>Delusions</u> of grandeur, and frantic activity to profound sadness, guilt, lowered self-esteem, fatigue, and suicidal ideation. Intervention techniques are planned based on the types of symptoms, client insight, and evaluated strengths and needs. For those with the capacity for insight, cognitive behavioral approaches have been successful in treating individuals with bipolar disorders. These approaches include <u>Relaxation therapy</u>, <u>Biofeedback</u>, <u>Stress management</u>, and <u>Cognitive behavioral therapy</u>. Additional approaches include skill training, education, self-management approaches, and occupation-based intervention to ensure maximal occupational performance related to work, leisure, education, and socialization.

Blindness. Loss of vision that, when corrected, is no better than 20/200. This term may also refer to a visual field deficit, which results in only 20 degrees of vision from the center of peripheral vision. Persons who are born blind are diagnosed with congenital blindness, whereas persons who are blind resulting from a trauma or sudden onset of a disease are referred to as *newly blind*. Causes include <u>Macular degeneration</u>, cataracts, diabetic retinopathy, <u>Multiple sclerosis (MS)</u>, conjunctivitis, a detached retina, glaucoma, or pressure on the optic nerve. According to the Centers for Disease Control and Prevention (2015), the leading causes of blindness and <u>Low vision</u> are age-related conditions such as cataracts, macular degeneration, diabetic retinopathy, and glaucoma.

Specific Interventions

- Provide mobility training in the home, work environment, and community; transportation alternatives to driving should be considered.
- Teach compensation techniques through the use of the other senses such as hearing or smell.
- Use magnifiers and other visual adaptive equipment; magnification programs are also available for computers.
- Educate the client on devices that can assist with learning such as audiobooks, podcasts, or a computer that is voice-activated and talks back to the user.

- Address emotional adjustment to the condition.
- Increase the client's self-esteem by completing activities that allow the client to be successful.
- Help the client reorganize the home to make functional activities easier (e.g., reorganize the kitchen to place all necessary items within easy reach).
- Increase socialization through community outings or support groups.
- Teach the client skills that will be required for return to work if applicable.
- Help the client develop new leisure interests.
- Instruct the client regarding assistive devices that can help in the home such as talking clocks, timers, etc.

Contraindications/Precautions

- Monitor the client's safety judgment.
- Inspect the home for hazards or dangerous situations.
- Educate the client on other impairments resulting from diabetes, such as decreased sensation and poor circulation, if blindness has occurred as a result of diabetic retinopathy.

Blood Pressure. The pressure of the blood moving through the circulatory system. The pressure of the blood during the heartbeat is referred to as the *systolic pressure*, while the pressure during the heart at rest is the *diastolic pressure*. Generally, a blood pressure of 120/80 (or less) is considered normal. High levels of blood pressure can indicate a number of medical conditions and may predispose someone to a stroke. Occupational therapists should learn to take a client's blood pressure and recognize the importance of maintaining normal blood pressure levels.

Body Dysmorphic Disorder. A condition marked by an individual's overfocus or preoccupation with a particular body part that to others appears fairly normal. The individual may be focused on weight or a specific part and continually check self in the mirror. This condition may coexist with <u>Obsessive compulsive disorder</u>, <u>Anxiety disorder</u>, or various eating disorders. Therapists may use <u>Cognitive behavioral therapy</u> and projective techniques with persons exhibiting body dysmorphia.

Body Image. An individual's subjective concept of his or her physical appearance based on conscious or unconscious feelings toward self.

Body Mechanics. How we use our bodies in daily activities. Education is designed to improve an individual's posture, stamina, and functionality. To prevent back or other injuries, the occupational therapist should educate the client on biomechanical principles. These principles assist a client in positioning him- or herself in postures that reduce the stress placed on the spine or other joints. Proper body mechanics may not only decrease pain or vulnerability to injury, but they also help the client conserve energy because it requires more energy to hold an unnatural position. Positions to be avoided include prolonged static flexion or repetitive flexion of the lumbar spine and lifting or carrying objects without maintaining the lumbar curve of the spine. Once the client understands the underlying principles, the therapist should observe the individual completing activities such as <u>Self-care</u>, therapeutic exercise, work, or transfers. The therapist should provide verbal cues and reminders to incorporate proper body mechanics into regular routines. As treatment progresses, the client should become more accustomed to the new positions, and he or she should be able to recognize and self-correct poor positions/patterns.

Principles

- Tilt the pelvis slightly anteriorly from neutral when sitting or standing for long periods to decrease low back muscle tension.
- When lifting objects, position oneself close to and facing the object to prevent reaching with the upper extremities or twisting of the trunk. Bend the knees when lifting from the ground.
- If a person needs to turn the body, turn with both lower extremities while keeping the trunk in line with the lower extremities. This helps prevent injury from twisting the trunk separately from the lower extremities.
- Use the hip flexor and extensor muscles to lower and raise the pelvis to pick items up from low surfaces while keeping the back straight and bending knees as needed. Do not bend at the spine to reach down to the floor.
- Incorporate rest or walking breaks into the routine each hour if the client has <u>Low back pain (LBP)</u> and is required to sustain static positions for extended periods.
- A client can place one foot on a short stool when standing at the bathroom sink, kitchen counter, etc. This tilts the pelvis slightly posteriorly to relieve pressure since prolonged standing can promote an overemphasized anterior <u>Pelvic tilt</u>.

- When sitting, the client should flex the hips and knees without flexing the spine. Desk chairs are positioned to allow 90 degrees between the hip and trunk.
- If the client is lifting a heavy object, the object should be brought close to the client's center of gravity. The client should also balance the weight of the object between both upper extremities (e.g., the client should not carry a heavy bookbag over only one shoulder).
- Work surfaces should be adjusted to the proper height to promote good posture and body mechanics. A client should have the ankles, knees, hips, and elbows near 90 degrees flexion. The wrists and the neck should be in the neutral position.

Body on Body Righting. A righting reflex. See <u>Reflexes and reactions</u>.

Body on Head Righting. Body righting in response to the head direction. See <u>Reflexes and reactions</u>.

Body Part Identification. The ability to identify the position of body parts on self or on other persons. See <u>Cognitive-perceptual deficits</u> for further discussion and treatment.

Body Scheme. The perceptual process of being aware of one's body and its integral parts. An individual with hemiplegia may experience difficulty with incorporating the affected site in <u>Activities of daily living (ADLs)</u> and can develop neglect. It is assessed by the ability to identify the position of body parts in relation to one another and to objects in the environment. Other neurological conditions may cause body scheme disorders. See <u>Cognitive-perceptual deficits</u> for further discussion and treatment.

Borderline Personality Disorder. A personality disorder characterized by unstable <u>Self-image</u>, difficulty with relationships, a feeling of emptiness, emotional dysregulation, and impulsivity. Emotional outbursts, sadness, fear, and suicidal ideation are frequently experienced. This disorder can lead to suicidality, self-harm, eating disorders, substance abuse, domestic violence, criminal behavior, and homelessness. In addition to medication, interdisciplinary approaches include <u>Dialectical behavioral therapy (DBT)</u>, <u>Cognitive behavioral therapy</u>, <u>Stress management</u>, and <u>Psychoeducational</u> approaches.

Boutonniere Deformity. A digit that demonstrates flexion of the proximal interphalangeal (PIP) joint with hyperextension of the distal interphalangeal (DIP) joint. This condition can result from disruption of the central slip that causes volar migration of the extensor mechanism, resulting in shortening of the oblique retinacular ligament.

Bowel Program. In addition to developmental disabilities, a number of conditions may cause bowel problems. Techniques used by occupational therapists may include the use of programs and schedules to facilitate independence, incorporation of adaptive aids and toileting techniques, and developing an interdisciplinary client-centered bowel program designed to maximize daily function. See also <u>Toileting</u> in <u>Self-care</u>.

Bradykinesia. Delayed or slowed movements that may result in impaired motion. A client with this deficit may demonstrate slow eye movements, decreased arm swing during ambulation, or decreased equilibrium or protective responses. A lesion in the basal ganglia may result in bradykinesia. Clients who have Parkinson's disease often demonstrate these symptoms; bradykinesia may also be seen in negative symptoms of <u>Schizophrenia</u>. See <u>Parkinson's disease</u> for treatment and further discussion.

Brain Injury. An insult to the brain, often causing cognitive and other damage. See <u>Traumatic brain injury</u>.

Bridging. To raise the hips in supine position in order to promote hip extension and activate the gluteal muscles.

Broca's Aphasia. Expressive aphasia. See <u>Aphasia</u> for more details.

Brunnstrom Approach. A motor control intervention developed by Signe Brunnstrom (1970), a Swedish therapist who emphasized synergic patterns (muscles working together) of improvement for patients recovering from a stroke. See <u>Motor control</u>.

Brushing. Various forms of brushing are used in occupational therapy. Historically, Rood (1962) hypothesized that using a soft-bristled brush at a very high frequency would help facilitate muscle tone. This type of brushing was used for 3 to 5 seconds, with 30 seconds between repetitions. The muscle responds best to the facilitation if the brushing is completed over the <u>Dermatome</u> that is innervated by the same segment that innervates the muscle (e.g., if facilitating the biceps, dermatome C5 should be brushed, as this is the primary segment that innervates the biceps). The best facilitation occurs while the brushing is being performed. Areas that have many free nerve endings should not be brushed, including the face, head, and ear. Results have shown that the effects last a very short period. Patricia Wilbarger (1995) also developed a brushing program used in sensory integration therapy. The program combines brushing over the skin (and sometimes clothes) paired with firm pressure and proprioceptive input. A particular type of corn brush is used within the protocol. Although more research is needed, many therapists use this in combination with other sensory integration interventions.

Contraindications/Precautions

- Avoid the use of brushing to the face of clients with spinal cord injuries or brainstem injuries since it could result in Autonomic dysreflexia.

- Within the Willbarger protocol (now called *Therapressure*), the stomach is not brushed. In addition, it is important to watch for autonomic signs of overstimulation.

See Motor control problems, Rood approach, and Sensory integration (SI)/sensory processing therapy for more discussion of brushing and Facilitation techniques.

Bulimia. An eating disorder marked by recurrent or continuous episodes of binge eating followed by compensatory behaviors to counteract the binge such as self-induced vomiting, fasting, and abuse of laxatives. The individual may also engage in excessive exercise. At times, individuals with Anorexia nervosa may later develop bulimia, or the reverse may be true. Researchers and clinicians attribute bulimia to biopsychosocial factors such as genetics, perfectionist personality patterns, social and societal expectations, family pressures, or Hypersensitivity to criticism. Depression and an overconcern about body shape frequently accompany bulimia. Other symptoms include menstrual disturbances, tooth decay, and dehydration. The first step in intervention is to protect the client's health and to remove the symptoms that are life threatening such as starvation and dehydration. Intervention should include a holistic approach to address physical, psychological, social-emotional, and spiritual issues. Interdisciplinary approaches include Cognitive behavioral therapy, Dialectical behavioral treatment (DBT), Family therapy, Group therapy, and expressive techniques.

Burn Hand Splint/Orthosis. The occupational therapist ideally evaluates the client within 24 hours of admission. In early stages, the therapist uses static splints and later works toward Active range of motion (AROM). A resting splint is fabricated to prevent a client from developing a Claw hand deformity following a burn to the hand, specifically the dorsal surface. The claw hand deformity results in hyperextension of the metacarpophalangeal (MCP) joints, flexion of the proximal interphalangeal (PIP) and distal interphalangeal (DIP) joints, and a flattened palmar arch. The resting hand splint should place the client's hand in 30 to 40 degrees wrist extension, thumb abduction to a functional position, 0 degrees PIP and DIP flexion, and 70 to 75 degrees MCP flexion. The prescribed schedule is for the client to wear the splint at all times unless the client is bathing or doing hand exercises. See Burns for further discussion and treatment.

Burns. An injury to the skin caused by fire, heat, friction, chemicals, and radiation. Burns are graded based on the amount of the body burned/affected, as well as how many layers of the skin (dermis) are affected. Burns range from superficial (first degree) to severe (fourth degree) burns affecting other tissues, tendons, and bones.

Specific Interventions

- Provide positioning devices to prevent contractures or pain; devices include a foam head donut (prevent neck flexion contracture), foam ear protector (prevent pressure on ear), arm trough (prevent shoulder adduction contracture), and foot board (maintain functional position of ankle).
- Fabricate splints as needed to prevent deformity and contractures; splints include a soft cervical collar (prevent neck flexion contracture), airplane splint (prevent shoulder adduction contracture), elbow conformer (prevent elbow flexion contracture), wrist cock-up splint (prevent wrist flexion contracture), C-splint (prevent tightening of thumb web space), abductor wedge (prevent hip adduction contracture), knee conformer (prevent knee flexion contracture), and foot-drop splint (maintain functional position of ankle).
- Use range of motion (ROM) exercises.
- Maintain positioning and implement postural control techniques.
- Implement fatigue management techniques.
- Complete activities that allow the client to demonstrate success and increase self-esteem.
- Assist the client with finding an alternative way to communicate, such as a communication board, if the client is intubated.
- Ensure edema management and wound care.
- As the client improves, teach techniques for safe transfers and functional mobility.
- Complete Self-care activities to maintain functional activity.
- Later in therapy, address skills that will be necessary for return to work such as Gross motor coordination and Fine motor coordination or muscle strength.
- Help the client develop new leisure interests.
- Address occupational performance in Activities of daily living (ADLs), Instrumental activities of daily living (IADLs), Work, Leisure, and socialization.

Contraindications/Precautions

- Monitor the skin for infection, and disinfect splints.
- Avoid the use of chemicals, which may irritate the skin.
- Observe the skin for areas of breakdown or areas where skin grafts have failed.
- Monitor ROM for changes that could be due to <u>Heterotopic ossification</u>.
- Observe for signs of peripheral nerve damage, which may result from compression.
- Monitor the scars and treat with scar pads, if needed, to prevent hypertrophic scarring.
- Monitor ROM to prevent contractures and provide assistive devices as needed; see recommendations provided earlier.

Buttonhook. A piece of adaptive equipment that is useful in assisting a client in buttoning a shirt independently. The individual places the hook through the buttonhole of the shirt, and then the client positions the hook around the button. While pulling the hook toward the buttonhole, the button is pulled through and the button is fastened. This tool is helpful for a client who has hemiplegia and must fasten buttons with one hand. See <u>Cerebrovascular accident (CVA)</u> for further discussion and treatment techniques for dressing.

C

CAM. An acronym for complementary and alternative medicine. Denotes interventions that are usually not taught in medical school such as herbals, <u>Acupuncture</u>, massage therapy, spiritual healing, and therapeutic touch. Current research is used to validate clinical intervention.

Cancer. Unregulated division and cell growth, which may invade surrounding tissue and metastasize to move to other areas of the body. Many types of cancer exist that can occur throughout the lifespan. The cause is unknown; however, lifestyle decisions such as tobacco use and excessive sun exposure may increase cancer risk. Unregulated cell growth disrupts the ability of organs to complete their normal functions. While it is important to monitor physician recommendations and client factors in interdisciplinary intervention, consideration should be given to maintain strength. A large systematic review and meta-analysis have shown positive effect sizes for physical activity during post-cancer interventions (Speck, Courneya, Masse, Duval, & Schmitz, 2010).

Specific Interventions

- Retrain and utilize remedial and adaptive strategies to address <u>Activities of daily living (ADLs)</u> and <u>Instrumental activities of daily living (IADLs)</u>.
- Complete activities to maintain muscle strength, range of motion (ROM), and endurance.
- Fabricate orthoses and provide positioning devices as needed to prevent contractures and deformity.
- Teach <u>Pain management</u>, <u>Stress management</u>, and <u>Relaxation therapy</u>.
- Instruct the client to use energy conservation and work simplification techniques when completing functional activities.

Stein, F., & Haertl, K.
Pocket Guide to Intervention in Occupational Therapy, Second Edition (pp 45-82).
© 2019 Taylor & Francis Group.

- Check the client's safety judgment and treat as needed.
- Encourage the client to become involved in support groups for socialization and emotional adjustment to the disease.
- Take the client on community outings to elevate mood and increase socialization.
- Assist the client with finding a new means of communication if needed.
- Ensure success by grading activities to the client's ability, which will help increase self-esteem.
- Address the client's ability to cope with the disease and problems resulting from its progression.
- Complete Self-care activities to maintain functional activity.
- Instruct the client on assistive devices, which can make functional activities easier; devices may be used for dressing, feeding, and tub or toilet transfers.
- Complete a home evaluation and give recommendations regarding modifications of the environment to increase the client's safety.
- Address end-of-life issues and collaborate on strategies to maintain meaning throughout the lifespan.

Contraindications/Precautions

- Know the client's medications being used, including radiation and chemotherapy, and possible side effects.
- Address fatigue and safety issues that arise in the course of the illness.

Cardiac Disease/Cardiac Dysfunction. A disorder that affects the function of the heart by an adverse condition of the blood, tissue, muscles, or vessels around the heart. Some cardiac dysfunctions include the following: *arteriosclerosis* (also referred to as *coronary artery disease*), a buildup of plaque on the coronary artery walls that decreases the amount of oxygenated blood being delivered to the heart, which results in ischemia of heart muscle; *myocardial infarction*, death of heart muscle, which may occur from ischemia of heart muscle and cause a decreased ability of the heart to pump blood; *angina pectoris*, chest pain, which often radiates to the left shoulder, jaw, neck, or down the left arm; and *valvular disease*, the state of valves becoming fibrous, which affects their ability to close completely and results in regurgitation of blood (heart murmur). Clients receive rehabilitation services for a variety of cardiac conditions, especially those who are recovering from a myocardial infarction or open heart surgery. Open heart surgery may be performed to complete coronary artery bypass graft, with the goal being to prevent a myocardial infarction by providing more blood to heart tissue if the client has arteriosclerosis. The use of balloon angioplasty (insertion of a long, thin catheter with a small balloon on the end) can help open a narrowing artery. Often, balloon angioplasties are accompanied by the placement of a stent to keep the vessel open and facilitate blood flow. A systematic review and meta-analysis of integrated exercise–based cardiac rehabilitation for those with coronary heart disease correlated with reduced mortality rates (Taylor et al., 2004).

Specific Interventions

- Coordinate care and suggestions with the physician and intervention team.
- Complete activities to maintain the client's endurance.
- Use resistive activities to maintain muscle strength.
- Instruct the client on energy conservation and work simplification principles.
- Teach <u>Relaxation therapy</u> and <u>Coping skills</u> and work on <u>Stress management</u>, as high stress may negatively affect heart conditions.
- Teach the use of good <u>Body mechanics</u>.
- Instruct the client to use adaptive techniques and/or assistive devices to make functional activities easier.
- Evaluate the client's home environment and provide adaptations as necessary.
- Set up a schedule for the client to follow when completing home management activities, which allows for periods of rest between activity.
- Complete job simulation if the client plans to return to work.
- Modify current leisure activities or explore new interests.
- Consider lifestyle modification and healthy lifestyle.

Contraindications/Precautions

- Talk with the physician and team about precautions specific to the client's diagnosis, comorbidities, and current medications taken.
- Overly stressful situations should be avoided.
- Initially, the client should use assistive devices rather than bending over to dress or pick up items.
- In early stages of rehabilitation, overhead reaching should be avoided.

- While completing isometric exercise, the client should be taught to exhale to avoid holding the breath.
- Hot, humid environments should be avoided.
- The client should not overexert while exercising.
- Cease activity if the following symptoms occur: a cold sweat, glassy stare, dizziness, angina or chest discomfort, fatigue, dyspnea, high systolic or diastolic blood pressure, irregular pulse, palpitations, or pain (especially in the legs).
- Clients who have had open heart surgery should not have resistance against shoulder motion, and they should also avoid horizontally abducting the upper extremities, which can pull the incision open.
- Be sure the client is educated on medications, contraindications, and proper use.

Carpal Tunnel Syndrome. A condition involving numbness and tingling along the pattern of the median nerve (the thumb, index, long, and lateral half of the ring finger). Symptoms may cause weakness, clumsiness, and discomfort. The cause is compression of the median nerve within the carpal tunnel, which occurs from a thickness of the transverse carpal ligament or inflammation of the tendons within the carpal tunnel, most often due to illness, repetitive use, or cumulative trauma. In addition to surgical repair for more severe cases of carpal tunnel, the following are common rehabilitative interventions.

Specific Interventions

- Address Edema and inflammation utilizing Icing and other techniques.
- Modify and adapt the task and environment to place the wrist in neutral position and reduce tendon tension and torque force.
- Use graded activities as tolerated to gradually increase the client's hand strength.
- Utilize splinting techniques; often, a neutral orthosis is worn at night.
- Practice coordination activities and tendon-gliding activities.
- Following surgery, also instruct the client to complete nerve-gliding exercises.
- Provide Friction massage to prevent adhesions at the scar site.
- Maintain upper extremity range of motion through exercises.

- Reeducate the affected hand with different textures and sensory stimuli.
- Educate the client on the condition and its cause to help prevent reinjury from repetitive movements.
- Teach the client to use joint protection principles and good <u>Body mechanics</u>.
- Complete a job site evaluation and make recommendations to prevent reinjury from repetitive trauma.
- Adapt tools to prevent tight grasp or bad positioning of the upper extremity.
- Explore other occupations and new leisure interests if necessary.
- Have the client wear a splint to help immobilize the wrist at work.
- Facilitate return to daily <u>Activities of daily living (ADLs)</u> and <u>Instrumental activities of daily living (IADLs)</u>.

Contraindications/Precautions

- Monitor for skin breakdown and pressure areas from the splint.
- Instruct the client that overuse of the affected hand can lead to tenosynovitis.

Case Management. A comprehensive system and interdisciplinary approach to addressing the needs of the client, often those with mental health conditions. The focus of case management includes evaluation, intervention, and monitoring of progress on goals. Case management also includes care coordination across teams, settings, and important persons (e.g., family members, education staff, group home staff, etc.).

Catecholamine. Derived from the amino acid tyrosine, it has a vital function in the brain of stimulating the nervous system, cardiovascular function, metabolic rate, temperature, and smooth muscles. It plays a key role in arousing the autonomic nervous system (sympathetic response). <u>Dopamine</u> and norepinephrine are catecholamines.

Categorization. The cognitive ability to sort objects into similar or different groups. It entails the ability to generalize and differentiate people, objects, concepts, emotions, and animals. Purposeful activities can be devised by the therapist to stimulate learning (e.g., games where the individual sorts pictures into categories or groups). Categorization is also used in health care related to the utilization of classification systems (e.g., diagnosis).

Catharsis. A term used by Freud to describe how repressed ideas or traumatic experiences are brought to the consciousness during psychotherapy. In general terms, it refers to the free expression of strong emotion, such as fear and <u>Anxiety</u>, which are released through intervention techniques (e.g., use of expressive media such as art, music, poetry, or <u>Dance</u>).

Catheterization. The procedure of inserting a long, flexible tube (catheter) into the body, often in the bladder, heart, artery, or vein. Occupational therapists are often involved in rehabilitation following catheterization, particularly in training related to urinary catheters and toileting.

Cerebral Palsy (CP). A group of neurological disorders disrupting movement that results from damage to the brain before, during, or shortly after birth. According to the Centers for Disease Control (2017a), CP is the most common motor disability in childhood.

Etiology and Epidemiology

The immediate cause of CP varies but may be due to a lesion in the brain usually caused by <u>Anoxia</u> or insufficient oxygen to a part of the brain. Additional causes may include poor cell migration, decreased myelination, faulty synaptic connections, and brain cell death. Current prevalence estimates worldwide range from 1.4 to over 4 per 1000 live births (Centers for Disease Control, 2017a). Prematurity and low birth weights are both risk factors for CP. With the increasing number of infants with low birth weight who live as a result of medical technology, the risk for CP has increased. It almost seems ironic that excellent neonatal care may be an indirect risk factor for CP. Usually, the first sign that brain damage may have occurred is the accumulation of bilirubin in the blood indicated by the presence of jaundice. Other causes of brain damage in the fetus are (1) chemical damage to the fetus from the mother; (2) intrauterine infection during the first trimester of pregnancy; and (3) trauma, poor nutrition, radiation, inadequate prenatal care, rubella, AIDS, toxoplasmosis (protozoan parasite), or sepsis (toxins in the blood) during the later stages of pregnancy and during labor and delivery.

Diagnostic Types

Classification of CP may be according to severity (mild, moderate, severe), <u>Topographical orientation</u> (quadriplegia, diplegia, hemiplegia, etc.), muscle tone (hypertonic/hypotonic), and motor function (spastic/nonspastic). Additional classifications include the following four types: spastic (about 70%), athetoid or dyskinetic (20%), ataxic (10%), and mixed. Clinicians also place CP into one of two categories: pyramidal or extrapyramidal. Pyramidal or spastic CP indicates that the lesion was in the motor cortex or corticospinal tract. Extrapyramidal or athetoid CP indicates that the lesion was in the basal ganglia. Ataxic CP usually indicates damage to the cerebellum, which controls posture and balance, running, writing, dressing, eating, playing musical instruments, and visual tracking of objects.

Major Areas of Disability and Resulting Effects

Depending on the type of CP, the following areas may be affected:

- **Cognition.** The cognitive effects of CP vary, and intelligence may be affected. For those with cognitive struggles, the following may be affected (only a partial list): problem solving, judgement, sequencing, decision making, language, memory, <u>Recognition</u>, organization, abstraction, and comprehension.

- **Epilepsy or Seizures.** Persons with CP have a much higher incidence of epilepsy or seizures than the general population.

- **Visual Impairments.** Cortical visual impairments often accompany CP and may include visual fatigues and unusual eye movements. Additional visual effects may include strabismus (lack of alignment of two eyes), <u>Nystagmus</u>, and <u>Hemianopsia</u>.

- **Impaired Hearing.** Frequently occurs in children with CP. May cause disability in learning and difficulty in social interactions.

- **Sensory and Perceptual Impairments.** The presence of <u>Astereognosis</u> and abnormal pain sensations may be present.

- **Hydrocephalus.** Hydrocephalus often accompanies CP and is manifested by increased cerebrospinal fluid in the brain. Hydrocephalus may lead to CP and may be accompanied by additional cognitive, visual, and neurological symptoms.

Specific Interventions

- Motor treatments designed to improve function
- Strengthening activities to improve occupational performance
- <u>Neurodevelopmental treatment (NDT)</u> has been a popular approach to intervention, although more research support is needed
- <u>Augmentative communication</u> aids such as talking computers and language boards
- Ambulation aids to increase functional mobility (e.g., wheelchair, walker)
- <u>Activities of daily living (ADLs)</u> assistive devices in eating, dressing, toileting, and grooming; additional <u>Assistive technology</u> as matched to the client's needs
- Remedial and adaptive techniques for ADLs and <u>Instrumental activities of daily living (IADLs)</u>

- <u>Leisure</u> and play activities to stimulate development and increase socialization skills
- Therapeutic riding and <u>Hippotherapy</u> to improve motor function and posture
- <u>Stress management</u> to help individuals to deal with resultant disabilities
- <u>Family therapy</u> and <u>Psychoeducational</u> therapy
- <u>Creative arts</u> therapy to help individuals express feelings
- Vocational exploration to help individuals actualize abilities

Additional information on interventions designed to improve motor performance in children can be found in Case-Smith, Frolek Clark, and Schlabach (2013).

Cerebrovascular Accident (CVA). Often referred to as a *stroke*, a CVA is a blockage of blood supply to any part of the brain, which may occur suddenly or gradually. The intensity may vary from very small CVAs, which are called *transient ischemic attacks* and result in very little change of function, to large strokes, which can result in profound and permanent loss of function. Conditions that may cause CVAs include arteriosclerosis, hypertension, heart disease, family history of stroke, or hypercholesterolemia. CVAs result in various symptoms depending on the size and location of the lesion that suffers from decreased blood supply. The general public should be taught the warning signs of a stroke, which, according to the National Stroke Association (2017), range from decreased sensation and motor ability to decreased memory and cognitive ability. The National Stroke Association teaches a simple screen the general public can perform, which includes the acronym FAST (*Face*: Ask the person to smile and notice if there is a droop on one side; *Arms*: Ask the person to raise both arms and notice if one drifts downward; *Speech*: Ask the person to talk and notice if there is slurring or garbled speech; and *Time*: If a stroke is suspected, call 911 immediately. Symptoms often follow a typical distribution depending on the hemisphere that incurred the lesion. Clients who have had CVAs on the left side of the brain often display right hemiplegia, <u>Apraxia</u>, <u>Aphasia</u>, <u>Hemianopsia</u> in the right visual fields, impaired right/left discrimination, memory deficits, and <u>Depression</u>. Clients who have had CVAs on the right side of the brain often display left hemiplegia, hemianopsia in the left visual fields, left neglect, impulsivity, difficulty with spatial relations and figure/ground, and decreased judgment. A lesion in either hemisphere can result in memory difficulty, decreased attention, and emotional <u>Lability</u>. The prognosis for the return of function often depends on when therapy is initiated, the site and extent of the lesion, and the rate of recovery of function (e.g., a client who recovers experiences no change for some time following the stroke).

Specific Interventions

- The use of constraint-induced movement has been shown to improve movement after stroke (Thrane, Friborg, Anke, & Indredavik, 2014).
- Use balance and postural training along with motor awareness.
- Increase independence with <u>Activities of daily living (ADLs)</u> and <u>Instrumental activities of daily living (IADLs)</u>.
- Utilize an orientation board or other tools to improve the client's orientation, and develop aids to assist the client with memory.
- Increase visual tracking and scanning; teach compensation techniques to look to the affected side if the client demonstrates a hemianopsia, or patch one eye to decrease double vision.
- Improve <u>Tactile sensation</u> and teach safety precautions for sensory loss.
- Assist the client in finding an alternative means to communicate if the client has aphasia.
- Promote proper positioning for safety in swallowing and good body alignment.
- Use techniques to manage pain and edema.
- Maintain range of motion (ROM) through passive ROM (PROM) of affected upper extremity; make sure the head of the humerus is approximated into the glenoid fossa to increase ROM and decrease pain with movement.
- Increase voluntary use of affected upper extremity.
- Improve muscle strength, motor planning, and coordination.
- Normalize muscle tone on the affected side through facilitation or <u>Inhibition techniques</u>.
- Increase endurance.
- Work on eating and feeding (including swallowing).
- Assist client with psychological adjustment to condition.
- Educate client and family members on condition/disease process.
- Complete a home evaluation and give recommendations for equipment to increase the client's accessibility and safety in the home.
- Explore vocational opportunities as needed.
- Assist client with finding <u>Leisure</u> activities.

- Complete activities to increase the client's body symmetry and balance.
- Fabricate a splint to prevent contractures/deformity and maintain skin integrity.
- Teach the client to complete inspection of the skin (if the client is wearing a splint) to prevent skin breakdown.
- If the client demonstrates neglect, instruct the client to use visual cues and reminders to remember to include the affected side during activities.
- Adapt the treatment environment to reduce distractions if the client has decreased attention.
- Complete right/left activities while identifying the side being used to increase a client's right/left discrimination.
- Give simple directions if the client is unable to follow complex directions.
- Assess client's abilities to complete ADL/IADL (e.g., managing finances) and address as necessary.
- Teach <u>Stress management</u> and <u>Relaxation therapy</u>.
- Instruct the client on assistive devices that may be used to increase the client's independence with <u>Self-care</u> activities such as feeding, dressing, grooming, and tub and toilet transfers.
- Have the client bend the unaffected leg under the affected leg, and use it to assist with swinging the legs off the bed to increase independence with transferring from supine to sitting.
- Complete a job site evaluation if the client plans to return to work.
- Address homemaking activities such as cooking and cleaning, especially if the client plans to return home alone.
- Work on handwriting if the affected upper extremity is also the dominant hand.

Contraindications/Precautions

- Monitor for symptoms of <u>Reflex sympathetic dystrophy (RSD) syndrome</u>.
- Observe the client's mood and watch for signs of depression.
- Measure ROM and fabricate splints to prevent contractures from developing abnormal tone.
- Do not allow the client to use abnormal postures and movements; train the client to attempt normal movement.

Chaining. A behavioral therapy and cognitive technique in which an activity is broken down into task intervals for the client to learn in a sequential manner. *Forward chaining* is carrying the task from the first step until completion. *Backward chaining* starts with the last step in the task and works backward in sequence to the first step. Chaining requires careful <u>Activity analysis</u>. When used in intervention, the therapist divides a complex skill into smaller, manageable components and teaches the client one step of the desired skill at a time. With time, the client learns all steps of a task, and the therapist slowly removes assistance from each step. The therapist may also chain backward so that the therapist assists the client throughout the activity until the final step is reached. The therapist allows the client to complete the final step until the client demonstrates success. The therapist will then remove assistance one step earlier so that the client completes the final two steps of the activity.

Chiropractic Care. A discipline of health practice that examines the relationship between the structure and position of the spinal column to the onset of diseases, pain syndromes, and neurophysiological effects. Chiropractors emphasize health prevention and maintenance, as well as treatment. The major intervention is spinal manipulation in which the chiropractor uses his or her hands or a special instrument called an *activator* to mobilize, adjust, manipulate, massage, or stimulate the client's spine. Chiropractic care has been shown to be quite effective in treating individuals with <u>Low back pain (LBP)</u> and other spine and neck ailments.

Chorea. Involuntary movement that occurs in quick, jerky, and irregular movements. The face and extremities usually demonstrate this deficit. Lesions of the basal ganglia may result in chorea; however, clients have also displayed this deficit following rheumatic fever.

Chronic Fatigue Syndrome (CFS). A condition marked by excessive fatigue without a known cause (e.g., another medical condition). CFS may also be accompanied by muscular pain, headache, and confusion. The symptoms may be so pronounced that it causes significant impairment in daily function. In addition to pharmacological interventions, <u>Stress management</u>, stretching, light exercise, and <u>Cognitive behavioral therapy</u> may be used.

Chronic Obstructive Pulmonary Disease (COPD). An overarching term used to describe various progressive lung diseases that result in obstruction of the small airways in the lungs that interfere with normal breathing. Diseases encompassing COPD may include asthma, emphysema, or chronic bronchitis. Asthma results in spasms of the airways, which reduce the size of the airways and make breathing difficult. Emphysema is a decreased elasticity in the alveolae and bronchioles, which causes the client to have difficulty with forced expiration. Chronic bronchitis is inflammation of the bronchi, which increases mucus secretions. Causes of this condition can include smoking, allergies, infections, obesity, or nervous system diseases that weaken muscles of respiration.

Specific Interventions

- Work with the interdisciplinary team and client to address healthy lifestyle changes.
- Increase the client's endurance through gradual resistive exercises.
- Complete exercises to maintain range of motion.
- Teach the client to use pursed-lip breathing to slow dyspnea; this technique consists of inhaling through the nose with the mouth closed and exhaling through the mouth with the lips formed in a small circle as if the client were going to attempt to whistle.
- For clients with oxygen, instruct the client on the use of oxygen and implications for daily activities.
- Instruct the client on principles of energy conservation and work simplification.
- Prevent the client from holding the breath when using force such as while pushing or pulling against resistance; holding the breath will increase the client's shortness of breath.
- Educate the client on good Body mechanics to help the client conserve energy during activities as poor posture requires more energy than good upright posture.
- Instruct the client on the possibility of decreased respiration due to chemicals, smoking, or other hazardous materials.
- Teach the client Stress management and Relaxation therapy.
- Encourage the client to join a support group for socialization.
- Provide the client with education regarding assistive devices, which may make functional activities easier.
- Complete a home evaluation, and make recommendations for equipment to increase the client's safety and mobility in the home.
- Complete a job site evaluation, and make recommendations as needed.

Contraindications/Precautions

- Avoid the use of hazardous chemicals and irritants that can cause difficulty with breathing.

- Monitor for dyspnea, and do not overfatigue the client while completing endurance training.
- Monitor safety for those who are on oxygen.

Circadian Rhythm. The awake, sleep, and activity cycle in animals during a 24-hour period. Individuals can track their circadian rhythm by recording the average hours of sleep needed during a 24-hour period and their activity level during the day. Knowledge of this rhythm is important to occupational therapists who work with clients on <u>Sleep hygiene</u>.

Claw Hand. A condition in which the metacarpophalangeal (MCP) joints hyperextend and the proximal interphalangeal (PIP) and distal interphalangeal (DIP) joints flex. This may result from an ulnar nerve palsy, which paralyzes the interossei and intrinsic muscles, or from a burn to the hand. Clients with claw hand often receive rehabilitation therapy. See <u>Hand injuries</u> and <u>Burns</u> for further discussion and intervention.

Client-Centered Therapy. A type of psychotherapy developed by Rogers (1951) that emphasizes the relationship between the client and the therapist and empowers the client to facilitate psychological growth. Concepts of client-centered therapy have been adopted widely in health care, including occupational therapy.

Clinical Observation. Informally, clinical observation is a method of observing and evaluating the client's verbal and nonverbal behavior in a treatment setting. Within sensory integration intervention, the term *clinical observations* is often used to refer to a formal set of structured observations to assess sensory integrative function.

Clinical Reasoning. The process used by clinicians to consider the client's condition and personal goals, assess needs, consider theory and evidence-based practice, and determine the intervention approach.

Clonus. Alternating contraction and relaxation of a muscle that results in a twitching movement or spasm.

Closed Reduction. The act of correcting a fracture without surgical intervention. The physician manipulates the fragments back into alignment without having to open the skin. The doctor then immobilizes the fracture with a cast or external fixator until healing occurs. An external fixator is hardware, such as rod, which is applied externally to pins that have been screwed into bone.

Co-contraction. This occurs when both the agonist and the antagonist muscles contract at the same time to achieve stability. Examples would include the co-contraction of the muscles of the neck so that a person's head is held upright or the co-contraction of the muscles in a person's trunk and lower extremities while the person is in a <u>Quadruped</u> position.

Codependency. An individual's <u>Addiction</u> that is shared with a significant other such as a spouse. Addictions such as alcohol, drugs, gambling, or smoking may be reinforced by the codependent individual. Individuals with codependency many times have low self-worth, difficulties in relating to others, please others at the expense of self, and may have a need to control others. <u>Cognitive behavioral therapy</u>, <u>Psychotherapy</u>, and <u>Creative arts</u> are effective treatment techniques.

Cognition. The mental activities of perceiving, thinking, reasoning, evaluating, remembering, planning, and making decisions. The act of cognition includes memory (perception, encoding, storage, and retrieval of information), attention, language, and executive functioning. It is assessed by the ability to process information in order to solve problems, draw conclusions, or retrieve data. See <u>Cognitive-perceptual deficits</u> for further discussion and treatment.

Cognitive Behavioral Therapy. Based on the cognitive behavioral frame of reference, cognitive behavioral therapy focuses on changing faulty and negative thought patterns. The major premise is that thinking influences behavior and vice versa. Therapy involves a skills training approach to intervention where the client learns to self-regulate symptoms. Within this form of intervention, it is most helpful if the client has the capacity for insight. <u>Stress management</u>, <u>Biofeedback</u>, mindfulness, <u>Relaxation therapy</u>, <u>Prescriptive exercise</u>, <u>Progressive relaxation</u>, and <u>Psychoeducational</u> approaches are used by the therapist to help the client learn techniques to reduce symptoms and to prevent the recurrence of the disease. Adherence to the intervention and readiness for change are important components in the treatment. The client is an active participant in therapy, and the therapist helps the client to monitor improvement.

Cognitive-Perceptual Deficits. Impairment of cognition or perception (the capacity to understand sensory experiences). A client with cognitive or perceptual deficits may demonstrate difficulty with <u>Activities of daily living (ADLs)</u> even though the sensory and motor systems of the client are functioning normally. In this case, the therapist should evaluate the underlying cognition and perceptual causes, which can also greatly affect an individual's ability to complete activities independently. A client who has difficulty with storing or processing information may be unable to remember the steps of bathing. Likewise, a client who cannot integrate sensory input with previous knowledge, which gives meaning to the input, may not be able to understand how to put on a shirt. Among others, deficits may be displayed in the following cognitive areas: <u>Attention</u>, <u>Orientation</u>, <u>Memory</u>, <u>Problem solving</u>, <u>Awareness</u>, <u>Sequencing</u> and organization, and <u>Executive functions of the brain</u>. The perceptual areas that may demonstrate deficits include <u>Visual foundation skills</u> (<u>Visual acuity</u>, <u>Visual fields</u>, and <u>Oculomotor function</u>), visual discrimination skills, <u>Body scheme</u>, <u>Right/left discrimination</u>, <u>Body part identification</u>, <u>Finger agnosia</u>, <u>Anosognosia</u>, <u>Unilateral neglect</u>, <u>Position in space</u>, <u>Spatial relations</u>, <u>Topographical orientation</u>, <u>Figure/ground perception</u>, and <u>Apraxia</u> (<u>Limb apraxia</u>, <u>Constructional apraxia</u>, and <u>Dressing apraxia</u>).

Approaches

- The *sensory-integrative/sensory processing approach* uses sensory input to help elicit the desired motor responses; however, this treatment requires a lot of time, and research is primarily focused on younger populations, a time when the brain is more plastic.

- The *neurodevelopmental approach* (Bobath, 1990) aims to develop perceptual abilities during its handling and retraining techniques. Many of the techniques, which are specific to this <u>Motor control</u> theory, provide sensory input, which can be utilized for perceptual functions. During <u>Bilateral clasped activities</u>, the client may be increasing awareness of a neglected limb, body scheme, or position in space. While weightbearing, the client may be retraining proprioception as well as facilitating muscle contraction.

- The *transfer of training approach* emphasizes that the practice of a particular perceptual task can be generalized to other tasks that require the same perceptual function. If a person practices pegboard designs to increase spatial relations, then those spatial abilities may carry over to a transfer activity (the client may be able to judge the location of the target chair with better accuracy).

- The *functional or task-oriented approach* is a common method of rehabilitation of perceptual skills. This approach is based on the principle that repetition and practice of perceptual functions will increase the client's independence. Rather than practicing specific skills in an unfamiliar environment, the therapist works with the client in his or her natural environment and educates the client on personal deficits in order to develop strategies to remediate and compensate for loss. For instance, the therapist may help the client establish a routine during dressing that will allow the client to compensate for unilateral neglect. As the client learns the routine, he or she becomes more independent with dressing. The therapist may also adapt the environment or objects being used by the client in order to increase independence. The room may be arranged to decrease distractions, or cues may be written and displayed.

General Intervention Considerations

- It is important to note that the underlying causes of the cognitive-perceptual deficits will determine prognosis. For clients with a brain injury, remedial techniques are often used with the expectation that the brain will heal and function will improve. With a client diagnosed with a progressive dementia (neurocognitive disorder), approaches may rely more heavily on adaptive and compensatory techniques.

- There are many newer <u>Assistive technology</u> and computer-based interventions designed to improve cognition and perception. Research is beginning to study the effectiveness of such approaches.

- Intervention techniques should be practiced since repetition can help increase learning. It is important to note that clients vary in their ability to generalize from one environment to another.

- Intervention may begin with a specific activity or in a specific environment; however, when possible, treatment should be generalized and applied during functional activities. Doing puzzles does not help the client to increase body part identification if that ability is never applied during dressing to help the client understand the orientation of clothing.

- During cognitive intervention, focus may be placed on the process the client uses rather than the specific task. While techniques are developed for a specific task (e.g., putting on a shirt), the cognitive-perceptual processes are also an area of focus.

- Intervention should begin at the client's level of ability and then increase in difficulty as the client improves so the client is always challenged.

- Interventions regarding ADLs and <u>Instrumental activities of daily living (IADLs)</u> should pay specific attention to safety and judgement.

Intervention of Specific Deficits

- **Attention.** The ability to focus on a task, person, or object without being distracted by other stimuli. Attention problems may occur after a <u>Traumatic brain injury</u>, or may accompany congenital and developmental conditions. Attention is integral to the client's ability to learn. Often, therapists see clients with attention issues in hospitals, rehabilitation facilities, and schools.

- ○ When done in a clinical setting, therapy should occur in an environment with few distractions. As the client improves, the environment can be gradually "normalized" until intervention is possible in the usual location, such as within the client's home.

- ○ Intervention may be simple and brief in the beginning, but the therapist may increase the complexity of the treatment activity, as well as the duration of treatment, as the client improves.

- ○ Computer activities, which send immediate feedback, may be an effective way to increase the client's ability to sit and work on a task.

- ○ Often, the use of meaningful activities capitalizing on client interests will maximize the client's willingness or ability to attend.

- ○ The therapist may also ask the client to complete activities that divide attention (e.g., the client is asked to sort a deck of cards according to color and face cards).

- ○ For children, often the therapist is addressing attention in a school setting; see also <u>Attention deficit disorder (ADD)</u>.

- **Orientation.** The ability to identify information about oneself and the environment, including name, place, date, and situation.

- ○ Staff members and family should orient the client to time, place, person, and situation whenever possible.

- ○ Visual aids can be used such as calendars or individualized orientation boards that list the date, place, person's name, and situation (if desired).

- ○ If needed, provide context (e.g., for those with an <u>Acquired brain injury</u>, in early stages, you may need to daily restate your name, the date, and location to orient the client).

- **Memory.** The ability to store information for immediate recall or retrieval at a later date. There are many types of memory; two often focused upon include declarative memory, which involves the conscious retrieval of facts, and procedural memory, which involves the ability to remember and carry out tasks. Clients may have more difficulty with one type or another. For instance, a person with

Alzheimer's disease may be able to tell you how to do the laundry, but if asked to wash a load of laundry, he or she may have significant difficulty.

- Approaches to intervention in memory are both remedial/restorative (e.g., for those recovering from a traumatic brain injury) and compensatory/adaptive (as used with someone who has a progressive dementia).

- Compensatory techniques often use daily reminders, adaptation, and task simplification. The client may use signs placed around the client's room or house to give reminders for activities such as turning off the curling iron, lights, or stove. A notebook may be used to take notes when the client learns a new task or receives new information. An alarm can be set to remind the client to take medication. The client's environment can be labeled to help the client locate items (e.g., kitchen cupboards can be labeled if the client cannot find items when cooking, or a sign can be placed near the bathroom door if room location is difficult).

- In recent years, there has been increased use of technological advances to facilitate memory and organization (e.g., watches can be set to remind a client to take his or her medications).

- The client can verbally rehearse information to help increase recall.

- Visual images can be used to help the client recall information.

- If the client needs to recall a larger amount of information, he or she can make up a story that ties the information together.

- Mnemonics is the use of letters contained in each word in a list that are then joined together as a word to help abbreviate a large amount of information (e.g., when using a fire extinguisher, the mnemonic PASS helps a person recall the following steps of use: *Pull* the pin, *Aim* at the base of the fire, *Squeeze* the trigger, and *Sweep* across the fire in short alternating strokes).

- The therapist may assist the client in developing motor routines to help the client retrieve information (e.g., the client always undresses in the same pattern and places jewelry in the same location).

- The PQRSTA method includes the following tasks: *Preview* material, *Question* what will be included, *Read* the material,

State what was read, and *Test* by *Answering* questions about the material.

- **Problem Solving.** The ability to apply current knowledge in order to create solutions when new problems or situations arise.
  - ○ The therapist should provide the client with various problems and puzzles to solve. Practice will help the client find helpful strategies. It is important to not only use paper–pencil tasks but also functional activities that replicate the daily occupational expectations for the client.
  - ○ <u>Chaining</u> may be used to break a complex problem into smaller, manageable components. If the client is attempting to balance a checkbook, the therapist can have the client complete one entry at a time and then check the client's work to catch errors while the client still has the problem in mind.
  - ○ Group treatment for problem solving may help the client find new strategies, as well as help the client generalize strategies to new situations.
  - ○ Asking the client to self-assess performance and give feedback can help facilitate personal insight.
  - ○ The client can be taught the process for problem solving as follows:
    - ■ Define the problem.
    - ■ Develop possible solutions.
    - ■ Choose the best solution.
    - ■ Execute the solution.
    - ■ Evaluate the outcome.
- **Awareness.** Awareness refers to the ability of a client to understand a situation or fact. Self-awareness includes the ability to understand and remember that one not only has personal strengths, but also may have deficits that limit performance in the affected areas.
  - ○ Feedback from the therapist, or peers if group therapy is used, is an effective means of helping the client gain awareness regarding behavior.
  - ○ The therapist may use role reversal to help the client see how behavior is viewed by others.
  - ○ Self-evaluation encourages the client to view his or her actions and behavior.

- Peer feedback may be used in group interventions.

- **Sequencing and Organization.** The ability to categorize and organize the steps of an activity; for instance, understanding the steps in order to complete a cooking task.

  - Use of visual photos or drawn pictures may be included in intervention to assess the client's ability to organize tasks. Similar teaching techniques may be used to facilitate completion of tasks.

  - Teach the client to associate new tasks to familiar tasks to facilitate learning and organization.

  - Start with a minimalistic structure and, as the client improves, increase complexity.

  - Facilitate self-verbalization techniques and audible reminders (e.g., first this, then this).

  - For adaptive approaches, provide external reminders, lists, and visual schedules.

  - For individuals who learn visually (e.g., often persons with <u>Autism</u>), the use of simple photos on a Velcro-affixed board can help an individual conceptualize the sequence for the task or the routine for the day.

- **Executive Functions.** Cognitive processes that govern several thought processes and are integral to cognition. Executive functions regulate and control our ability to plan ahead, sequence, self-monitor, self-evaluate, problem solve, and maintain inhibition when necessary. Additional skills include <u>Concept formation</u>, abstraction, and decision making.

  - In addition to strategies listed in other cognitive components in this section, it is important to work with the client on safe problem solving. The use of scenarios, role play, and video may be helpful. For instance, if working with a client who has impulse control issues paired with poor insight, the use of video scenarios and alternatives discussion may be helpful.

  - When using written directions, have the client read the directions out loud and verbally explain the thought process related to the scenario described.

  - Be sure to monitor and adapt the environment for safety when working with clients who have poor judgment.

  - Use scenario planning to discuss alternatives.

- **Visual Foundation Skills.** These skills are composed of visual acuity, visual fields, and oculomotor function. *Visual acuity* is the ability to focus on objects both at near and far distances. A person with intact *visual fields* must be able to see objects in each of the four quadrants of vision with each eye. *Oculomotor function* is movement of the eyeball, which is caused by the muscles attached to the eye. The four parts of oculomotor function include range of motion, pursuits, convergence, and alignment.

  ○ A client with decreased visual acuity may first benefit from a pair of corrective lenses and should be seen by a physician. If a client has continued acuity issues, adaptive techniques are used.

  ○ The therapist can help adapt the environment to increase a client's ability to see. The client can identify the objects used in the environment that create the most difficulty, then the therapist can make adaptations to increase the background contrast (e.g., if a client is unable to see the edge of steps, the therapist can outline the edge of the step with brightly colored tape or paint). Therapists can also provide guidance for placement and organization in addition to assistive technology such as lighted magnifying glasses.

  ○ Used enlarged objects and print.

  ○ Teach the client about computer adaptations for visual loss—talking books and software may be advisable.

  ○ Provide intervention in a natural context/environment.

  ○ For safety, the use of prechopped items for cooking and predictable kitchen and home organization is advised.

  ○ An increase in illumination may increase the client's ability to see objects; however, the therapist should attempt to avoid an increase in glare or shadows. Recessed lighting increases shadows and should not be used. The best source of illumination is fluorescent lighting and halogen lamps. When reading, the recommended lamp is the 50-watt halogen desk lamp.

  ○ Patterned backgrounds decrease acuity; highly patterned objects such as rugs, bedspreads, placemats, countertops, and furniture should be modified or replaced with solid-colored items.

  ○ A client with a visual field cut should be trained to turn the head to the affected side in order to see the missing field.

Rehabilitation should focus on the client's speed when scanning to the affected side, as well as the client's ability to scan the entire scope of the affected area. This type of compensation is particularly important if the client wants to resume driving.

o   The therapist can provide the client with specific techniques to help with reading. A green line drawn on the left margin (GO) and a red line on the right margin (STOP) can help the client identify where the text of a line starts or stops. A client who has difficulty staying on the line while reading can place a ruler or straight edge below the line.

o   If a client has problems keeping text on the line while writing, the client should be taught to focus on the pen tip constantly to ensure the writing does not cross a line.

o   Activities that require scanning can help increase the client's visual attention. Treatment for attention and scanning is most effective when the client is required to touch or name the object. Objects can be enlarged on a screen to facilitate scanning and head turning.

o   Matching activities help increase visual attention, as the client must identify similar or contrasting details.

o   The client can practice all of these skills, but the client should then practice applying those skills in more functional circumstances. The client can practice scanning when getting clothes out of the closet. Visual acuity may be practiced in the community (e.g., while crossing a busy street or searching for items in a grocery store). The client may attempt to read the newspaper or look up telephone numbers using compensatory techniques for a visual field cut.

o   Clients with visual field neglect may need additional adaptive techniques, and the family/caregivers should be educated to promote safety in the case of a client's absence of awareness.

*   **Visual Discrimination Skills.** The ability to recognize different forms in order to recognize objects and their meaning. Persons with learning disabilities such as <u>Dyslexia</u> may have poor visual discrimination, as may others due to brain injury.

o   Have the client start with matching and sorting simple objects and work toward everyday functional objects.

o   The use of tactile cues may be helpful to facilitate visual discrimination.

- ○ Label items and provide visual cues.
- ○ Organize the environment so that the client may be able to distinguish items by location.
- **Body Scheme.** The ability to identify the position of body parts in relation to one another and to objects in the environment.
  - ○ Puzzles of the human body may help the client learn the arrangement of body parts in relation to one another.
  - ○ Bilateral activities can be helpful, especially when one side is more affected than the other.
  - ○ Use client cueing.
  - ○ Sensory stimulation to the affected extremities helps the client increase awareness of the affected side.
  - ○ For those with neglect, education of the client and family is important in order to ensure safety.
  - ○ <u>Sensory integration (SI)/sensory processing therapy</u> interventions are often used with persons who have sensory integrative dysfunction in order to increase awareness.
- **Right/Left Discrimination.** The ability to differentiate between the right and left sides of the body.
  - ○ The client who is not able to spontaneously identify right and left will need to learn compensatory techniques, such as using the wedding ring to help identify the left side of the body.
  - ○ Activities that stress the differentiation of right from left may help train the client in this skill. The client can be asked to identify body parts on the left or right side of the body. The client can also be asked to find objects located on the right or left side of a page or activity.
  - ○ Sensory input can be increased to the right or left side of the body while asking the client to identify the side.
- **Body Part Identification.** The ability to identify the position of body parts on oneself or on other persons.
  - ○ The therapist can touch one of the client's body parts and then ask the client to verbally identify which part was touched.
  - ○ The therapist can then name a specific part of the body and ask the client to touch the desired part.

- **Finger Agnosia.** The inability to name or identify a specific finger when asked to discriminate between fingers, usually during a sensory evaluation.
    - Rubbing the client's affected dorsal surface of the forearm and hand, as well as both the dorsal and ventral surfaces of the fingers (usually completed for minimum of 2 minutes), helps increase the client's awareness of the fingers.
    - Deep pressure (again completed for usually a minimum of 2 minutes) can be applied by placing a hard, rough cone in the client's hand. This pressure sensation may help the client identify his or her fingers.
    - See additional techniques under body scheme in this section.
- **Anosognosia.** The inability to perceive that one is ill, such as unawareness of hemiplegia following a lesion.
    - If a client consciously denies a condition or illness, intervention may be difficult.
    - As the client recovers, increase sensory stimulation, verbal cueing, and activities that focus on the client's condition.
    - Continually educate the client and caregivers to ensure maximal safety.
- **Unilateral Neglect.** The inability to sense or perceive stimuli that are presented on the side of the client's body that is contralateral to the site of the brain lesion (e.g., the client who has had a right Cerebrovascular accident [CVA] may not dress his or her hemiplegic left arm or turn toward the left to look for food on the left side of the plate).
    - Intervention may begin with the practice of visual scanning tasks. The client can complete cancellation tasks, which require the client to cross out a particular letter or symbol in a list of random letters/symbols. The activity could then proceed to crossing out a particular word in a paragraph. The task can be graded so that the final step requires the client to cross out a particular letter in a paragraph.
    - Activities that focus on the affected extremity may help increase awareness. Weightbearing, handling, verbal cueing, and repetitive tasks may help call attention to the neglected side.
    - The therapist and other staff should approach the client from the affected side to help the client learn to turn toward that side.

Also, the client's room can be rearranged to force the client to turn toward the affected side to watch television or to see who is entering the room.

- ○ Occasionally, a client who has left neglect may have a patch placed over his or her right eye to further encourage the client to look to the affected side.

- ○ If using an adaptive approach, items should be placed on the unaffected side and the therapist should also position on that side so the client is able to see everything easily during treatment.

- ○ The therapist may need to draw a green line on the left side of the page or a red line at the right margin of the page to help cue the client when or where to return to the next line while reading. Without these cues, the client most likely will miss part of the text and be unable to understand the material being read.

- ○ Be sure caregivers are educated in order to ensure safety.

- **Position in Space.** The ability to understand terms that define position (e.g., over, under, above, beneath, beside, in front of, in back of) and then apply those positions in relation to self in the environment.

- ○ The client may complete activities that require spatial abilities such as pegboard designs, block designs, or puzzles. Then, the client can answer questions about objects, such as which block is under, over, above, below, beside, and so on.

- ○ Functional activities that can help increase the client's sense of position include organizing a closet or cupboard while following the therapist's directions to place certain items in certain places.

- **Spatial Relations.** The ability to determine the position of objects in relation to each other or to oneself.

- ○ Walking along a path may help the client orient him- or herself to other objects.

- ○ The therapist can ask the client questions about the client's self in relation to other objects in the room.

- ○ For those who have difficulty with visual spatial relations such as lack of <u>Depth perception</u>, a consult with an eye specialist is advised.

- **Topographical Orientation.** The ability to move from one location to another without assistance.
  - ○ The therapist can place markers or cues along a path to help the client learn routes from one place to another (e.g., a client who is in a rehabilitation unit can use different colored signs to find his or her way to occupational, speech, or physical therapy). The therapist may also draw a simple map of the hospital floor or wing, which the client can follow between therapy clinics. In a long-term care setting, the therapist may place a colored piece of tape on the floor from the dining room to the client's room to help the client find the way back from meals independently.
  - ○ Once the client increases these skills, the therapist may attempt the use of verbal maps or instructions to help guide the client to new locations.
  - ○ The client benefits from the memorization of routes that are used the most often.
  - ○ If the client's difficulty with topographical orientation stems from visual deficits or neglect, then treatment should begin with those deficits.
  - ○ Portable GPS may be used to help orient the client to the environment.
- **Figure/Ground Perception.** The ability to discriminate between an object and its background.
  - ○ Intervention may begin by having the client locate objects in pictures taken from magazines and books. This activity should be graded according to the client's ability to prevent the client from becoming frustrated. As the client improves, the activity can be made increasingly difficult. (The *Where's Waldo* books [Candlewick Press] are excellent final activities for figure/ground perception.)
  - ○ Scanning activities such as word search puzzles can help the client learn to identify words within a complex background.
  - ○ It is important to move from paper/pencil activities toward a functional approach (e.g., locating grocery items in the store).
  - ○ The therapist may need to adapt the client's environment so that the background is simple and objects that are difficult for the client to see are brightly marked.

- **Apraxia.** A perceptual deficit that hinders clients from completing functional or purposeful movement. The client may have normal sensory, motor, and coordination skills or may suffer apraxia as a result of brain damage. See also <u>Apraxia</u>.

  ○ A client with ideomotor or ideational apraxia may benefit from the therapist manually guiding the client's limbs while completing an activity. This method is often referred to as *hand-over-hand*.

  ○ Increased tactile and proprioceptive stimulation may facilitate the proper motor movements.

  ○ Chaining is the act of dividing complex activities into smaller, manageable components. The client can learn each small step of an activity separately, and then combine the small steps into a larger activity once the client has demonstrated competence with each small step.

  ○ Visualization of the desired motion or activity may assist the client with motor planning.

  ○ Verbal instruction may be used minimally, but the client may not understand due to <u>Aphasia</u>.

  ○ Intervention should occur in the environment where the desired activity is usually completed (e.g., the steps of cooking should be practiced in a kitchen area rather than at a table in an outpatient clinic).

  ○ Clients who have demonstrated constructional apraxia may benefit from visual cues when constructing or drawing designs.

  ○ The therapist can have the client copy block or pegboard designs, and the therapist should increase the difficulty of the designs as the client improves.

  ○ Functional activities should be used whenever possible because learning may be task-specific in some cases, particularly with individuals who have a brain injury. A client with constructional apraxia can practice making a sandwich or folding laundry and putting it back into the dresser and closet.

  ○ Clients who have dressing apraxia benefit from learning a specific pattern of dressing. The therapist can then teach the client to use visual cues such as the zipper of pants or the label in a shirt to help orient clothing. Through repetition, the client will learn dressing. The client should then use different clothes while using the same visual cues to help orient the clothing so that the technique can be generalized to all pants and/or all shirts.

- o Individuals may have difficulty performing ADLs such as dressing, grooming, or bathing.

- o Use the remedial or transfer of training approach where the therapist works with the client on using compensatory movements.

- o Neurodevelopmental methods are also used by therapists in improving dressing skills. In general, therapists use functional and adaptive approaches to help the client be as independent as possible in performing <u>Self-care</u> activities.

- **Astereognosis.** The inability to identify objects through touch or <u>Tactile sensation</u>.

  - o Intervention should begin while allowing the client to touch and feel an object while looking at it. The next step is blocking the client's vision while the client continues to feel the object so the client cannot use visual cues for identification. The final step involves placing a pad or towel on the table while the client continues to feel the object so the client is not able to use auditory cues for identification.

  - o As the client demonstrates progress, the client should be asked to identify features of the objects without visual cues. Objects that have opposite or very dissimilar traits should be presented to the client (e.g., the client can learn to discriminate between a rough and smooth texture).

  - o The next step involves the identification of an estimated number of objects (e.g., the client is asked to place his or her hand in a bowl and estimate how many marshmallows are in the container).

  - o The client can learn to discriminate between large and small objects hidden in a container of sand. Another discrimination task may require the client to differentiate between two- and three-dimensional objects.

  - o The final step of intervention occurs when the client selects a small object from a collection of several objects and is able to identify the object with vision blocked.

- ○ Intervention may also progress in the following manner:
  - ■ Visual examination of the object
  - ■ Tactile examination with the unaffected hand while observing
  - ■ Tactile examination with both hands while observing
  - ■ Tactile examination with the affected hand while observing
  - ■ Tactile examination with the unaffected hand with vision blocked
  - ■ Tactile examination with both hands with vision blocked
  - ■ Tactile examination with the affected hand with vision blocked.
- ○ After the client is able to successfully identify various objects using this method, two objects can be hidden in a tub of rice or sand. The client is then asked to retrieve a particular object from the tub.

Cognitive Therapy. First conceptualized by Beck (1976), this is defined as a primarily verbal therapy that helps the client to examine his or her thoughts, impulses, and feelings that are contributing to a disorder. Cognitive therapy is related to current-day <u>Cognitive behavioral therapy</u> as it emphasizes that the way people cognitively structure a situation (how they think) determines how they feel and behave (e.g., if a person interprets a situation as dangerous, he or she may feel anxious and prepare to protect him- or herself). Behavioral techniques are used by cognitive therapists to help clients develop new approaches in dealing with everyday activities by helping them to monitor their behavior and to try out new behaviors.

Cogwheel Rigidity. A type of muscular rigidity characterized by arrhythmic relaxation and contraction of muscles during passive movement. When moving a body part that has cogwheel rigidity, the part may be difficult to move at first, causing the muscle to start and stop (looking somewhat like a ratcheted motion), but then both agonist and antagonist muscles will relax so that movement is easier. However, the muscle <u>Co-contraction</u> will again occur, making movement difficult. This contracting and relaxing will occur many times while the therapist moves the part through its range of motion, so that movement feels like it keeps "catching." See <u>Rigidity</u> and <u>Lead pipe rigidity</u> for further discussion. Cogwheel rigidity may be caused by certain conditions such as <u>Parkinson's disease</u> or may be a side effect of certain medications such as traditional neuroleptics.

Color Agnosia. The inability to name or identify a color. See <u>Cognitive-perceptual deficits</u> for intervention techniques for similar perception disorders.

Colostomy. A surgical opening in the abdomen in order to bring the colon through a stoma (opening) in order to divert stool and waste to a bag that is externally managed. Occupational therapists may be part of a team that facilitates education and management of the colostomy.

Coma. Marked by prolonged unconsciousness caused by a number of factors such as brain trauma; drugs and alcohol; or conditions such as stroke, diabetes, or other illness. Persons in a coma demonstrate varying levels of unresponsiveness. The *Glasgow Coma Scale* is a tool used extensively over the past 40 years (Teasdale et al., 2014) to assess level of consciousness based on eye opening and verbal and motor response. Based on the ratings and other assessments, therapists plan interventions to include <u>Positioning</u>, sensory stimulation, <u>Range of motion (ROM)</u>, and safety (e.g., assuring proper skin care).

Community Mental Health Center (CMHC). Originally an outgrowth of the Community Mental Health Center Act of 1963 (Mental Retardation Facilities Construction Act, 1963). The CMHC was conceptualized as an alternative to long-term <u>Institutionalization</u> for individuals with mental illness. CMHCs provide five basic mental health services: inpatient hospitalization when needed, outpatient care, <u>Partial hospitalization</u>, emergency mental health services, and consultation and education to community groups and agencies. In recent years, the Centers for Medicare and Medicaid Services (2014) established specific conditions for participation in CMHCs. In 2016, certified community behavioral health clinics were established to extend community-based mental health care.

Community Support Program (CSP). An initiative of the National Institute of Mental Health in response to the <u>Deinstitutionalization</u> of individuals with chronic mental illness, CSP supplied funds to public hospitals, <u>Community mental health centers (CMHC)</u>, and county and social service agencies to provide comprehensive services, including psychosocial rehabilitation to those with chronic mental illness. <u>Community support system (CSS)</u> was a major thrust of CSP.

Community Support System (CSS). A model designed to meet the needs of individuals with mental illness, such as health and dental, housing, income support, entitlement (Medicare, Medicaid), and employment, through a case management approach.

Complementary and Alternative Medicine (CAM). Complementary medicine refers to health-related techniques outside of the mainstream scientific or Western medicine along with conventional techniques. Some distinguish it from <u>Alternative medicine</u>, which may be used to denote methods used instead of traditional approaches. Complementary medicine approaches include techniques such as relaxation therapies, <u>Tai chi</u>, <u>Yoga</u>, reiki, massage, humor, and therapeutic use of vitamins and herbs.

Compression. Techniques used to help reduce and control edema due to certain health conditions or an injury such as a sprain. Compression may include the use of prefabricated compression garments such as compression socks, or may utilize wrapping techniques. See <u>Edema</u>.

Concentric Contraction. See <u>Contraction</u>.

Concept Formation. The cognitive ability to organize and classify information to form thoughts and ideas, such as the concept of an object (e.g., plane), values (e.g., altruism), norms, and beliefs. Concept formation is a higher-order cognitive ability that entails learning, memory, and generalization. In recent years, strategies have been developed to facilitate the development of concept formation. Group activities such as <u>Values clarification</u> and Socratic discussion can be used to clarify and facilitate concept formation.

Conduct Disorders. A psychosocial disorder that is characterized by persistent antisocial behaviors infringing on the rights of others or societal norms. Often, conduct disorders include behaviors such as aggression toward others, destruction of property, theft, dishonesty, and illegal violation of rules. The behaviors have a significant negative effect on interpersonal relationships, school achievement, and ability to work. A similar disorder, oppositional defiant disorder, often includes symptoms of angry and resentful behavior, poor <u>Self-control</u>, argumentativeness, defiance, and vindictiveness. Oppositional defiant disorder may result in sexual acting out, illegal drug use, delinquency, and running away from home. There is limited research to support the effectiveness of interventions for conduct disorder; therefore, a comprehensive approach should be used (Frick, 2001), which includes parental and caregiver training (Scott, 2007).

Specific Interventions
- Sports programs that allow individuals to express feelings in a socially accepted activity
- <u>Social skills</u> training that develops empathy and compassion toward others

- <u>Prescriptive exercise</u> that is meaningful to the child or adolescent and can be incorporated into his or her everyday life
- <u>Stress management</u> to help individuals develop relaxation strategies
- <u>Family therapy</u> to engage the family in the dynamics of treatment
- Nutritional and diet education
- Volunteer work in the community to develop compassion for others and a sense of responsibility
- Upward Bound and other similar programs to challenge individuals and create opportunities for cooperating with others in hiking, camping, and mountain climbing
- <u>Creative arts</u> therapy to help individuals express feelings in a nonjudgmental environment
- Role play, video feedback, and scenario discussions to encourage insight and provide opportunity for individual and collective feedback

Constructional Apraxia. See <u>Apraxia</u>.

Context. The *Occupational Therapy Practice Framework, Third Edition* (American Occupational Therapy Association, 2014) indicates that our social and physical environment occur within a context that may include cultural, physical, personal, social, temporal, and virtual contexts. Therapists consider the context in the occupational therapy process when planning evaluation and intervention. For instance, when working with a client who has a chronic mental illness, intervention plans will consider whether the client is likely to move to a group home, a board and care facility, or an independent apartment.

Contingency Management. A group of techniques used in <u>Behavior therapy</u> in which the client establishes a contract with the therapist to modify a behavioral response by shaping the consequences of that response (e.g., the client will receive a token for positive interpersonal communications). This type of intervention is often used in substance abuse, particularly in the earlier stages of treatment.

Continuous Quality Improvement (CQI). A systems approach built upon concepts of <u>Quality assurance</u> in order to improve the quality of care of an organization, hospital, or agency. In this approach, the system rather than the individual is the prime focus, and data are used to identify areas for improvement. Creativity, leadership, and achievable and measurable goals are emphasized in this approach.

Contraction. An increase in the tone of a muscle, which may or may not result in the shortening or lengthening of the muscle.

Types of Contractions

- **Isotonic Contractions.** A contraction that results in movement of a body part. Isotonic contractions can be further classified as follows:
  - ○ **Concentric Contractions.** A muscle contraction that results in shortening of the muscle fibers that are contracting and motion in the direction of the muscle's pull (e.g., when the biceps contracts, the fibers pull upward [toward the shoulder], resulting in the shortening of the muscle, which causes the forearm to be pulled toward the shoulder [elbow flexion]).
  - ○ **Eccentric Contractions.** A muscle contraction that results in elongation of the muscle fibers that are contracting and motion in the opposite direction from the muscle's direction of pull (from what is normally expected during a contraction). For example, when the biceps contracts, the expectation would be a shortening of the muscle, which would cause elbow flexion. However, if the elbow is already flexed against gravity (such as when the client is sitting upright), the biceps performs an eccentric contraction to return the elbow to full extension. The triceps do not need to actively complete extension since gravity would normally pull the arm into extension if the biceps was not contracting. Instead, the biceps continues contracting while slowly lengthening to slowly lower the elbow into extension.
- **Isometric Contractions.** A contraction that does not result in movement but is usually completed for the stabilization of a body part or object.

Contracture. An abnormal shortening of soft tissue or connective tissue that limits range of motion (ROM) at a joint and may cause disability. Contractures may be a result of injury or disability. Positioning to maintain ligament and muscle length and passive ROM (PROM) should be used to help prevent contractures; however, contractures may be unavoidable in some instances due to some disease processes. In that case, positioning should be used so that the contractures occur in a functional position so that the client is still able to complete functional activities in the presence of limited ROM. The functional position of the hand is slight wrist extension (10 to 30 degrees) with the thumb abducted and slightly flexed and the fingers flexed through partial ROM. This allows the client to <u>Place and hold</u> items in the affected hand or use the hand to assist in activities such as dressing. If the hand contracts while fully flexed, the client will develop sores in the palm from the fingernails, and cleansing the hand will be very difficult. If the hand contracts while fully extended, the client will not be able to use it to assist with holding or stabilizing objects.

Contraindication. A condition or previous diagnosis that makes a specific type of treatment dangerous or counterproductive. For example, a client who has hemiplegia may benefit from <u>Neuromuscular electrical stimulation (NMES)</u> to help reeducate the affected muscles. However, if the client has a pacemaker, the electrical current can cause failure of the pacemaker to respond to cardiac problems. In the case of a client who has both hemiplegia and a pacemaker, NMES should not be used. Contraindications for treatment are listed following treatment techniques throughout the text.

Contrast Bath. A type of <u>Hydrotherapy</u> that is used to help decrease edema and <u>Hypersensitivity</u> through immersion of the affected extremity or the body into alternating warm and cold baths. See <u>Edema</u> for more information.

Controlled Breathing. Learning to use abdominal muscles in breathing slowly with the aim of reducing stress and <u>Anxiety</u>.

Coordination. The ability to control muscle contractions to produce smooth movement with appropriate speed, rhythm, muscle tone, postural tone, and accuracy. To produce controlled movement, the client must have the appropriate muscles contracting to move a body part, as well as to stabilize the joint. The client may have difficulty with coordination if there are perceptual deficits with proprioception, position in space, <u>Body scheme</u>, or spatial relations. Coordination may be further subdivided into <u>Gross motor</u> and <u>Fine motor coordination</u>. Gross motor coordination is the ability to control the contraction of large muscles and groups of muscles to complete large, less specific movements. Fine motor coordination is the ability to control the contraction of small muscles to complete fine, precise movements. Bilateral coordination refers to the ability to synchronize movement from both sides of the body. Following is a list of treatment methods to help a client increase the control of movements.

Specific Interventions

- **Gross Motor**
  - The use of activities that require large motor movements
  - Sliding or tossing bean bags toward designated targets

- ○ Light homemaking tasks such as making a bed or setting a table
- ○ Folding laundry
- ○ Reaching for items above the head
- ○ Playing catch
- ○ The use of obstacle courses
- ○ Cardiovascular training with increased complexity (be sure there is medical clearance)
- ○ Pulleys—this activity is especially good for teaching the client bilateral coordination with both upper extremities
- ○ Placing and removing items from shelves
- ○ Light cooking activities that involve opening containers, cutting, and stirring
- ○ Large tabletop board games like giant checkers
- ○ Karate or martial arts
- ○ For those with <u>Sensory integration (SI)</u> difficulties, often sensorimotor/SI activities are incorporated into the treatment protocol
- ○ See <u>Range of motion (ROM)</u> treatment methods

- **Fine Motor**
  - ○ Manipulating coins
  - ○ Theraputty with small objects in putty to be removed
  - ○ Tying shoes
  - ○ Buttoning buttons
  - ○ Pegboard activities
  - ○ Lacing
  - ○ Cutting
  - ○ Writing
  - ○ Board games, including checkers, dominoes, Operation (Hasbro), and Perfection (Hasbro)
  - ○ Puzzles
  - ○ Opening containers
  - ○ Making necklaces/bracelets
  - ○ Needlework or knitting
  - ○ Crafts such as making tile trivets or painting
  - ○ Dialing a telephone

Coping Skills. An individual's ability to self-regulate stress and master the environment. Stress management is an example of a coping skill where the individual becomes aware of the stressors that trigger symptoms and the copers that are helpful in reducing the symptoms. <u>Stress management</u> techniques include <u>Relaxation therapy</u>, <u>Biofeedback</u>, <u>Cognitive behavioral therapy</u>, skill training, and <u>Prescriptive exercise</u>.

Coronal plane. Division of the body from head to feet into front and back portions. See <u>Anatomical position</u>.

Course. The predicted stages of an illness based on clinical observations of the illness and epidemiological studies of stages in an illness (e.g., <u>Alzheimer's disease</u> has a progressive course where the individual often deteriorates in predictable stages).

Creative Arts. The creative arts include the use of art, music, <u>Dance</u>, drama, poetry, crafts, and other expressive media as therapeutic and purposeful activities for the client. In designing a creative arts therapy program, the therapist should consider the interests of the client, goals of intervention, cognitive level, and feasibility of implementing the modality. In general, the creative arts should allow the client to express his or her feelings, attitudes, and problems in a free, uncensored environment. The creative media should enable the client to be spontaneous (e.g., in drawing a dream, acting out a personal conflict, expressing emotion through dance, or creating a poem expressing a feeling). The therapist tries to guide and encourage the client to use the creative media in a meaningful way. The interpretation of the client's finished product can be done jointly with the client. It can help the client in gaining insight into conflicts and emotional problems by tying together the process of completing the creative expression and the client's attitude toward the product. Although the arts may be used in a variety of <u>Frames of reference</u>, they are particularly integral to the <u>Psychodynamic/Object relations</u> frames of reference. The creative arts have also been an important area for occupational therapists to embed physical goals such as coordination, muscle strength, range of motion, and perceptual motor into a purposeful activity.

Crepitus. A creaking or grating sound and feeling that occurs under the skin or at a joint during movement. This sensation often accompanies movement at arthritic joints.

Crisis Intervention. A 24-hour service that provides short-term immediate help for those with imminent mental health concerns who need emotional or physical assistance (e.g., if someone is in danger of harm to self or others). The service is designed to meet the needs of and decrease stress on the client or family members. Problems such as a loss of job, broken friendships, drug-related problems, or criminal offenses can many times put the individual into a crisis. A case manager or mental health professional can provide support by linking the individual to resources in the community. Telephone hotlines open and accessible to the individual can be extremely important in alleviating a crisis. Ideally, a client is offered additional support following the time of crisis.

Criterion. A standard that is used to measure performance. For instance, an assessment that is criterion-based may have the therapist check a box if a client successfully performs a skill (e.g., paying a bill).

Criterion-Referenced Test. A test based on standards of performance, competence, or mastery, rather than on comparison to a normative group.

Crossed Extensor Reflex. A withdrawal reflex of the lower limbs. See Reflexes and reactions.

Crossing the Midline. The ability to move the arms and legs across the body, coordinated with one's eyes in controlled, goal-directed actions. Examples include putting on one's socks and shoes, buttoning one's shirts, playing checkers, doing a picture puzzle, playing the piano, and assembling parts.

Cruising. To walk or shuffle along while holding on to objects. This is often the final stage babies go through prior to walking. Safety is a priority as the child starts to cruise.

Cryotherapy. The application of cold temperature through compressed ice packs or sprays to relive pain, reduce spasticity, and reduce tissue swelling, such as in sprains to muscles or ligaments. See Physical agent modalities (PAMs) for further discussion and treatment.

Cubital Tunnel Syndrome. This condition results from compression of the ulnar nerve within the cubital tunnel, which is formed by the ulnar collateral ligament, trochlea, medial epicondylar groove, and triangular arcuate ligament. The client may complain of severe pain, decreased grip and pinch strength, or decreased Fine motor coordination. Repetitive elbow motion that requires constant grip may result in this condition. Rest, anti-inflammatory medication, and modalities such as ultrasound, which decrease swelling around the nerve, may be applied as conservative treatment or as adjunct treatment following surgery to release the cubital tunnel. The client should receive ergonomic education, including avoiding direct pressure on the medial elbow and placing the elbow in extension at night to help decrease the stress to the affected area, which has occurred from cumulative trauma.

Culture-Free Test. A test that is not culturally biased and can be administered across cultures.

Cumulative Trauma Disorders. Conditions caused by cumulative wear and tear to the muscles, joints, tendons, and nervous tissue. Causes may include overuse, poor positioning, or repetitive stress. Interventions may include postsurgical rehabilitation, education on ergonomics and positioning, and remedial and adaptive strategies to address <u>Activities of daily living (ADLs)</u>, <u>Instrumental activities of daily living (IADLs)</u>, <u>Work</u>, and <u>Leisure</u> activities.

Cylindrical Grasp. See <u>Grasp</u>.

D

Dance. Movement using a series of rhythmical motions and steps. It is a good form of exercise and expression of emotions. Dance may take a variety of forms, from prescriptive and choreographed to free-flowing and expressive. Some health care facilities hire dance therapists to facilitate healing through dance movements.

Dance Therapy. The use of dance or movement as a carefully guided tool to promote healing through cathartic release, self-awareness, and emphasis on mind–body integration. Therapy may take place individually or occur within a dance therapy group that seeks to promote social interaction and social awareness.

Day Treatment Centers (DTCs). Previously referred to as *day hospitals*, these were established in the United States in the 1950s for individuals who were discharged from mental hospitals and could potentially benefit from a period of transitional services. DTCs are licensed and provide comprehensive treatment, including medication management, counseling, group therapy, and occupational therapy. The occupational therapist plays an important role in the DTCs in helping individuals in the performance areas of <u>Work</u>, <u>Self-care</u>, and <u>Leisure</u>. A guiding philosophy of the DTC is to treat the individual as a member of the community where he or she lives.

Deafness. The inability to hear verbal language and sound, either through congenital conditions or acquired via trauma or medical illness. Deafness may also denote profound hearing loss, particularly with respect to loudness, pitch, or both. Occupational therapy approaches will vary based on the client and circumstances under which deafness occurs. For those completely deaf, it is helpful for the therapist to understand sign language. The use of visual information and pictures may also augment other strategies. Additional intervention techniques include the following:

Stein, F., & Haertl, K.
Pocket Guide to Intervention in Occupational Therapy, Second Edition (pp 83-95).
© 2019 Taylor & Francis Group.

- Address any <u>Developmental delays</u> secondary to congenital causes of deafness
- Use of <u>Sensory processing</u> techniques to address secondary sensory processing difficulties
- Psychosocial intervention for adjustment difficulties, particularly those who have acquired deafness and previously had normal hearing
- Use of <u>Assistive technology</u>
- Use of positioning for communication (e.g., address individual face on, particularly those who are able to read lips)
- Provide environmental adaptation and activity compensation as appropriate

Debridement. An intervention method used to remove dead tissue and foreign matter from a healing wound. Methods used in debridement include surgical, chemical, and other modes in order to rid the wound of dead tissue. Hand therapists often work with traumatic injuries that require debridement. See <u>Hand injuries</u> for further discussion and treatment.

Decubitus Ulcer. A pressure sore that arises from remaining in a position too long. These ulcers and sores are often in the place of a bony prominence such as at the elbows, knees, and sacrum. For instance, clients who require total or maximal assistance for bed mobility or repositioning in a wheelchair can develop pressure areas on the sacrum or heels of the feet. Prolonged pressure results in decreased circulation to an area, which then causes sores or open areas of the skin. Equipment such as air mattresses/cushions, water cushions, or gel cushions to help relieve pressure may help prevent sores. Bony prominences may also be padded for protection. Special boots or elbow pads may be used while the client lies in bed. Clients who are specifically at risk are clients who have a spinal cord injury that has resulted in decreased sensation in the lower extremities. If a client is able to push up from the armrests of the wheelchair or roll from one side to the other, the client should be instructed to relieve pressure 1 minute for every 30 minutes if possible. Otherwise, nursing staff should set up a schedule to turn the client while the client is in bed to help prevent ulcers.

Deep. Toward the middle of the body. See <u>Anatomical position</u>.

Deep Tendon Reflexes. A reflex that occurs in response to muscular stretching. See <u>Reflexes and reactions</u>.

Deinstitutionalization. The process of discharging individuals from large state or county hospitals into community facilities such as <u>Day treatment</u>

centers (DTCs) or supportive housing such as Halfway houses, group homes, and residential treatment centers. Initial deinstitutionalization of persons with mental illness occurred in the 1960s. While the goal of facilitating community integration was positive, unfortunately, there were too few programs available at the time, resulting in increased homelessness and rehospitalization.

Delirium. A decrease in cognitive abilities, often marked by significant confusion and fairly sudden onset. Delirium may arise from a variety of causes, including high fever, drugs, infection, surgery, or a serious metabolic shift. If delirium is suspected, contact the physician immediately.

Delusion. A false belief not based in reality, such as believing that people are reading one's mind, food is being poisoned, or people are plotting against the individual.

Dementia. A term now classified under "neurocognitive disorders" in the DSM-5 (American Psychological Association, 2013). Historically, *dementia* has been a broad term that refers to chronic disorders (often progressive) of the brain. Symptoms of dementia may include memory loss, confusion, disorientation, personality deterioration, and a complete breakdown in Self-care functions. Alzheimer's disease, Pick's disease, Huntington's chorea, and organic brain syndrome associated with alcoholism can lead to dementia. Whereas some types of dementia such as Alzheimer's disease often begin with cognitive symptoms prior to motor difficulties, subcortical dementias such as Parkinson's disease and Huntington's often begin with motor/praxis problems and later progress to memory loss and other cognitive difficulties. Occupational therapy interventions are specific to the type of dementia and subsequent symptoms and effects on occupational performance. In addition to working to maintain current cognitive function and self-care, adaptive and compensatory techniques are used. Evaluation of the client's functioning level and home evaluation are often key to developing a strategy for potential decrease in function over time. Caregiver education is a prominent part of occupational therapy intervention. See Alzheimer's disease for additional information.

Dependent Personality Disorder. Describes an individual with an extreme need to be taken care of by another individual. The disorder usually begins in childhood and is characterized by passivity, submissiveness, indecisiveness, poor self-confidence, and a need to be nurtured and supported.

Depression. A term classified under "depressive disorders" in the DSM-5 (American Psychological Association, 2013). Depression may take on several forms and may be characterized as mild, moderate, or severe.

Symptoms of depression include eating dysfunction, sleeping disturbance, fatigue, low self-esteem, inability to concentrate, difficulty in making decisions, feelings of hopelessness, loss of libido, and sadness. Depression may be situational or clinical and may be episodic or chronic. See also <u>Dysthymic disorder</u>. Although feelings of depression are universal, it is diagnosed as an illness when it interferes with an individual's ability to work or attend school, engage in <u>Leisure</u> activities, attend to <u>Self-care</u> activities, and maintain family and social relationships. Approximately 25% of a given population will experience some type of depression sometime during their lifetime. Certain types of depression are considered to have a biological cause that is linked to the depletion in the body of the neurotransmitter <u>Serotonin</u>. Precipitating factors implicated in depression are related to loss, such as the death of a close friend or relative, loss of a job, financial loss, divorce or separation, disabling illness or disease, school or work failure, or inability to achieve personal goals. Predisposing factors can include genetic predisposition, such as personality traits where the individual is unable to deal with severe environmental or personal loss.

Course of Illness

Bouts or episodes of depression can last for weeks, months, or years. A vicious cycle of depression can occur when the depression "feeds upon itself" by dragging the individual into deeper and deeper holes where suicide can be a real threat to the individual. The vicious cycle starts with sleep disturbances that can cause fatigue and low energy levels, leading to an inability to work or attend school, causing further withdrawal from social interactions that can lead to a deepening of the illness accompanied by low self-esteem, <u>Anxiety</u>, and suicidal ideation.

Specific Interventions

Intervention during each episode of depression is critical to prevent the downward spiral that accompanies the course of the illness. A holistic approach is recommended, including medication, exercise, nutrition, <u>Creative arts</u>, individual or group counseling/psychotherapy, vocational counseling, <u>Stress management</u>, <u>Relaxation therapy</u>, <u>Cognitive behavioral therapy</u>, leisure, occupation-based approaches, vocational counseling, and support, which are integral to intervention.

Suggested Guidelines for Occupational Therapy (Stein & Cutler, 2002)

- The cognitive behavioral approach emphasizes individuals learning and applying stress management skills, relaxation therapies, exercise, and leisure occupation in their everyday schedules. The therapist works with the individual in designing realistic goals and helps the individual to monitor compliance to the therapeutic program.

- Consider cultural values and interests of the individual in designing a therapeutic program.
- Use activities and creative media to increase self-esteem, express and channel anger, build lifelong leisure interests, and help the individual to gain self-insight.
- Establish a stress management program for the individual to identify symptoms that are triggered by situations that provoke stress and coping activities that reduce stress.
- Research supports the use of exercise-related interventions in depression (Bridle, Spanjers, Patel, Atherton, & Lamb, 2012). Establish an exercise program with the client considering his or her physical fitness, sports or exercise interests, intensity, and frequency and duration of exercise. Consider the feasibility of doing exercise in the individual's home, neighborhood, or sports center.
- Consider using <u>Role playing</u> or adopted <u>Psychodrama</u> with client in rehearsing stressful or anxiety-provoking situations or as part of group therapy sessions.

Depth Perception. The ability to determine the relative distance between one's self and an object. This skill is particularly important in driving a car. See <u>Cognitive-perceptual deficits</u> for further discussion and intervention.

Dermatome. An area of the skin innervated by a specific spinal nerve root. For example, the C4 spinal root provides sensation to the area of skin over the shoulders, across the chest from near the clavicle to an imaginary line drawn horizontally between the highest point of the axillae, and a corresponding area over the superior part of the back above the scapulae.

Desensitization. A method of treatment used with clients who are hypersensitive to help increase the client's tolerance of uncomfortable, irritating stimuli. See <u>Sensory deficits</u> and <u>Hypersensitivity</u> for specific treatment methods.

Developmental Delay. A condition identified when a child is behind expected physical, cognitive, and <u>Developmental milestones</u>. Persons with developmental delay may go on to achieve normal development, yet in other situations, especially when paired with a developmental condition, the individual may have lasting developmental disabilities.

Developmental Disability. This term was established once the U.S. Congress passed the Developmental Disabilities Services and Facilities Construction Amendments of 1970 (Haertl, 2014). Although there are varying definitions, a developmental disability is typically chronic, attributable to a physical or mental impairment prior to 22 years of age, and results in substantial functional and/or adaptive impairment. Common developmental disabilities include (but are not limited to) <u>Intellectual disability</u>, <u>Cerebral palsy (CP)</u>, <u>Down syndrome</u>, <u>Learning disability</u>, <u>Attention deficit hyperactivity disorder (ADHD)</u>, <u>Autism</u>, <u>Spina bifida</u>, and hearing and vision disorders. Interventions are habilitative and rehabilitative and are aimed at the specific condition and resulting effects on occupational performance. The following are examples of remedial and adaptive approaches.

Remedial

- Use of skill training to increase performance in <u>Activities of daily living (ADLs)</u>, <u>Instrumental activities of daily living (IADLs)</u>, <u>Work</u>, <u>Leisure</u>, socialization, and <u>Coping skills</u>
- Sensory and perceptual motor approaches
- Cognitive skill training in preparation for school and work
- Range of motion, positioning, and mobility training

Adaptation/Compensation

- Provide <u>Assistive technology</u>/adaptive equipment as needed
- Assess and adapt the environment as needed for maximal performance
- Educate and train caregivers and service providers

Developmental Milestones. Physical, cognitive, mental, and performance skills expected of infants, toddlers, and children at a certain age. Typically, there is a range of "normal development" at which time a specific skill such as crawling, walking, and talking is developed. Charts of expected development are found in most clinics and are widely available on the internet. See <u>Appendix C</u> for specific milestones.

Developmental Test. A measure of a client's performance in age-related tasks such as language, perceptual-motor, social, <u>Self-care</u>, emotional, and ambulation.

Dexterity. The ability to use the body in a coordinated and purposeful manner. When using this term, most therapists refer to the ability of the upper extremity to manipulate objects. Dexterity may be subdivided into manual or gross dexterity, which is the movement of the arm and hand to work in larger patterns and with larger objects; and finger or fine dexterity, which is the movement of the fingers in small patterns or with small objects. For similar terms and treatment, see <u>Coordination</u>, <u>Gross motor coordination</u>, and <u>Fine motor coordination</u>. Mental dexterity refers to a sharp, flexible mind that is able to think quickly.

Diabetes. Specific diseases that alter how the body uses glucose and produces or utilizes insulin. Type 1 diabetes usually occurs in the younger years (often before age 25) resulting in dependence on outside sources of insulin. Type 2 diabetes results in decreased sensitivity to insulin; persons with obesity are at a higher risk. Whereas type 1 requires insulin, type 2 may or may not require insulin and may be managed with other medications, diet, and exercise. Occupational therapy interventions often focus on client lifestyle, medication management, and psychosocial adjustment.

Diadochokinesis. The ability to perform antagonist movements in succession. An example of diadochokinesis is the rapid supination and pronation of the arms.

Diagonal Patterns. Patterns of movement used within Voss's (1967; Voss, Ionta, & Myers, 1985) framework of proprioceptive neuromuscular facilitation to help remediate motor control. A flexion and extension component are added together to produce a diagonal movement, which imitates movement that occurs during functional activities. See <u>Motor control</u> problems and <u>Proprioceptive neuromuscular facilitation (PNF)</u> for further discussion of diagonal patterns.

Dialectical Behavioral Therapy (DBT). A specific type of cognitive behavioral intervention originally developed for persons with <u>Borderline personality disorder</u> (Linehan, 1993). The intervention has since been used with a number of populations, including persons with <u>Depression</u>, <u>Addictions</u>, <u>Eating disorders</u>, and <u>Anxiety disorder</u>. The program includes specific skill training exercises, often in a group setting, and an individual counselor. Occupational therapists may be trained to administer DBT groups. Given the emphasis on occupation-based practice, it is important to pair the skills learned with strategies to improve occupational performance.

Diathermy. The use of electrical current to induce heat used to relieve pain, increase circulation, and facilitate healing and mobility in musculoskeletal conditions.

Diathesis. A predisposition or vulnerability to a specific disease, disorder, or condition. A stress diathesis refers to the precipitating episode of symptoms that leads to a disease through a stressful event or stressors in the environment.

DIP. Acronym for distal interphalangeal.

Diplegia. Paralysis of two extremities.

Diplopia. Double vision.

Disability. A physical or mental restriction of the ability to perform an activity in the manner or within the range considered normal for a human being. These human activities include movement, interaction, thought process, and other everyday activities in daily life. A psychiatric or physical disability results from the symptoms of an illness such as Aphasia, Hemiplegia, Dysphagia, auditory impairment, Delusions, or Hallucinations that can prevent an individual from engaging in everyday human activities.

Discourse Analysis. The study of language as communication through the forms and mechanisms of verbal interaction.

Dislocation. An abnormal separation of bones that limits motions at the joint and therefore prevents functional activity.

Dissociation. A detached mental and emotional state that may manifest in the individual continuing to operate in day-to-day situations amidst periods of lack of conscious memory of the present. Dissociation occurs on a continuum; mild dissociation may include daydreaming and brief states, whereas significant dissociation may be manifested in major psychiatric dissociative disorders. Dissociation may arise after significant stress or trauma.

Dissociative Identity Disorder. A complex psychological condition marked by two or more distinct personalities; gaps in the recall of everyday events; and impairment in social, occupational, and other functioning that is not due to a broad cultural or religious practice, nor attributable to substance abuse (American Psychological Association, 2013). This disorder, previously often referred to as Multiple personality disorder, may lead to severe self-harm and suicidal behaviors. Occupational therapy intervention often includes expressive and creative therapy, Dialectical behavioral therapy (DBT), Cognitive behavioral therapy, Stress management, and discharge planning.

Distal. Farthest point from, as in the distal portion of the hand. See Anatomical position.

Dopamine. A Catecholamine neurotransmitter that occurs naturally in the brain and affects arousal in the autonomic nervous system. An overabundance of dopamine has been implicated as a factor in the etiology of Schizophrenia. A paucity of dopamine is associated with Parkinson's disease and Tardive dyskinesia. L-dopa, the precursor of dopamine, is used in the treatment of Parkinson's disease. Medications that block the action of dopamine are used to treat schizophrenia.

Dorsal Splint/Orthosis. An orthosis that is applied to the dorsal surface of the forearm, hand, and/or fingers. This type of splint may be used as a static application to immobilize the wrist without compressing the carpal tunnel, or as a base for hardware, which will produce a dynamic application to substitute for extensor muscles in the case of extensor <u>Tendon repair</u>.

Dorsiflexion. A joint motion at the ankle that results in the toes being pulled upward toward the knee. This is ankle joint extension, which is often mislabeled as flexion. See <u>Appendix F</u> for the normal range of this motion.

Down Syndrome. Down syndrome is an <u>Intellectual</u> and <u>Developmental disability</u> marked by a chromosomal abnormality most often characterized by three copies of the 21st chromosome, often referred to as *trisomy 21* and resulting in a wide range of intellectual abilities and disabilities (Haertl, 2014). Early sensory programs, motor activities, special education, and vocational preparation are critical aspects of <u>Habilitation</u> programs for these individuals. In addition to compromised intellect, other associated conditions include a variety of medical problems, low muscle tone, and coexisting mental health concerns. The cause is unknown; however, the age of the person's mother is associated with this condition. Mothers who are 40 years of age or older have a higher incidence of children with Down syndrome.

Specific Interventions

- Provide proper positioning, beginning from birth.
- Educate the parent on developmental needs and home-based strategies.
- Use sensory-based interventions from birth on through childhood.
- Increase the strength of antigravity muscles to assist with trunk control, posture, range of motion, and stability.
- Complete activities to increase both <u>Gross motor coordination</u> and <u>Fine motor coordination</u>.
- Promote the use of both hands and playing at midline for <u>Bilateral integration</u>.
- Apply different textures to decrease <u>Tactile defensiveness</u> and increase sensory stimulation.
- Provide proprioceptive stimulation through joint compression, playing "wheelbarrow," bouncing on a ball, or weighted objects.

- Increase vestibular stimulation with scooterboard, swing, or rotational devices such as a merry-go-round to also help decrease gravitational insecurity.
- Provide auditory input.
- Complete activities to increase the client's equilibrium and righting reactions necessary for balance and protection.
- Educate the client or the client's parents on a home program for follow-through.
- Complete <u>Self-care</u> activities to increase the client's self-esteem and independence.
- Work on oral motor development to increase feeding and dental hygiene ability.
- Address areas of <u>Activities of daily living (ADLs)</u>, <u>Instrumental activities of daily living (IADLs)</u>, <u>Work</u>, <u>Leisure</u>, and socialization in order to improve occupational performance.

Contraindications/Precautions

- Be aware that the occipitoatlantal or atlantoaxial joints (C1–C2 joints) may be at risk for subluxation or displacement.
- Watch for ligament laxity.
- Contact sports may be contraindicated.
- Be aware that the client may have heart problems such as congenital heart disease, which can affect endurance.
- Be aware of coexisting conditions.
- Be prepared since the client may be at risk for seizures.
- Allergies or asthma may also be a risk factor for particular activities.
- The client may also demonstrate ear problems that can affect hearing and/or balance, as well as vision problems, which can affect function.

Dream Therapy. A method of using dreams, as in <u>Psychoanalysis</u>, to gain access to the unconscious by examining the content of dreams. Using a dream diary is helpful in this process. The use of dreams and the dream state to accomplish physical and emotional healing involves both interpretation and the active participation of the client in the dream process.

Dressing. An <u>Activity of daily living (ADL)</u> that is essential to an individual's self-care. See <u>Self-care</u> for specific adaptive techniques, <u>Assistive technology</u> for adaptive equipment, and specific diagnoses/conditions for further discussion and treatment.

Dressing Apraxia. See <u>Apraxia</u>.

Drunkorexia. A newer identified mental health disorder marked by significant binge drinking paired with disordered eating such as restriction of food or bingeing and purging. This pattern can cause significant physical and mental health problems.

Duchenne Muscular Dystrophy. A genetic disorder that results in general weakness and wasting of the skeletal muscles that control the pelvis and upper and lower proximal extremities. Persons with this type of muscular dystrophy usually do not live longer than 20 to 25 years of age. The cause of Duchenne muscular dystrophy is a sex-linked recessive gene, which is carried on the X chromosome. Additional types of muscular dystrophy that have been identified include myotonic, Becker, limb-girdle, facioscapulohumeral, congenital, oculopharyngeal, distal, and Emery–Dreifuss.

Specific Interventions

- Complete activities to maintain <u>Gross motor coordination</u>.
- Fabricate orthoses and recommend positioning devices to prevent deformity.
- Use exercise for strength and endurance—it is important to coordinate with the physician on the types of exercise most appropriate for the client. Often, the use of low-impact exercises such as swimming are advised.
- Preserve muscle strength, especially at the large joints, which are responsible for ambulation, as well as range of motion.
- Provide activities to maintain <u>Fine motor coordination</u> and dexterity.
- Educate the client on work simplification and energy conservation principles.
- Recommend power equipment such as power wheelchairs when needed.
- Consult the client and family on diet restrictions to assist the client with easier chewing and swallowing.
- Complete a home evaluation and make recommendations for equipment to increase safety and mobility in the home.
- Encourage the client to attend support group meetings for socialization and emotional adjustment to the disease.
- Instruct the client on assistive devices to increase independence with <u>Self-care</u> activities.
- Explore <u>Leisure</u> skills to help the client feel productive.

Contraindications/Precautions
- Avoid exposure of the client with persons who have respiratory infections or colds
- Communicate changes in respiration or signs of respiratory distress to the physician

Dynamic Splint/Orthosis. Fabricated in order to increase mobility at a joint. See <u>Splints/orthoses</u>.

Dynamic Systems Theory. Originally developed in mathematics, dynamic systems theory acknowledges the complexity of factors that affect a system. Dynamic systems theory seeks to study and understand the concept of change. This theory has been applied to psychological concepts, sensory integration, and motor development.

Dysarthria. Difficulty with the production of speech. A client who has dysarthria may display slurred speech, a nasal tone, a difference in pitch of voice, or explosive speech. This deficit may result from a cerebellar lesion.

Dysdiadochokinesia. Difficulty in completing quick alternating movements, such as supination/pronation or elbow flexion/extension, in a smooth and rhythmic manner. A complete inability in completing this movement is adiadochokinesia. This deficit results from a cerebellar lesion. Treatment should focus on compensatory techniques to allow the client to complete necessary functional activities.

Dyskinesia. Abnormal, impaired motor movements and coordination, as seen in conditions such as <u>Parkinson's disease</u>. Dyskinesia may also be a result of external factors such as the movement disorders found as a result of neuroleptic use, as seen in <u>Tardive dyskinesia</u>.

Dyslexia. A neurobiological learning disorder resulting in difficulty with reading, writing, and word and letter interpretation. Occupational therapists work in tandem with the team to address learning issues and often may address additional coexisting <u>Sensory processing</u> difficulties.

Dysmetria. The inability to accurately complete the range of motion needed to reach a target. Rather than a problem with the range, the client is unable to judge or coordinate movement to the desired position. This deficit in coordination displays itself when a client is asked to touch a target such as the therapist's finger, the client's own nose, or an object resting on the table. A cerebellar lesion may result in this type of incoordination. Treatment should focus on compensatory techniques to allow the client to complete necessary functional activities.

Dysphagia. Difficulty swallowing, which may be a result of congenital, developmental, or acquired conditions. Occupational therapy interventions are often done in conjunction with other team members and include individualized compensatory approaches, adapted mealtime routines and diet, positioning, preparatory exercises, and reinforcement of strategies to prevent aspiration and promote swallowing (Avery, 2011).

Dyssynergia. The inability to accomplish a smooth and complete movement. A client with this deficit will demonstrate many small and jerky motions rather than one total movement. This deficit results from a cerebellar lesion, and treatment should focus on compensatory techniques to allow the client to complete necessary functional activities.

Dysthymic Disorder. A chronically depressed mood occurring over a period of at least 2 years in which the individual experiences the symptoms of depression for most of the day. See <u>Depression</u>.

Dystonia. A motor disorder characterized by stiffening in muscles and sudden contractions or "jerky" movements of the arms, neck, or face. It involves a peculiar twisting movement of the trunk or proximal musculature, which can result in odd posture and muscle spasms. This deficit is a type of <u>Athetosis</u>, and it results from a lesion in the basal ganglia. It is sometimes a side effect of long-term usage of antipsychotic drugs. See <u>Coordination</u> for specific treatment suggestions.

E

Eating Disorder. Psychological disorders marked by a disturbance in eating patterns. <u>Anorexia nervosa</u> and <u>Bulimia</u> are two of the most common types. See specific eating disorders for interventions.

Eccentric Contraction. The lengthening of muscle fibers while under load. See <u>Contraction</u>.

Echolalia. Repetitive, meaningless vocalizations, often mimicking others in the area or sounds made from the radio or TV. Echolalia may accompany many developmental, psychiatric, and clinical conditions.

Edema. A condition involving excessive fluid in the tissues, which results in inflammation. Conditions such as kidney disease, congestive heart failure, and cirrhosis may cause edema (also referred to as *swelling*), along with other conditions and injury to a localized area, as in the case of a broken bone. When tissue is injured, white blood cells rush to the site of injury to help control infection. This inflammatory response causes swelling, or edema, in and around the affected area. The edema may continue due to damaged structures, immobility, or overuse of the affected limb/area. Mild edema following an injury such as a sprained ankle is often treated with the RICE treatment: Rest, Ice, Compression, and Elevation. More serious edema may be treated by a physician with prescribed medications such as diuretics along with rehabilitation. Untreated edema may result in adhesions and pain, causing reduced range of motion and an impact on functional mobility.

Specific Interventions

- **Elevation.** The client should elevate the affected part above the heart to facilitate return of the fluid to the lymph system (e.g., a client who has hemiplegia often demonstrates edema in the affected upper extremity). When the client is lying in bed, the affected upper

Stein, F., & Haertl, K.
Pocket Guide to Intervention in Occupational Therapy, Second Edition (pp 97-105).
© 2019 Taylor & Francis Group.

extremity should be elevated on pillows. If two pillows are available, one should be placed under the entire forearm with the second placed only under the hand. This creates a better incline for the arm toward the heart. If only one pillow is available, the therapist can place the pillow under the entire forearm and double the distal end of the pillow over itself so that the pillow beneath the client's hand is at a greater incline. The client should also have the upper extremity supported while sitting. If the client is in a wheelchair, an elevated arm trough, which slides onto the armrest of the wheelchair, can be used. If this special equipment is not available, a pillow can again be propped under the affected extremity. Special inclined cushions can be purchased to place in a nonelevating arm trough or for use in a hand clinic during treatment.

- **Contrast Baths.** By placing the affected limb in alternating temperatures of water, vasodilation and vasoconstriction occur successively. The action of the blood vessels creates a mechanical pump, which helps push the increased fluid out of the affected area. The recommended temperatures for the water range from 96° to 111°F for the warm water and 36° to 65°F for the cold water. Treatment typically begins with a warm water soak for 3 minutes. The client is then encouraged to immerse the limb in the cold water for 30 to 60 seconds. Treatment should alternate between the 3-minute warm soaks and 1-minute cold soaks for the duration of treatment, up to 20 to 30 minutes. Treatment should conclude with a final soak for 3 minutes in the warm water. This treatment may also be effective with clients who are hypersensitive or those who have <u>Reflex sympathetic dystrophy (RSD) syndrome</u>. The cold water immersion may be painful. It is the writer's experience that clients tolerate the treatment better if the therapist immerses one hand as well. The therapist is then able to identify with the client's discomfort and empathize on a personal level.

Contraindications/Precautions

See <u>Physical agent modalities (PAMs)</u> for general guidelines when using heat and cold. Clients who have small vessel disease from diabetes, Burger's disease, and arteriosclerotic endarteritis should not complete this treatment.

- **Retrograde Massage.** (Note, lymphatic drainage techniques have replaced many of the retrograde massage techniques in the clinic.) This technique is for a client who has hand, wrist, or forearm edema. The therapist can passively move the fluid toward the heart through massage. The client should elevate the hand, either on an inclined cushion or by simply setting the elbow on a table and holding the hand straight up from the elbow. The therapist often uses lotion (watch for skin sensitivity) and applies equal pressure with both hands to either side of the forearm, while slowly and firmly pressing in a proximal direction from the wrist to the elbow. After the forearm looks less swollen (maybe 8 to 10 strokes), the therapist should massage the palm and dorsal surface of the hand by starting at the metacarpophalangeal (MCP) joints and pushing proximally toward the wrist. Again, the therapist should use both hands while applying equal pressure to either side of the hand. Once the hand demonstrates decreased edema, the therapist should place circumferential pressure around the finger while massaging from the fingertip toward the MCP joint. Each finger is massaged individually, and then the therapist can use both hands to apply pressure to the dorsal and volar surfaces of the four digits at the same time. The thumb is completed separately. After the fingers show improvement, the therapist should again massage the hand in the manner described. Finally, the forearm should be massaged to force the last of the moveable fluid from the area toward the heart. This method is based on the physical principle that fluid moves from an area of greater concentration toward an area of lesser concentration. Fluid will not be able to move from the fingers to the hand if the hand already has an increased concentration of fluid. However, if the extra fluid is moved from the hand, then the fluid in the fingers will physically want to move from the fingers (high concentration) to the hand (lesser concentration). Likewise, if the forearm contains increased fluid, it will not accept more fluid. Therefore, the fluid should first be removed from the forearm, then the hand, and finally the fingers. However, the fluid from the fingers should not be allowed to remain in the hand, and massage should be completed to force that fluid from the hand to the forearm and then back to the heart. (*Special Note*: Manual edema mobilization is similar to retrograde massage but follows the lymphatic pathways and follows a proximal to distal pattern.)

○ Precautions: It is important to work closely with the health care team to ensure there are not acute injuries that would be harmed by massage. Caution should also be taken with those who have heart conditions, as they may not handle fluid being pushed toward the heart.

- **Compression.** The application of snug garments or a wrap to an edematous extremity also helps push extra fluid from the limb toward the heart. If using a wrap such as Coban, the wrap should begin distally and work proximally to promote flow of the fluid back toward the heart. Care should be taken so that the area is not wrapped too tightly; this may decrease blood flow to the area. A client with hand and finger edema can wear an Isotoner glove throughout the day. The therapist should use the opposite glove and turn it inside out to apply it to the affected hand. For example, a client who has hemiplegia may demonstrate edema in the right hand. The therapist would order a left glove and then turn it inside out and place it on the right hand. This prevents the seams of the glove from indenting the edema, and it provides a more uniform pressure to the fingers. Finally, specially ordered garments can be purchased to provide compression to an edematous limb. For example, a client with breast cancer may demonstrate moderate to severe edema in the entire upper extremity nearest the cancer site. The client can be measured for a JOBST or other compression garment, which compresses the entire limb from the wrist to the shoulder. An Isotoner glove then may also be applied to prevent fluid from pooling in the hand.

- **Active Motion.** Movement of the affected area increases blood flow, which helps the removal of extra fluid. The therapist should stress that slight wiggling movements are not beneficial. The client must complete full range of motion, or as close as possible, to receive maximum benefits with edema control.

- **Ice.** Vasoconstriction occurs from the application of cold. When dilated blood vessels at a site of injury are quickly caused to constrict, a natural pumping effect occurs, which helps move extra fluid back toward the heart.

Types of Edema

- **Brawny Edema.** Edema lasting over 3 months, often brawny in color. Tissues are fibrous and hard when palpated.

- **Pitting Edema.** On <u>Palpation</u>, this type of swelling will be soft and indent with pressure. Pitting edema is often present 2 days to 3 weeks post-injury.

Electrical Stimulation. Applying an electrical stimulus to help facilitate muscular control, decrease spasm, or reduce pain.

Electroconvulsive Therapy (ECT). A procedure designed to administer small electric currents that trigger a seizure in order to achieve the desired therapeutic benefit. The procedure is done under general anesthesia and muscle relaxants. Despite some controversy, a meta-analysis demonstrated the effectiveness of ECT for <u>Depression</u>, and it outperformed some common other methods used for intervention (Pagnin, de Queiroz, Pini, & Cassano, 2008). ECT is endorsed by the American Psychiatric Association and is most often used in affective disorders. It is generally started at a dosing of two to three times per week for a few weeks. Individuals may then be put on maintenance ECT for a certain period. Therapists must adhere to general health requirements prior to and post-ECT treatment. For instance, clients are not able to eat or drink in the hours prior to ECT. In addition, there is often a period of cognitive shift and memory lapse immediately following ECT; therefore, cognitive tests and interventions should not be done immediately after ECT.

Electroencephalograph (EEG). An instrument for detecting and recording the electrical potential produced by the brain cells. Brainwave activity is recorded indicating alpha, beta, delta, and theta rhythms, which describe the range of cycles per second of the amplitude of the signal. An individual producing alpha waves (8- to 12-second waves) is usually in a very relaxed state, whereas beta waves (15 to 30 seconds) are indicative of normal consciousness. EEG is used in <u>Biofeedback</u> training.

Electromyograph (EMG). An instrument to record the electrical activity of muscles by applying surface electrodes (transducers) or needle electrodes into the muscle. Along with the EMG, an oscilloscope and amplifier are used in <u>Biofeedback</u> to record muscle activity (e.g., the frontalis muscles in <u>Relaxation therapy</u>).

Electronic Health Record (EHR). Electronic version of a client's medical record. Hospitals often have specific electronic health systems that therapists need to learn. Increasingly, other nonhospital-based settings are also using EHR.

Endorphin. A polypeptide component found naturally in the brain that acts as a natural analgesic by binding to opiate receptor sites. Some researchers have found that endorphins are produced by aerobic exercise such as jogging and fast walking.

Endurance. Musculoskeletal and cardiopulmonary ability to engage in a motor activity over time. Intervention plans to increase endurance require prolonged effort in walking, movement, or working in an occupation. Graded activity programs are used to increase endurance. Occupational and physical therapists often use techniques aimed at increasing endurance. It is important to remain in close communication with the physician and be apprised of any health-related precautions.

Specific Interventions

- Use of exercise equipment such as treadmills, upper extremity ergometers, stationary bikes, and elliptical machines. Conditioning involves gradual increase in time or intensity.
- Occupational craft-based activities may work to increase endurance (e.g., sanding on an incline).
- Occupation-based activities such as cooking, yardwork, gardening, laundry, dressing, and cleaning can also increase endurance.

Energy Conservation. A treatment technique that provides the client with procedures to reduce energy expenditure during activities. First, the client should be made aware of the energy required for particular activities; if the therapist wishes to be very specific, metabolic equivalent tables may be used to provide the client with the exact amounts of energy required for activities. The client should then be instructed on principles and techniques that will help the client conserve energy while completing tasks. This allows the client a higher quality of life by allowing the client to maintain independence with a greater number of tasks. If the client is not aware of these methods, he or she may run out of energy early in the day and require help with any functions throughout the rest of the day. Clients who have <u>Cardiac dysfunctions</u>, pulmonary conditions, or poor endurance can benefit from these principles. See <u>Metabolic equivalent (MET)</u> for additional information.

Specific Interventions

- Use of planned schedules to decrease energy expenditure
- Use of <u>Activity analysis</u> and compensatory and adaptive techniques
- Use of rest breaks before and after activities
- Wear comfortable shoes and clothing
- Home modification
- Rest breaks prior to fatigue
- Collaboration with the work site to perform work-related tasks during high-energy times of the day

Epilepsy. A chronic neurological disorder marked by recurring seizures. Causes may be congenital or acquired. In addition to <u>Relaxation therapy</u> and <u>Coping skills</u>, therapists address <u>Self-care</u> and additional areas of occupational performance needs.

Equilibrium Reaction. Enables the body to recover balance. See <u>Reflexes and reactions</u>.

Ergonomics. The principle of fitting the job or environment to the worker or homemaker. The occupational therapist using ergonomics considers the tools; equipment; seating; dials; lighting; colors; and placement of furniture, appliances, and other parts of the environment in preventing work injuries and enhancing function. The physical and psychological characteristics of the individual are considered in environmental adaptation. The therapist works with the client to facilitate ergonomically correct positions such as seating position, use of an ergonomically correct computer and mouse, and consideration of placement of work and home furniture. See Stein, Soderback, Cutler, and Larson (2006).

Ergonomic Job Analysis

Analysis of a work site or a specific job, including the tasks, demands, equipment, and skill sets needed. Therapists often evaluate the client's skills, condition, and needs, along with the specific demands of the job.

Risk Factors

Variables related to performing a job that can potentially lead to injuries, illnesses, or diseases. These factors can include the environment (e.g., extreme temperature, poorly designed tools, an uncomfortable chair, work methods such as using poor lifting techniques, undue or continual stress, and repetitive motions).

Ethnoscience. The study of the characteristics of language as culture in terms of lexical and/or semantic relations.

Etiology. Examination of the cause or causes of an illness or disease. There are predisposing and precipitating factors that lead to the onset of a disease. Some conditions have specific causes, such as Lyme's disease. Other physical and mental health conditions may have multiple causes. For instance, the presence of obesity along with other physiological and hereditary factors may predispose someone to <u>Diabetes</u>. Most mental illnesses have multiple risk factors such as genetic, physiological, developmental, psychological, and sociological factors that can predispose a vulnerable individual to mental illness. Stress and sudden losses can precipitate an episode of mental illness in an individual who is vulnerable.

Evaluation. In a broad sense, evaluation includes an analysis of an individual's behavior, characteristics, aptitudes, and present functioning gained through specific tests, clinical observations, and procedures that can be used for treatment planning or discharge recommendations. The American Occupational Therapy Association (AOTA; 2014) identifies evaluation as a key part of the occupational therapy process. Evaluation considers client and family wishes along with individual needs (e.g., cognitive, physical, psychological, social-emotional, etc.). The process is occupational in nature and focuses on developing an <u>Occupational profile</u> and then assessing occupational performance (AOTA, 2014). Goals and interventions are developed from the evaluation process.

Eversion. Turning outward, as in turning the foot outward at the ankle. See <u>Anatomical position</u>.

Evidence-Based Practice. Utilization of the best evidence (e.g., meta-analysis and systematic research reviews) along with clinical expertise and client values.

Executive Functions of the Brain. Higher-level cognitive tasks such as abstraction, sequential organization, motor planning, and decision-making. See also <u>Cognitive-perceptual deficits</u>.

Exercise. See <u>Prescriptive exercise</u>.

Expressed Emotion (EE). A concept related to a family's psychological interactions with a family member who has a mental illness (e.g., a diagnosis of <u>Schizophrenia</u>). The criteria for high EE are based on factors such as negative comments about the family member, personal criticism, dissatisfaction with the individual's behavior, lack of warmth expressed toward the individual, and constant worry about the individual. A study analyzing aggregate data from 25 studies on EE found an "overwhelming" link between EE and relapse (Bebbington & Kuipers, 1994). Family psychoeducation has been used to educate families about mental health conditions and promote positive socialization.

Extension. Movement involving straightening, for instance, increasing the angle of a joint. See <u>Anatomical position</u>.

Extensor Synergy. An automatic pattern of movement that may occur when a client with hemiplegia attempts the motion of extension, such as elbow or knee extension. The stereotypical pattern for the upper extremity combines the following motions: scapular abduction and depression, shoulder adduction and internal rotation, elbow extension, forearm pronation, and wrist and finger extension. The stereotypical pattern for the upper extremity combines the following motions: hip adduction, extension, and internal rotation; knee extension; ankle plantarflexion and inversion; and toe flexion. See <u>Motor control</u> problems for treatment methods.

Extensor Thrust (Reflex). Spinal-level reflex that results in leg extension following pressure to the sole. See <u>Reflexes and reactions</u>.

External Rotation. Turning outward from the midline of the body. See <u>Anatomical position</u>.

Extinction. Elimination or inhibition of behavior by not reinforcing the behavior.

Extrapyramidal Side Effects (EPSE). Medication/drug-induced effects often caused by psychiatric medications that produce movement disorders. Types of EPSE include cogwheeling (jerky feeling within the muscles of a limb), akathisia (feeling of restlessness), tremors, and the more serious and more permanent <u>Tardive dyskinesia</u>, which causes movement issues particularly in the face and limbs.

F

Facilitation. The act of increasing or supporting. Often used when referring to a client who demonstrates low muscle tone. See <u>Motor control</u> problems for applications of facilitation.

Facilitation Techniques. Techniques that help increase the tone of a muscle so that it is able to contract and cause movement. Some examples include <u>Brushing</u>, <u>Stroking</u>, <u>Tapping</u>, and <u>Vibration</u>. See <u>Motor control</u> problems for more examples.

Falls Prevention. A systematic approach to preventing falls, applying intrinsic (within individual) and extrinsic (environmental) interventions. Some people are more vulnerable to falls than others, particularly those who have neurological conditions or the elderly. About 30% to 60% of people older than 65 years of age will have an accidental fall, and of these falls, 10% to 20% will cause serious injury such as <u>Hip fractures</u>, hospitalization, or even death (Gillespie et al., 2012). Falls may lead to fearfulness of leaving home and can lead to <u>Depression</u>. Most falls are caused by accidents. Some reasons people fall:

- Muscle weakness causing instability when walking
- Losing balance on a ladder
- Joint pain when standing
- Dizziness from high blood pressure or side effects of medication
- Sudden loss of consciousness
- Temporary confusion, as in dementia
- Changing one's position quickly when standing up
- Visual problems, especially in people wearing bifocals who may miss a step when climbing stairs
- Walking or navigating on ice and unsteady surfaces

Stein, F., & Haertl, K.
Pocket Guide to Intervention in Occupational Therapy, Second Edition (pp 107-114).
© 2019 Taylor & Francis Group.

Occupational therapists use functional exercise and occupations to increase strength and balance and provide adaptations to activities and the environment. Examples include the following:

- Place handrails in a shower or bathtub to prevent falls.
- Remove throw rugs.
- Increase lighting in halls and other important spaces.
- Change water faucets that are difficult to use.
- Add railings to steps.
- Lower kitchen cabinets that are hard to reach.
- Adjust bed height.
- Move furniture that obstructs the walking path.
- Buy stable ladders and foot stools. For excessive height (e.g. roofs), have someone else do the task.
- Take extra precaution on slippery surfaces.

Therapists may also work with the client to improve flexibility, coordination, muscle strength, and balance. Clients should also be taught proper <u>Body mechanics</u>. Assistive devices may also be used along with <u>Prescriptive exercises</u> such as <u>Tai chi</u>, <u>Yoga</u>, weight lifting, use of the stationary bike, and swimming and water exercises.

For more information, see the Centers for Disease Control's online brochures and website in <u>Appendix I</u>.

Family Therapy. The process of treating an individual by focusing on the dynamics in the family. In this process, the communication patterns of the family are emphasized, as well as the relationships between family members. Therapists try to assist the family by providing insight into the dynamics of interactions and by helping family members to develop healthy and honest communication. <u>Role playing</u> can be used in facilitating this process.

Feeding/Eating. An <u>Activity of daily living (ADL)</u> that is essential to an individual's self-care. Whereas feeding relates to the meal setup and bringing food to the mouth, eating relates to manipulating food within the mouth and swallowing (American Occupational Therapy Association, 2014). See <u>Self-care</u> for specific adaptive techniques, <u>Assistive technology</u> for adaptive equipment, and specific diagnoses/conditions for further discussion and treatment.

Feldenkrais Method. A motor therapy that involves learning new patterns of movement to enhance the communication between the brain and body. The method includes lying on one's back, sitting, or standing while becoming aware of each movement. The therapist or instructor may use massage to reduce stress or muscular tension. The purposes of this method are to reduce joint pain, improve joint mobility, increase muscle coordination, and improve posture.

Festinating Gait. Gait that is characterized by small, shuffling steps, which propel the client's body forward in an increasing rate. Clients who have a lesion in the substantia nigra often demonstrate this deficit. See <u>Parkinson's disease</u> for treatment and further discussion.

Fetal Alcohol Syndrome (FAS). An overarching term that denotes developmental disorders caused by a pregnant mother who consumed alcohol (Mukherjee, Hollins, & Turk, 2006). FAS disabilities may cause physical, psychological, behavioral, and <u>Intellectual disabilities</u>. Often, persons with FAS have facial characteristics that include small head, eyes, and jaws; a wide, flat nose bridge; and lack of a groove between the lip and the nose. *Fetal alcohol effects* is a term used to denote a milder form of this disorder. Occupational therapy intervention focuses on the manifested symptomatology, including use of behavioral, sensory, and cognitive techniques. Additional focus is placed on skill training in order to maximize occupational performance.

Figure/Ground Perception. The ability to discriminate between an object and its background. For instance, a client who has difficulty with figure/ground perception may be unable to find a white piece of paper lying on top of a white bedsheet. See <u>Cognitive-perceptual deficits</u> for further discussion and treatment.

Fine Motor Coordination. The ability to control the contraction of small muscles to complete fine, precise movements. Examples of functional activities using fine motor skills are crocheting, tying shoelaces, opening up a can, and handwriting. See <u>Coordination</u> for treatment methods.

Finger Agnosia. The inability to name or identify a specific finger when asked to discriminate between fingers, usually during a sensory evaluation. See <u>Cognitive-perceptual deficits</u> for further discussion and treatment

Flaccidity. A decrease in <u>Muscle tone</u>, also referred to as <u>Hypotonicity</u>, and often present immediately following a stroke or as a result of other motor and neurological conditions. The client often has a large range of motion available passively; however, very little, if any, active motion can be observed. The client may be at danger for <u>Subluxation</u> of the head of the humerus if the low muscle tone continues for any length of time. See <u>Motor control</u> problems and <u>Cerebrovascular accident (CVA)</u> for treatment methods. See also interventions under specific causes of the individual's flaccidity.

Flashback. Recurrence of a traumatic event, memory trace, emotion, or perceptual experience. It may be present in individuals with <u>Post-traumatic stress disorder (PTSD)</u>.

Flexion. Bending movement that decreases the angle of a joint. See <u>Anatomical position</u>.

Flexor Synergy. An automatic pattern of movement that may occur when a client with hemiplegia attempts the motion of flexion, such as elbow or knee flexion. The stereotypical pattern for the upper extremity combines the following motions: scapula adduction and elevation, shoulder abduction and external rotation, elbow flexion, forearm supination, and wrist and finger flexion. The stereotypical pattern for the lower extremity combines the following motions: hip flexion, abduction, and external rotation; knee flexion; ankle <u>Dorsiflexion</u> and inversion; and toe extension. See <u>Motor control</u> problems for intervention methods.

Flexor Withdrawal. A withdrawal reflex at the spinal level that protects the body from harm. See <u>Reflexes and reactions</u>.

Fluidotherapy. The application of a dry heat modality consisting of cellulose particles held in a container and moved in air. The turbulence of the mixture generates a thermal effect when objects are immersed in the medium. It uses convection to transfer heat to superficial physiological tissues. See <u>Physical agent modalities (PAMs)</u> for further discussion and treatment.

Forensic Psychiatry. The application of psychiatry and psychosocial practice to individuals who have committed a crime or are incarcerated for an illegal offense. Often, persons with mental illness are in traditional jail and prison systems, and there are also specialized forensic programs and hospitals that treat individuals with mental health conditions who have committed crimes. Occupational therapists working in correctional institutions, psychiatric intensive care units in prisons, or community facilities for individuals on probation employ various activities to engage the individual in everyday occupations. The purposes of these programs are to foster community living skills, such as in preparation for <u>Work</u>, literacy, social skills, communication, <u>Stress management</u>, and anger management. In recent years, there has also been an increased emphasis at looking at coexisting conditions such as sensory problems or <u>Addictions</u>. The overall purposes of these programs are to promote self-worth, individual responsibility, and self-regulation. Individual and group therapy techniques are employed to achieve these goals.

Form Constancy. The perceptual process of being able to recognize an object in various positions, sizes, and environments. Reading letters and numbers and identifying objects depend on this skill. This process is also dependent upon <u>Object permanence</u>.

Fracture. The damage to cartilage or bone, often as a result of an accident or trauma. Some conceptualizations consider a fracture to be hairline and a break to be a complete break to a bone. A closed fracture is an injury that does not pierce the skin. An open fracture occurs when the skin is pierced by the bone. Typically, intervention includes immobilization, slow return to mobility and function, and, in many cases, planned rehabilitation intervention.

Fragile X Syndrome. A chromosomal developmental condition affecting males. Fragile X is the most common inherited <u>Intellectual disability</u> in males and is marked by symptoms including an altered appearance (large head and prominent forehead), intellectual disability, and often behavioral difficulties. Occupational therapy interventions often focus on the manifesting symptomatology. For instance, if a client has cognitive deficits that limit <u>Self-care</u>, skill training will be adapted to the client's functional level. If the client demonstrates social deficits, <u>Social skills</u> training may be implemented.

Frame of Reference. Based on a theoretical model or theory that generates specific evaluation and intervention techniques in clinical practice. The following are common frames of reference used in occupational therapy:

- **Psychodynamic/Object Relations.** Based on the work of Freud (1937) and expanded upon by occupational therapist Ann Mosey (1970), this frame of reference helps explain mental processes, socializations, and behavior by acknowledging the role of the conscious and unconscious processes. Expressive and projective techniques are often used in evaluation and intervention.

- **Behavioral.** Grounded in the work of traditional psychological theorists such as Watson (1913) and Skinner (1938), the behavioral frame of reference emphasizes how learning results from observation and experience. Concepts of conditioning, shaping, and modeling are areas of focus, and individuals may be placed on behavioral programs or <u>Token economies</u> to encourage positive reinforcement. Traditional behaviorism was sometimes criticized for its lack of focus on the thought process, but in recent years, the behavioral theories and frames of reference have evolved. Evaluation and intervention often include observation and checklists, and the focus is on what the client does (observable behavior). Intervention includes modeling, shaping, <u>Reinforcement schedules</u>, token economies, and <u>Desensitization</u>.

- **Cognitive Behavioral.** This frame of reference builds on the work of Beck (1976) and Bandura (1977). Emphasis is placed on the interrelationship between thinking and behavior. Emphasis also is placed on addressing cognitive distortions (faulty thoughts). When applying this frame of reference, it is helpful for the client to have the capacity for insight. Evaluation often includes self-reports, inventories, and, at times, skill-based tests. Intervention utilizes individual and group therapy, <u>Dialectical behavioral therapy (DBT)</u>, insight-oriented techniques, homework, and direct feedback.

- **Cognitive Disability.** This frame of reference was originally developed by Claudia Allen (1985) and formulated for chronic mental health populations. Initially, it emphasized the baseline cognition of clients and identifying when a client has a capacity for learning and skill training and when adaptation and compensation should be used. Clients are given a screen called the *Allen Cognitive Lacing Screen* and may be tested with an additional Allen-based test/evaluation. Theressa Burns (2018) later adapted the frame of reference for those with dementia. Although her levels originally corresponded to the Allen levels, in recent years, her *Cognitive Performance Test* has evolved to have its own levels. A new manual published in 2018.

- **Sensory Integration and Sensory Processing.** Based on the work of A. Jean Ayres (2005), the sensory integration frame of reference follows concepts of neuroscience. Dr. Ayres emphasized the importance of the vestibular, proprioceptive, and tactile senses, which she identified as *proximal senses*. Focus in this frame of reference includes evaluation and intervention early in life when the brain is more plastic, working with clients who have modulatory or discriminatory issues, and developing a "sensory diet" in order to ensure an individual gets proper daily sensory input. Special training in these techniques is highly recommended.

- **Occupational Behavioral/Model of Human Occupation (MOHO).** Originated by Mary Reilly (1974) as the occupational behavioral frame of reference and expanded to the MOHO (Gary Kielhofner, 1985), these frames of reference emphasize the role of occupational engagement and occupational performance in health. Emphasis is placed on habits, routines, and roles and how they contribute to or inhibit health. The MOHO further discusses the systems view of the individual into a hierarchy of subsystems including volition, <u>Habituation</u>, and performance. Evaluation includes MOHO-based assessments in addition to role analysis and activity configurations that track time use and life balance. Interventions focus on skill training, role and life balance, and occupational performance in one's natural environment.

- **Motor Control and Motor Learning.** Historical concepts built on the work of Bobath (1990) and Rood (1962) in identifying neuro-maturational patterns of performance. Research has questioned the application of traditional <u>Neurodevelopmental treatment (NDT)</u> approaches, and, in recent years, motor learning and task performance as identified by Mathiowetz and Bass-Haugen (1994) have proposed a contemporary task-oriented approach utilizing function-based motor learning. Goal orientation includes assisting clients in developing cognitive and motor strategies in natural environments. Newer elements of this approach also use constraint-induced movement in order to encourage use of an affected limb after conditions such as a stroke.

Friction Massage. A type of deep tissue/connective tissue massage. See <u>Massage</u>.

Function. The degree of a client's independence in occupational performance such as in <u>Activities of daily living (ADLs)</u>, <u>Work</u>, and <u>Leisure</u> activities.

Functional Capacity Assessment (FCA). Comprehensive and systematic approach that measures the client's overall physical ability, such as muscle strength, endurance, joint range of motion, ambulation, sitting, standing, and lifting, most often as it relates to work activities. FCAs may be job-specific or may be general in order to match the client with a specific type of work or task. Examples of FCAs are the *Isernhagen Work System Functional Capacity Evaluation Procedures, Baltimore Therapeutic Equipment, Key Functional Capacity Assessment*, and *Blankenship System* (De Baets et al., 2018).

Functional Electrical Stimulation (FES). A term used for <u>Neuromuscular electrical stimulation (NMES)</u> while applying the current to a client during the attempt of functional activities. See <u>Physical agent modalities (PAMs)</u> for further discussion and treatment of NMES.

Functional Position. A position that allows a person to complete necessary functional activities, even if that position is fixed so that movement is limited to that single position. Functional positioning relates to everyday occupational performance and may include positioning of all the limbs and body, such as in seating, lying, or positioning of the hands and feet. See <u>Functional position of the hand</u>.

Functional Position of the Hand. A client should be positioned so that he or she has some functional use of the hand, even though the hand has limited range of motion (ROM). The most functional position of the hand is slight wrist extension (10 to 30 degrees) with thumb abduction and slight flexion and finger flexion through partial ROM. If the hand contracts while fully flexed or extended, the client will not be able to use the hand for any activities. If the hand contracts in this partially flexed position, then the client has the opportunity to use the hand to hold or stabilize items or assist with functional activities such as dressing. The Intrinsic plus position is another recommended position for immobilization. In this position, the metacarpophalangeal (MCP) joints are flexed to 60 to 90 degrees while the proximal interphalangeal (PIP) and distal interphalangeal (DIP) joints are fully extended. This helps prevent shortening of the musculoskeletal unit (e.g., ligaments, tendons, muscle belly), which would cause the client to lose the ability to cup the palm/hand. If a client has some shortening of the muscles and is not able to compositely flex at the MCP, PIP, and DIP joints through partial ROM, this position may be more achievable since flexion is occurring only at the MCP joints in this position.

G

Galvanic Skin Response (GSR). The change in the electrical resistance of the skin reflecting the individual's emotional state. What is being measured is the conductive pathway of a sweat gland, which is associated with an individual's sympathetic response. The GSR is traditionally used in "lie detector" tests.

General Systems Theory. A model of understanding the relationships between people and organizations and between parts and wholes (von Bertalanffy, 1950). General systems theory discusses differences between closed and open systems and dynamics of external factors that may influence a system.

Generalization. A cognitive ability to apply learned concepts and behaviors to new situations such as using tools, driving different cars, adapting to social situations, and engaging in a sport. Generalization is important in applying basic skills in Self-care, Leisure, and Work activities.

Gestalt Therapy. A form of humanistic psychotherapy developed by Perls (1969) that emphasizes the client's awareness of the perceptual environment and the "here and now." The approach also emphasizes the therapist–client relationship, client factors, and context.

Global Aphasia. The most severe form of aphasia, affecting the ability to read and write. See Aphasia.

Global Assessment of Function (GAF) Scale. This was the fifth axis on the five-axis system of the DSM-IV-TR (American Psychiatric Association [APA], 1994). The scale grades a client's functioning from 1 to 100, with 1 indicating that the client is a persistent danger to self or others and a rating of 100 indicating that an individual is functioning at a superior level in a wide range of activities, has many positive qualities, and has no symptoms. The scale is based on a mental health–mental illness continuum (APA, 1994). The axis system is no longer used in the DSM-5 (APA, 2013).

Stein, F., & Haertl, K.
Pocket Guide to Intervention in Occupational Therapy, Second Edition (pp 115-120).
© 2019 Taylor & Francis Group.

Goal Attainment Scaling (GAS). An evaluation tool used originally for mental health settings to describe the personal goals of clients on five possible levels of outcome for each goal (e.g., a client can identify lack of assertiveness as a personal problem, and a mutual goal is developed). Levels rated often include +1: somewhat better; +2: much better; 0: achievement of goal as expected; -1: somewhat worse than expected; and -2: much worse (Turner-Stokes, n.d.). This type of measurement is helpful for tracking rehabilitation outcomes.

Graded Motor Imagery. A newer technique used in rehabilitation that incorporates a number of motor reeducation techniques. The technique involves neuroscience education, left–right discrimination, sensory training, mirror therapy, and visualization of movement techniques to facilitate neuroplasticity. The technique involves graded techniques that integrate motor and visual processing. This is often used in <u>Pain management</u>, rehabilitation, <u>Neuropathy</u>, and hand therapy.

Graphesthesia. The ability to identify numbers, letters, or symbols traced on the skin with vision blocked. Asking the client to report which items are traced on the client's palm or fingertips with a dull pencil or instrument while blocking the client's vision can test this perceptual skill.

Grasp. The act of positioning the hand so that objects are held against the palm and the palmar surface of the fingers. According to Feix, Romero, Schmiedmayer, Dollar, and Kragic (2015), the definition of grasp is as follows: "every static hand posture with which an object can be held securely with one hand irrespective of the hand orientation" (p. 2). Most grasp patterns include the thumb in opposition to help complete this task.

When a client with a condition such as <u>Hemiplegia</u> is just beginning to regain hand motion, grasp is sometimes referred to as *mass* or *gross grasp* since a specific pattern is not seen. Rather, the client is simply beginning to flex the fingers in order to hold objects. Specific grasp patterns that can be observed in clients with normal muscle tone and coordination include the following:

Types of Grasp

- **Cylindrical Grasp.** Grasp that uses the thumb to oppose against a cylindrical object so that the object is held against the palm and palmar surface of the fingers. The fingers flex at each joint to curve around the surface of the object being held. This grasp is used when holding a soda can or handle of a hammer.
- **Spherical Grasp.** Grasp that uses the thumb to oppose against a round object to hold it against the palm and palmar surface of the

fingers. This grasp differs from the cylindrical grasp since the ring and small fingers flex more around a round object, which helps to cup the palm. This grasp is used when holding a baseball or apple.

- **Hook Grasp.** Grasp with the fingers that does not include the thumb. The metacarpophalangeal (MCP) joints of the fingers are extended (or may be hyperextended), while the proximal interphalangeal (PIP) and distal interphalangeal (DIP) joints are flexed. This grasp is used when holding the handle of a suitcase or briefcase. This hand position may also be observed following nerve damage to the upper extremity or during the return of muscle tone to the upper extremity after a stroke.

- **Intrinsic Plus Grasp.** Grasp that uses the thumb to oppose near the ring and small fingers to help hold an object against the palm and palmar surface of the fingers. All fingers flex at the MCP joint while fully extending at the PIP and DIP joints. This grasp is used when holding a plate or book.

Grasp Reflex. Primitive reflex also known as the <u>Palmar grasp reflex</u>. The infant closes the hand around an object placed in the palm. See <u>Reflexes and reactions</u>.

Gravitational Insecurity. Fear beyond that which is normal with ordinary body movement or when feet are off the ground. This condition often occurs in persons with <u>Sensory processing</u> difficulties.

Grief. Deep sadness or sorrow after an event, often following the death of a loved one. Occupational therapists work in grief and bereavement through addressing stress and coping, caregiver training following a death (e.g., if a caregiver never cooked or handled the finances prior to the death of a spouse), and through legacy and life review techniques to help honor the deceased loved one.

Grooming. An <u>Activity of daily living (ADL)</u> that facilitates an individual keeping neat and clean. Activities of grooming include tasks such as taking care of one's hair and brushing teeth. See <u>Self-care</u> for specific adaptive techniques, <u>Assistive technology</u> for adaptive equipment, and specific diagnoses/conditions for further discussion and treatment.

Gross Motor Coordination. The ability to control the contraction of large muscles and groups of muscles to complete large, less specific movements when engaging in everyday activities such as walking, running, and bicycling and in sports such as swimming, tennis, and basketball. See <u>Coordination</u> and <u>Range of motion (ROM)</u> for treatment methods.

Group Dynamics. The study of the factors and conditions that affect the actions in a group (e.g., the building of group cohesion and leadership functions).

Group Home. A residence for persons who often have physical, developmental, or mental illnesses. There are state and federal regulations governing the type of group home, policies followed, and number of residents allowed at the home.

Group Therapy. The applications of group methods to help clients gain insight, learn skills, prepare for employment, express feelings, and try out new behaviors. It is appropriate with almost all clients, including those with psychosocial and physical disabilities and cognitive deficits. The therapist should consider the following factors in establishing a group:

- Group goals are identified by the therapist and clients, such as stress management, prevocational preparation, creative expression, Pain management, and prevention of work injuries.

- The structure for the group is established considering the number of clients in the group, number of sessions, length of each session, and area where group therapy will take place.

- An administrative contract is established where the therapist gains the approval for group therapy from the administrator and interdisciplinary team.

- Clients are selected for group therapy considering age, gender, diagnosis, individual goals, and client motivation and fit for the group.

- Therapeutic leadership style is considered.

- Group therapy methodology is designed (e.g., type of group, modalities used, educational, task based, etc.)

- Media and modalities used in group therapy are selected according to client needs, such as arts and crafts, Dance, music, poetry, cooking, computers, prevocational training, and skill training.

- The effectiveness of group therapy is determined through psychometrics, self-reports, and family and staff clinical observations.

Occupational therapists often deliver group therapy in social skills, Stress management, Creative arts and Leisure activities, anger management, Assertiveness training, employment preparation, and addressed Activities of daily living (ADLs) and Instrumental activities of daily living (IADLs) skills.

Guiding. A treatment technique used by Bobath (1990) to help a client relearn normal movement while the therapist places his or her hand on the client's arm and helps move it through patterns. See <u>Motor control</u> problems and <u>Neurodevelopmental treatment (NDT)</u> approach.

Guillain-Barré Syndrome. A condition that causes demyelination of peripheral nerves and results in muscle weakness and sensory loss. <u>Hemiplegia</u> and <u>Hemiparesis</u> occur in an ascending manner, but remyelination may occur, which causes the condition to descend. The onset lasts for 1 to 3 weeks, followed by a plateau period when no change occurs, followed by remyelination, which can take up to 2 years. The cause is unknown, but a virus may be responsible for the attack of peripheral nerves by the immune system.

Specific Interventions

- Maintain range of motion (ROM), both passively and actively, as paralysis descends.
- Utilize nonresistive activities for strengthening until the client is able to demonstrate muscle strength of 3/5 (see <u>Manual muscle test [MMT]</u>), then the client may begin gentle and graded resistive activity.
- Fabricate splints to prevent deformity from atrophy of muscles.
- Complete activities for <u>Bilateral integration</u> and coordination.
- Increase endurance by slowly increasing the time during which the client participates in therapy.
- Provide sensory stimulation as the sensation returns.
- Educate the client on progression of the disease and expectations for treatment.
- Instruct the client on principles of energy conservation and work simplification.
- Teach joint protection principles.
- Train the client to use <u>Stress management</u> and <u>Relaxation therapy</u> as needed.
- Stress the importance of avoiding fatigue as it may trigger a setback in recovery.
- Encourage the client to join a support group for socialization and adjustment to the disease.
- Retrain <u>Self-care</u> activities using compensatory techniques and assistive devices as needed.
- Complete a home and/or job site evaluation, and provide recommendations to modify the environment for increased independence with activities.

- Explore new <u>Leisure</u> interests as needed.
- Address pain.

Contraindications/Precautions

- Monitor the skin for redness over bony prominences, which could result in pressure sores.
- Discontinue activity if the client becomes fatigued.
- Prevent substitution of muscles that are not the <u>Prime movers</u> for a motion during strengthening or ROM.
- Provide equipment to maintain proper positioning.
- Stop at the point of pain when completing passive ROM.

Gustatory Sensation. Receiving, discriminating, localizing, and interpreting taste mainly through the receptors on the tongue.

H

Habilitation. The development of function in the performance areas such as <u>Work</u>, <u>Leisure</u>, and <u>Self-care</u> by an individual with a <u>Developmental disability</u> such as <u>Autism</u> or <u>Cerebral palsy (CP)</u>. In some cases, adults with chronic mental illness who have not developed functional abilities are taught these competencies for the first time and are considered to be habilitated rather than rehabilitated.

Habituation. Refers to the daily adaptive behavior or routines of an individual as described in the <u>Model of Human Occupation (MOHO)</u>.

Halfway House. A supportive housing environment in which clients are provided a structured and supportive setting in preparation for community living. Frequently, clients are given communal responsibilities for maintenance and household tasks such as kitchen or yard duties.

Hallucination. A false perception of a sensation, such as seeing, hearing, or smelling, that does not exist in reality. The individual with a hallucination is unable to distinguish between the real and the imagined sensation. Hallucinations, particularly hearing voices, is common in psychotic disorders such as <u>Schizophrenia</u>.

Hand Injuries. The treatment of hand injuries is very specific and specialized; therefore, hand injuries are briefly discussed. For more specific protocols, the therapist may refer to various references, including the *Indiana Hand Center Protocol* (Cannon, 2001) or the two-volume set, *Rehabilitation of the Hand and Upper Extremity* (Skirven, Osterman, Fedorczyk, & Amadio, 2011a, 2011b). The therapist should take extreme caution to talk to the physician for his or her preferred protocol or plan of treatment as physicians and treatment protocols often change with advances in surgical techniques. Some approaches tend to be more conservative, whereas others are aggressive. All need to be customized to

Stein, F., & Haertl, K.
Pocket Guide to Intervention in Occupational Therapy, Second Edition (pp 121-130).
© 2019 Taylor & Francis Group.

the client's individual injury, rate of healing, and aptitude. The therapist should also consult the physician about precautions and contraindications to treatment; however, many protocols and more-detailed hand references are specific with treatment to prevent injury during the healing process. *Please remember when reading the following material that this is a general treatment guide for hand therapy, which was taken from only a few references since so many varying protocols exist. Please consult further resources when treating specific injuries.*

Types of Injuries

- **Joint Injuries.** Treatment should stress gentle exercise within the client's tolerance of pain. Exercise should not increase pain or edema; however, if <u>Edema</u> does occur, ice massage or Coban wrapping may help decrease swelling, or manual edema mobilization may be used. (Note: This requires extra training.) The therapist should be careful to prescribe exercise for the unaffected part of the hand and the upper extremity to help maintain ligament length and prevent joint contracture and joint stress during healing. For stiff joints, prolonged gentle stretching techniques are recommended.

- **Ligamentous Injuries.** The most common type of this injury affects the proximal interphalangeal (PIP) joint. Treatment should balance immobilization vs guarded <u>Active range of motion (AROM)</u> to prevent loss of motion. Immobilization may be required for a period of time due to instability. After the splint is removed, the affected finger may be taped to an adjacent finger to help protect the affected joint while it continues to strengthen.

- **Volar Plate Injuries.** This type of injury is usually caused by hyperextension at a joint. If the injury is not treated properly, the joint may heal with a <u>Swan neck deformity</u>. The affected finger should be immobilized with a splint to hold the joint in 20 degrees of flexion for up to 2 weeks, with instruction on range of motion for uninvolved joints. Next, depending on the injury, a dorsal blocking splint may be fabricated and worn by the client for 1 to 2 more weeks to prevent full extension of the weak joint.

- **Dislocations.** The joint most commonly dislocated is the PIP joint. A dislocation that results in a volar plate injury should be treated in the manner listed earlier. If the proximal interphalangeal joint is dislocated in flexion, then the joint should be splinted in extension. An injury of this type often requires surgical intervention.

Handicap. A disadvantage for an individual, resulting from an impairment or a disability that limits or prevents the fulfillment of a normal role depending on age, sex, social, and cultural factors. A physical or psychiatric handicap is the inability to perform normal role functions as a student, worker, husband, wife, father, or mother or to engage in <u>Work</u> and <u>Leisure</u> activities, or be independent in <u>Self-care</u> or social functioning. Although the term is still used, many prefer the term *disability* or "different ability."

Handling. This term was originally often used in neurodevelopmental treatment (NDT) related to the therapist's use of his or her hands to assist the client with movement patterns. When necessary, the therapist facilitates active movement or tone, inhibits abnormal movement or tone, reeducates muscles to complete normal movement patterns, and realigns joints. Present-day use of handling also refers to the importance of safe handling techniques for patient care. See <u>Motor control</u> problems and <u>Neurodevelopmental treatment (NDT)</u> for more treatment techniques.

Health. The overall physical, mental, psychological, and spiritual wellness of an individual.

Health Insurance Portability and Accountability Act (HIPAA). U.S. law that mandates the security and privacy of certain health care information.

Health Maintenance Organization (HMO). A prepaid group health care program that provides diagnostic treatment services, ambulatory care, hospitalization, and surgery with an emphasis on prevention.

Heart Disease. See <u>Cardiac disease/cardiac dysfunction</u>.

Hemianesthesia. A complete loss of sensation to either the right or left side of the body.

Hemianopsia. A condition in which a client has no vision in half of the visual field of one or both eyes. If the client has had a <u>Cerebrovascular accident (CVA)</u> in the occipital lobe, it can result in a homonymous hemianopsia—the client is blind in the corresponding fields in both eyes (e.g., a client who has a left homonymous hemianopsia has a sensory loss resulting in loss of vision in the left half of the visual field with both eyes; thus, the left eye cannot see to the far left, and the right eye cannot see to its left, which would include the area slightly to the left and center of the client). See <u>Cognitive-perceptual deficits</u> and <u>Visual foundation skills</u> for treatment of visual deficits.

Hemiballism. Involuntary movement that occurs as rapid gross motor movements, which are violent and forceful. The extremities display this deficit as flinging movements, usually on only one side of the body. Lesions of the subthalamic nucleus may result in hemiballism.

Hemiparesis. Weakness of half of the body, usually resulting from an insult to the brain.

Hemiplegia. Paralysis of one side of the body, which usually occurs following an insult to the brain.

Herbal/Botanical. A method of using forms of plants for prevention and treatment of illnesses.

Heterotopic Ossification. The formation of bone in locations where bone does not normally form, such as soft tissue surrounding a joint. Symptoms that may signal ossification include localized pain, redness or warmth, edema, and rapidly decreasing range of motion (ROM) at a joint. Joints that seem to be at higher risk of involvement include the shoulder, elbow, hip, and knee.

Specific Interventions
- Include <u>Active range of motion (AROM)</u> throughout the available range, positioning, and splinting, or passive ROM (PROM) only to the point of pain.
- Surgery may be necessary to free a joint and increase ROM.
- Clients who may be at increased risk of heterotopic ossification are those with burns, <u>Traumatic brain injury</u>, or spinal cord injury.

High-Voltage Galvanic Stimulation (HVGS). A physical agent modality that uses electrical current to treat pain and edema, improve circulation, reeducate muscles, reduce muscle guarding, decrease atrophy/increase strength, or heal wounds. See <u>Physical agent modalities (PAMs)</u> for further discussion and treatment.

High-Voltage Pulsed Current (HVPC). This modality may also be referred to as *high voltage-galvanic stimulation* (HVGS). See <u>Physical agent modalities (PAMs)</u> for further discussion.

Hip Fracture. Femoral neck and intertrochanteric hip fractures are the most common fractures for those over 50 (Altizer, 2005; Lareau & Sawyer, 2010). Hip fractures are often treated with surgery and may or may not involve a hip replacement. Occupational therapy following hip surgery often focuses on reinforcing hip precautions and helping clients with <u>Activities of daily living (ADLs)</u> and <u>Instrumental activities of daily living (IADLs)</u>. Typical movement restrictions following surgery include no hip flexion beyond 90 degrees, avoidance of hip rotation, no crossing the operated leg over the other, and no adduction of the operated leg (Maher, 2014). Additional adaptations are often made for ADLs. See <u>Self-care</u>.

Hippotherapy. Intervention with the help of the horse to strengthen, stretch, and relax the muscles; enhance the motor coordination of the rider; improve posture; and attain psychological goals such as increased self-esteem, body image, and <u>Self-concept</u>. The rationale for its use as a therapeutic modality is that the horse's movement produces a smooth, rhythmical pattern to the rider. Therapeutic riding programs have been used successfully with clients having diagnoses such as <u>Multiple sclerosis (MS)</u>, <u>Traumatic brain injury</u>, stroke, learning disabilities, orthopedic disorders, <u>Spina bifida</u>, <u>Intellectual disability</u> and <u>Developmental disability</u>, juvenile delinquency, <u>Cerebral palsy (CP)</u>, <u>Autism</u>, and mental illnesses.

Histrionic Personality Disorder. Characteristic of individuals who are prone to exaggerate, act out or demonstrate feelings, and show explosive personality reactions. In this disorder, the individual strives for excitement and surprise in relationships with others. Others characterize individuals as vain, self-centered, demanding, and shallow.

Holistic Medicine. A comprehensive approach to treatment considering the physical, social, psychological, spiritual, and economic needs of the client. Holistic methods include diet therapy, exercise, <u>Stress management</u>, and <u>Relaxation therapy</u>, as well as traditional treatments.

Home Evaluation. Prior to a client's discharge from the hospital to home, an occupational therapist should evaluate the client's home to provide recommendations for equipment to be installed and adaptations to be completed. A variety of formal and informal assessment tools are available to assist with evaluation. When possible, the physical therapist should accompany the occupational therapist so that all areas are addressed. The client and a caregiver, when applicable, should accompany the therapist. The client may be asked to demonstrate <u>Transfer/mobility</u> and other <u>Self-care</u> activities to show the therapist if the current environment is acceptable. The therapist should also ask the client and caregiver what the routine was prior to the injury and what the expectations are for the routine when the client returns home. While demonstrating ambulation or transfers, the caregiver can be given recommendations to assist the client if needed. The therapist should measure entry ways and ensure adequate space for mobility devices. Recommendations should be given to simplify tasks, remove obstacles, or widen pathways throughout the home. After the evaluation is completed, the therapist generally meets with the client and caregiver(s) to present recommendations. A list of problem areas, adaptations to solve those problems, and recommendations for equipment to increase the client's independence should be given to the client and caregiver. Following is a list of areas that should be assessed during the home evaluation:

Components of the Home Evaluation

- Overview of the home environment and the client's ability to perform <u>Activities of daily living (ADLs)</u> and <u>Instrumental activities of daily living (IADLs)</u> within the home
- The client's mobility status and devices used (wheelchair, quad cane, etc.)
- Type of home and number of levels within the home, including basement when applicable
- Access from the driveway and/or the garage to the house
- Number of steps at entrance to the home, the steps' dimensions, and if railing is installed
- Ramp location and dimensions if applicable
- Size of the threshold at the entrance
- Size of door at entrance and the direction it opens
- Type of floor covering in rooms used by the client
- If living room arrangement is conducive to client's mobility status
- Height and firmness of furniture used by client
- Dimensions of hallways and if sharp turns are necessary when entering various rooms
- Door dimensions of bedroom and direction it opens, including threshold height
- Type and height of bed, including client's ability to transfer to/from bed
- Space in bedroom, including room for wheelchair or hospital bed if needed
- Accessibility of dressers and closet
- Door dimensions of bathroom and direction it opens, including threshold height
- Dimensions of tub, type of water barrier (curtain vs glass doors), and if shower head is available
- Dimensions of door and height of threshold if walk-in shower
- Height of sink and type of faucets
- Height of toilet, toilet paper location, or location near cabinet-type sink to assist client with standing, including client's ability to transfer
- Availability for grab bar installation if not currently installed

- Door dimensions of kitchen and direction it opens, including threshold height
- Height of stove, location of oven, location of controls, and accessibility
- Height of sink, type of faucets, and availability for wheelchair to fit beneath if applicable
- Accessibility, type, and location of cupboards
- Accessibility and location of all major kitchen appliances
- Accessibility and locations of necessary switches and outlets
- Height of kitchen table and countertops
- Door dimensions of laundry room and direction it opens, including threshold height
- Dimensions and number of steps to laundry facilities
- Accessibility and type of washer
- Accessibility and type of dryer
- Location of any throw rugs
- Location of phone
- If client has an emergency call system or list of emergency numbers
- Location of mailbox
- Location of thermostat
- Notation of any unsafe situations like sharp-edged furniture, non-insulated hot water pipes, or imperfect floors
- Notation of cluttered areas
- If client has a fire extinguisher and its location
- List of equipment the client currently has
- List of problem situations and areas to be rectified
- Recommendations for adaptations to be made
- Recommendations for equipment to be purchased

Homeopathy. A school of medicine founded by Dr. S.C.F. Hahnemann (Haehl, 1922) in the late 18th century based on the theory that large doses of drugs that produce symptoms of a disease in healthy people will cure the same symptoms when administered in very small amounts. This is loosely based on the theory that "like cures like." Homeopathic physicians use natural remedies of specially prepared plants and minerals to boost the body's defense mechanisms and healing processes.

Homeostasis. Refers to the state of dynamic equilibrium that internal body organisms strive to maintain through feedback mechanisms and regulatory functions. Cannon (1932) described the processes in the body in maintaining normal values such as heart rate, blood pressure, salt, water, blood sugar, and hemoglobin. Homeostasis also refers to the body's reaction to disease, such as T-cell production to fight infection.

Homogeneous. Refers to like characteristics such as age, gender, or intelligence.

Homolateral Limb Synkinesis. A manifestation of certain hemiplegia disorders resulting in a mutual dependency between limbs causing the same action in both affected extremities (e.g., if the client tries to flex the affected upper extremity, then the lower extremity also involuntarily flexes). See <u>Motor control</u> problems.

Hook Grasp. The fingers hook around an object. See <u>Grasp</u>.

Horizontal Plane. Dividing the body between upper and lower parts. See <u>Anatomical position</u>.

Horticulture. The science and art of gardening and cultivating fruits, vegetables, flowers, and plants. Horticulture is used as a therapeutic modality in occupational therapy.

Hot Packs. A physical agent modality that uses conduction to transfer heat to superficial physiological tissue. See <u>Physical agent modalities (PAMs)</u> for further discussion and treatment.

Humanism. A system of beliefs and a theory of knowledge that emphasizes the inherent value of humans. Humanism embraces the acceptance of diverse cultural values, capacities, and achievements of human beings. Intervention focuses on unconditional acceptance of the individual, even when a behavior is unacceptable. It is also related to the humane treatment of individuals with mental illness during the 19th century termed <u>Moral treatment</u>.

Humanitarianism. The promotion of social betterment through social action groups that provide aid, welfare, and opportunities to those in poverty or survivors of wars and natural disasters.

Humor. Any communication that leads to laughing, smiling, or a feeling of amusement by any of the interacting parties. Humor can be used as a stress-reducing method in treatment. There is some evidence that humor stimulates neuropeptides and endorphins that can relieve pain. Mosey (1986) identified humor as relevant to conscious use of self in practice.

Huntington's Disease/Huntington's Chorea. A hereditary disease resulting in the progressive degeneration of nerve cells in the brain causing an abnormal movement disorder, behavioral shifts, and often dementia. Individuals live 10 to 15 years beyond initial symptoms. Huntington's chorea refers to irregular and involuntary movements of the trunk and limbs that result from degeneration of the basal ganglia.

Hydrotherapy. A physical agent modality that uses water in the context of therapy. Uses may include varying temperatures (hot or cold) in addition to the use of water in motion such as in a therapeutic whirlpool. This type of therapy may be used in treating individuals with pain, increasing Range of motion (ROM), decreasing stress, enabling exercise, and increasing blood circulation. See Aquatic therapy and Physical agent modalities (PAMs) for further discussion and intervention.

Hyperextension. A joint motion that may or may not be beyond the normal range of joint motion in extension, but it is beyond the normal alignment of the body parts (e.g., some hyperextension can occur within the curvatures of the spine [Lordosis or Kyphosis], which would be greater than the normal alignment of the spine but would not be beyond the normal range of motion available in the spine).

Hypersensitivity. A condition in which normal stimuli cause pain or discomfort. A client who has had a crushing injury, nerve injury, burn, or other injury may be vulnerable to this condition. The client often guards the extremity to protect it from painful situations; however, this causes decreased use of the extremity, which leads to impaired function. A client with this condition is often treated through Desensitization or sensory-based approaches.

Hypertonicity. Muscle tone that is greater than normal tone and inhibits the client from completing voluntary movements. Also referred to as Spasticity, hypertonicity can occur in clients with various Upper motor neuron disorders, including Parkinson's disease, Multiple sclerosis (MS), Traumatic brain injury, Spinal cord injury, cerebrovascular accident (CVA), Cerebral palsy (CP), or brain tumors. An increase in Deep tendon reflexes, as well as a demonstration of Clonus, helps determine a diagnosis of hypertonicity. Hypertonicity can be graded on the following scale.

Grades of Hypertonicity

- **Severe.** Presence of a strong Stretch reflex and *strong* resistance to passive range of motion (PROM) (PROM may not be possible), as well as possible presence of clonus
- **Moderate.** Visible stretch reflex and PROM is possible but slow

- **Minimal.** Stretch reflex can be palpated but very little resistance to PROM (if any), and <u>Active range of motion (AROM)</u> may be possible with movement against the spastic muscles occurring more slowly than normal.

<u>Inhibition techniques</u> may help decrease the muscle tone and make movement easier. See <u>Motor control</u> problems and <u>Cerebrovascular accident (CVA)</u>, as well as other cross-referenced disorders listed earlier, for treatment methods.

Hypnotherapy. Treatment by inducing an alternative state of consciousness in which the individual feels relaxed and with little pain. Has been used successfully in some cases to decrease smoking, for obesity, and in substance abuse. Practitioners should be specially trained in using this technique.

Hypothalamic-Pituitary-Adrenocortical Axis. Refers to the complex interactions that occur in the autonomic nervous system that involve neurotransmitters and hormonal secretions. It plays an important role in the <u>Stress reaction</u> and in maintaining the health of the individual in homeostatic reactions.

Hypothesis. A statement that predicts results and is testable. An example of a hypothesis is aerobic exercise lowers blood pressure in middle-aged sedentary males.

Hypotonicity. Muscle tone that is less than normal and inhibits the client from completing voluntary movements. Also referred to as <u>Flaccidity</u>, hypotonicity often occurs in clients who have suffered a <u>Stroke</u>/cerebrovascular accident (CVA). Facilitation techniques may help increase muscle tone and produce a contraction so that movement is possible. See <u>Motor control</u> problems and <u>Cerebrovascular accident (CVA)</u> for treatment methods.

I

Icing. A method used to facilitate <u>Muscle tone</u> or to facilitate recovery from an injury in order to reduce pain or swelling.

Contraindications/Precautions

- If there is an injury with pain and inflammation, often ice is used with elevation. A soft cloth or covering may be used in order to prevent skin irritation from excessive cold.
- Icing should not be completed along the client's midline, especially to clients with spinal cord injuries at level C4–C5, as this may result in <u>Autonomic dysreflexia</u>.
- Icing should also not be applied above the client's neck to the trigeminal nerve area (except if using ice in the mouth), to the pinna of the ear, or behind the ear.
- Ice that is applied to the left shoulder may cause heart arrhythmia or angina, so this technique should not be used when working with clients who have cardiovascular problems.

See <u>Motor control</u> problems and <u>Rood approach</u> for more discussion of <u>Facilitation techniques</u>.

Ideational Apraxia. Unable to conceptualize movement such as in <u>Activities of daily living (ADLs)</u> . See <u>Apraxia</u>.

Ideomotor Apraxia. Unable to carry out motor tasks such as in <u>Activities of daily living (ADLs)</u>. See <u>Apraxia</u>.

Imagery. A relaxation technique that involves visualizing relaxing scenes with the eyes closed. Many practitioners recommend that the client rotate his or her eyes inward and upward as a warm-up technique before visualizing colors, objects, abstract ideas, and significant people in the client's life.

Stein, F., & Haertl, K.
Pocket Guide to Intervention in Occupational Therapy, Second Edition (pp 131-135).
© 2019 Taylor & Francis Group.

Imitation Synkinesis. A technique developed by Brunnstrom (1970, 1996) that involves completing a desired movement with the unaffected extremity while trying to complete that same movement with the affected extremity as a means of facilitation (e.g., if the client is trying to flex the affected shoulder, then he or she will flex the unaffected shoulder simultaneously).

Impairment. Any loss or abnormality of physiological, psychological, or anatomical structure or function such as <u>Blindness</u>, deafness, <u>Astereognosis</u>, mental condition, or lack of pain sensation. The World Health Organization's (2017) definition of impairment is "a problem in body function or structure." For instance, a psychiatric impairment may include a phobia, <u>Delusion</u>, <u>Hallucination</u>, severe <u>Anxiety</u>, or <u>Depression</u>.

Incoherence. Incomprehensible speech or thinking.

Independence. The extent to which one can manage his or her daily requirements and function apart from others (e.g., the ability to dress self, maintain one's finances, and navigate from one place to another). Within rehabilitation, independence is often broken down into levels such as minimum, moderate, and maximum assistance.

Independent Living Assessment/Evaluation. Assessment tools used to measure a client's ability to perform <u>Activities of daily living (ADLs)</u> and <u>Instrumental activities of daily living (IADLs)</u>. Several tools are available depending on need and population. Examples include the *Barthel Self-Care Index, Functional Independence Measure, Kohlman Evaluation of Living Skills,* and *Performance Assessment of Self-Care Skills.* Areas assessed vary based on the tool and may include observation, checklist, interview, and environmental assessment. See Asher (2014) for a comprehensive list of assessment tools.

Inhibition. The act of decreasing or suppressing. Often used when referring to a client who has high <u>Muscle tone</u>. See <u>Motor control</u> problems for applications of inhibition.

Inhibition Techniques. Techniques that decrease the tone of a muscle so that the distal attachment of the muscle and its body part are able to move in the opposite direction (e.g., the goal of inhibition to high tone in the biceps is the extension of the elbow [the forearm is the distal attachment of the biceps, and extension is the opposite action/direction of the biceps]). Inhibition is used to help a spastic muscle relax so that the antagonistic muscle can complete its action as well. Techniques that help decrease high tone include pressure, rocking, and rolling. See <u>Motor control</u> problems for more examples.

Initiation of an Activity. The cognitive ability to begin an activity on one's own. This can become impaired in clients who are depressed, in clients who have severe <u>Intellectual disabilities</u>, and in individuals with brain damage. Therapists can help clients to initiate an activity by using forward or backward <u>Chaining</u> or work on sequencing. This enables the client to complete or participate in the activity, such as in dressing.

Innate Intelligence. The inherited biological aptitudes and abilities of an individual.

Instinctive Avoiding Reaction. A forward or upward movement of a client's affected arm results in the involuntary extension and/or hyperextension of the client's fingers and thumb. See <u>Motor control</u> problems.

Instinctive Grasp Reaction. Similar to the <u>Grasp reflex</u>, the client's affected hand flexes or closes involuntarily when it comes into contact with a stationary object. The client will not be able to actively extend his or her fingers in order to release the object on command. See <u>Motor control</u> problems.

Institutionalization. Placement in an institution for reasons such as mental health care or for punishment purposes. Over time, institutionalization may be used to refer to an insidious process where, over many years, an individual living in an institution, (e.g., a state mental hospital or prison) develops apathy, flattened affect, hopelessness, dilapidated appearance, and dependency on others and the institution.

Instrumental Activities of Daily Living (lADLs). According to the American Occupational Therapy Association (2014), IADLs are "[a]ctivities to support daily life within the home and community that often require more complex interactions than those used in ADLs" (p. S19). Examples of IADLs include care of self and others (e.g., children/pets), communication management, driving, financial management, health maintenance and home management, meal preparation, religious expression, safety, and shopping. See <u>Assistive technology</u> and specific diagnoses/conditions for further discussion and intervention.

Intellectual Disability. The variety of intellectual disabilities are categorized under "neurodevelopmental disorders" in the DSM-5 (American Psychiatric Association, 2013) and involve deficits in general mental or cognitive abilities such as planning, problem solving, reasoning, abstract thinking, and learning. The disorder arises during development (often in utero or congenital) and includes both intellectual and adaptive functional deficits. Occupational therapists work with individuals based on their diagnoses and subsequent effects on occupational performance. Typically, therapists use both remedial/restorative and adaptive approaches based · on individual needs. See also <u>Developmental disability</u>.

Intelligence. The capacity to comprehend and understand based on innate and learned skills. There are several theories of intelligence focused on general intelligence (e.g., capacity for verbal, spatial, and mathematical skill), as well as theories of multiple intelligence focused on aptitude in a number of areas, such as the capacity for a number of mental functions including but not limited to musical, verbal, mathematical, interpersonal, intrapersonal, etc. Psychologists often administer intelligence tests in order to obtain an intelligent quotient, which compares a client to the norm. One must be cautious to ensure the reliability and validity of the tools used, particularly when working with clients from other cultures or those with limited ability to focus on the task.

Intention Tremor. A client with this deficit demonstrates small involuntary rhythmic movements at one or more joints when attempting voluntary movement. While the client is at rest, tremors will decrease or may disappear. Once the client attempts movement, tremors will reappear and may hinder the client's ability to complete the desired tasks. This deficit results from a cerebellar lesion, and clients who have multiple sclerosis often demonstrate intention tremors. See <u>Multiple sclerosis (MS)</u> for treatment and further discussion.

Interdisciplinary Team. Individuals from different disciplines who work cooperatively in generating intervention goals in collaboration with the client.

Interests. Psychological constructs that include an individual's choice in engaging in activities such as sports, reading, music, films, theater, arts and crafts, cuisine, and table games. The motivation to engage in activities depends on the opportunities available to the individual, the ability to do the activity, and the pleasure related to the activity. Occupational therapists can help clients to widen their repertoire of interests by exploring and teaching various activities.

Interference Current (IFC). This modality may also be referred to as <u>Interferential electrical stimulation</u> and involves two alternating currents used for the electrostimulation of nerves. See <u>Physical agent modalities (PAMs)</u> for further discussion.

Interferential Electrical Stimulation. A physical agent modality that uses electrical current to treat pain and edema. See <u>Physical agent modalities (PAMs)</u> for further discussion and treatment.

Internal Rotation. Turning a limb toward the midline of the body. See <u>Anatomical position</u>.

Interpersonal Skills. Verbal and nonverbal communication as a part of social skills, and knowing how to initiate a conversation, express support of another, show humor, problem solve, and demonstrate <u>Self-control</u>. The use of interpersonal skills requires an individual to shift contexts, for instance, relating to others in a business context vs relating to friends.

Interphalangeal. Between the joints of the fingers and toes. See <u>Hand injuries</u>.

Intervention. With respect to occupational therapy, intervention relates to skilled services provided to facilitate occupational participation and enhance health, participation, and well-being (American Occupational Therapy Association, 2014). The intervention process utilizes information from the <u>Occupational profile</u> and evaluation in order to work collaboratively with the client to develop goals and establish an intervention plan.

Intrinsic Motivation. The internal motivation to achieve or perform an activity without external rewards (e.g., an artist will continue painting without expecting any reward or praise). Individuals with intrinsic motivation often have an internal <u>Locus of control</u>.

Intrinsic Plus Grasp. See <u>Grasp</u>.

Intrinsic Plus Position. This position places the intrinsic muscles in an optimal position to help prevent atrophy and preserve the length of the proximal interphalangeal (PIP) and metacarpophalangeal (MCP) collateral ligaments. A hand that has atrophy of the intrinsic muscles will lose its ability to cup the palm/hand. This position places the MCP joints in flexion to near 90 degrees while allowing full extension of the PIP and distal interphalangeal (DIP) joints.

Iontophoresis. A physical agent modality that uses electrical current to drive ions, which are contained within topical medications, into underlying tissue for the purpose of promoting wound healing or reducing pain, muscle spasm, calcium deposits, infection, scar tissue, or edema. See <u>Physical agent modalities (PAMs)</u> for further discussion and treatment.

Isometric Contraction. Exercise involving the muscle and joint staying the same length. See <u>Contraction</u>.

Isotonic Contraction. Constant tension during lengthening and shortening of a muscle. See <u>Contraction</u>.

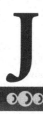

J

Job Burnout. A debilitating condition caused by chronic <u>Occupational stress</u>, which results in depleted energy, lowered resistance to illness, job dissatisfaction, pessimism, increased inefficiency, and absenteeism.

Job Coach. A counselor or therapist who provides support to the employed client.

Joint Compression. A technique that can be used to either facilitate or inhibit <u>Muscle tone</u>. When heavy joint compression is applied, the joint receives more force than it regularly supports. For instance, through the act of pushing downward on the client's shoulders, the therapist manually assists a client who is prone on elbows. The client is receiving more force through the shoulder joint than the shoulder usually supports when the client is in this position. This technique facilitates <u>Co-contraction</u> of muscles around the joint. If light joint compression is applied, meaning the same or less force is applied than the joint is used to supporting, inhibition occurs. The main application of this type of compression occurs when a client with hemiplegia lies supine and the therapist approximates the head of the humerus. See <u>Motor control</u> problems and <u>Rood approach</u> for further discussion of <u>Facilitation</u> and <u>Inhibition techniques</u>.

Joint Mobilization. A technique in which the therapist passively moves a joint to its accessory motions prior to voluntary movement of that joint to achieve maximum range of motion (ROM). Accessory motion, sometimes referred to as *joint play*, is nonvoluntary movement that occurs at the joint as the bones glide over one another. If the bones are not gliding or rotating as they should, both passive and active ROM/movement will be hindered. Accessory motions include rotation, anterior-posterior glide, lateral glide, flexion and extension tilt, and distraction. A therapist must know the orthokinematics of the joint being treated before attempting to

Stein, F., & Haertl, K.
*Pocket Guide to Intervention in Occupational
Therapy, Second Edition* (pp 137-140).
© 2019 Taylor & Francis Group.

restore joint play. Passive movement to promote each accessory motion at a joint should be completed for 30 to 60 seconds prior to ROM if the client demonstrates impaired movement. Mobilization is appropriate for clients with limited ROM caused by a tight joint capsule, pain, meniscus displacement, tight ligaments, muscle guarding, or adhesions (Norkin & Levangie, 1992).

Contraindications/Precautions

- Passive accessory motion should not be applied when a client has hypermobility, infection, inflammation, effusion, osteoporosis, degenerative joint disease, unhealed fracture, or <u>Rheumatoid arthritis</u>. Care should be taken if a client has malignancy of the site being treated, excessive pain, or total joint replacement.

Techniques

- **Rhythmic Oscillations.** The bones are passively moved through either a small or large range of movement, at a rate of two to three oscillations per second. This type of mobilization may be used for clients who complain of pain.

- **Sustained Stretch or Distraction.** The bones are passively moved through the entire available range of movement and held in that position. Tiny oscillatory movements may be applied at the limit of the range. This type of mobilization is used when accessory motion is tight and limits the client's functional ROM.

Examples

- **Metacarpophalangeal (MCP) Joint.** This joint is able to complete three motions: flexion/extension, abduction/adduction, and rotation. Before mobilization begins, the therapist must decide which way the moving bone glides at the articular surface. The head of the metacarpal is convex, and the base of the proximal phalanx is concave; therefore, the base of the proximal phalanx moves on the metacarpal and glides in the same direction as the physiological motion being completed. Each MCP receives mobilization individually.

  ○ **Distraction.** This is the first movement to be completed since the intra-articular space must be large enough to allow any ROM at the joint. The therapist should firmly hold the metacarpal bone with one hand while using the other hand to grasp near the base of the proximal phalanx while the MCP is slightly flexed. The therapist gently pulls the phalanx distally to distract the joint.

- ◦ **Flexion/Extension.** Again, the therapist firmly holds the meta-carpal bone with one hand and the base of the proximal pha-lanx on the dorsal and volar surfaces with the other hand while slightly flexing the MCP. The client's hand is usually pronated during the procedure. The therapist gently pushes downward, while slightly distracting the joint, to produce a volar glide. Then, the therapist allows the bone to relax back to its original position. Volar glide helps increase flexion of the MCP. To increase extension at the MCP, dorsal glide is completed. The therapist begins mobilization with the same grasp as in the volar glide. The therapist gently pushes upward on the base of the proximal phalanx to produce a dorsal glide. The proximal phalanx is then allowed to relax back to its previous alignment.

- ◦ **Abduction/Adduction.** The therapist holds the metacarpal bone and proximal phalanx with the same method used during flexion/extension, except the proximal phalanx should be held on the radial and ulnar surfaces. The therapist then slightly distracts the joint and gently pushes toward the radius, while the hand is pronated, to produce a radial glide. This glide helps increase ROM when completing abduction with the index and adduction with the ring and small digits. The joint should be allowed to relax back to its starting position. To help increase adduction with the index and abduction with the ring and small digits, the therapist should gently push the proximal phalanx toward the ulna. Again, the joint is allowed to relax and return to its starting position.

- ◦ **Rotation.** The therapist continues to hold the metacarpal bone and proximal phalanx in the manner described earlier. The therapist then gently oscillates the base of the phalanx in a circle in one direction. The therapist should then complete cir-cular motions with the phalanx moving in the opposite direc-tion since rotation can occur in either direction.

- • **Wrist (Radiocarpal) Joint.** This joint completes two motions: flexion/extension and radial/ulnar deviation. The proximal row of carpal bones is convex, so they move on the concave surface of the radius and radioulnar disk. As the carpal bones glide downward (toward the volar surface of the arm), the wrist is extended. During flexion at the wrist, the proximal carpal bones glide upward/dorsal-ly. In this case, the accessory motion occurs in a direction opposite of the physiological movement.

- ○ **Distraction.** The therapist should palpate the wrist to grasp the proximal row of carpal bones with one hand while holding the distal radius and ulna with the other hand. The therapist places the palms over the dorsal surface of the client's wrist with the index fingers and thumbs as close together as possible while holding the proper structures. The therapist should stabilize the radius/ulna while gently pulling the hand outward from the wrist. The hand is then allowed to relax back to its previous position. This increases the intra-articular space, which will increase all ROM.

- ○ **Flexion/Extension.** The therapist grasps the wrist using the same method that was used for distraction. The therapist slightly distracts the joint and gently pulls the proximal row of carpal bones upward (toward the dorsal surface of the arm) while the forearm is either pronated or in neutral. The hand relaxes back to its starting position. This dorsal glide helps increase wrist flexion. For extension, the proximal row of carpal bones is pushed in a volar direction to produce a volar glide, using the earlier positioning of the therapist and client's hands.

- ○ **Radial/Ulnar Deviation.** The therapist and client begin in the same position as noted earlier; however, the therapist's palms are placed over the radial side of the wrist with the fingers wrapped around the ulnar side of the wrist. The therapist slightly distracts the joint and gently lifts the proximal row of carpal bones toward the radius. The hand should relax back to its starting position. Radial glide increases ulnar deviation. For radial deviation, the therapist pushes the proximal row of carpal bones toward the ulna to produce ulnar glide. The therapist always allows the joint to return to its original position unassisted.

K

Key Points of Control. Specific areas of the body used by the therapist during <u>Handling</u> to help control movement patterns. The main key points used for controlling proximal movement include the shoulder, pelvis, and spine/ribcage. When controlling distal movement patterns, the hand and foot are key points. See <u>Motor control</u> problems and <u>Neurodevelopmental treatment (NDT)</u> for further discussion of this type of treatment.

Kinesthesia. A perceptual process or ability to understand and perceive the direction, amount, and position of movement in space (e.g., one's ability to throw a ball or use a hammer depends upon kinesthesia).

Kinetic. Relating to motion. Within the human body, kinesiology is the study of <u>Body mechanics</u> and human motion. The kinetic chain refers to the interlocking muscular, nervous, and joint systems that are used to produce movement. For instance, the cervical spine connects to the thoracolumbar spine, which connects to the pelvis, hips, knee, foot, and ankle. Damage to one area often affects the others. Therapists use knowledge of open and closed chain movement to design rehabilitation programs.

Klinefelter Syndrome. A male with this syndrome has three sex chromosomes, XXY. The person may develop primary male characteristics; however, he will most likely be infertile and develop few, if any, male secondary sex characteristics such as facial hair, etc. The person may also demonstrate learning disabilities in the areas of reading and verbal comprehension.

Kyphosis. A concave curvature of the spine that may result from pathology or posterior pelvic tilt. See <u>Pelvic tilt</u>.

Stein, F., & Haertl, K.
Pocket Guide to Intervention in Occupational Therapy, Second Edition (p 141).
© 2019 Taylor & Francis Group.

L

Lability. Undergoing continuous change. *Emotional lability* refers to rapid changes of mood such as an individual laughing one minute, crying the next, and then becoming angry. Various psychiatric and neurological conditions may cause emotional lability (e.g., stroke, mood disorder, brain injury).

Labyrinthine Righting. A reflex that corrects the position of the body to bring the head into the upright position. See Reflexes and reactions.

Lateral. Away from the midline. See Anatomical position.

Lateral Prehension. This prehension pattern is composed of opposition of the thumb to the radial side of the index finger (either the middle or distal phalanx). This pattern is used when turning a key or holding a fork.

Lateral Rotation. Turning away from the midline of the body. See External rotation.

Laterality. Ability to use one side of the body, or single hand or foot in purposeful activities such as eating with a fork, kicking a soccer ball, writing with a pencil, tossing a baseball, or using a screwdriver.

Lead Pipe Rigidity. This type of rigidity is characterized by constant resistance to movement in any direction with no relaxation of the agonist or antagonist muscles occurring. This Hypertonicity is uniform so that the same resistance is felt at any point in the affected joint's range of motion (ROM). See Rigidity and Cogwheel rigidity for further discussion.

Learning. Cognitive ability to acquire new concepts and behaviors. Learning can occur through trial and error, such as in walking, riding a bicycle, and playing a musical instrument. Learning also involves memory, as in learning how to read, rehearsing multiplication tables, and reciting a poem. In addition, learning involves imitation, as in social skills and dancing. Learning can also include the formation of religious beliefs, values, ethical behavior, and occupational interests.

Stein, F., & Haertl, K.
Pocket Guide to Intervention in Occupational Therapy, Second Edition (pp 143-149).
© 2019 Taylor & Francis Group.

Learning Disability/Specific Learning Disorder. Often referred to as a *learning disability*, the current DSM-5 (American Psychiatric Association, 2013) has now developed a category of specific learning disorders, which refers to difficulties using academic skills as evidenced by the presence at of at least one symptom, including (1) inaccurate, slow, or effortful reading; (2) difficulty understanding what is read; (3) difficulties with spelling; (4) difficulties with written expression; and (5) difficulties with numbers and mathematical reasoning. This type of disorder often affects a person's ability to interpret visual and auditory stimuli and to integrate information processed by the brain. Difficulties result in spoken and written language, reading, calculating numbers, spelling, attending, and motor planning.

Related Disabilities

- **Attention Deficit Hyperactivity Disorder (ADHD).** Symptoms of inattention, hyperactivity, and impulsiveness that interfere with an individual's ability to learn, work, and engage in interpersonal and leisure activities.

- **Developmental Aphasia.** Difficulty in understanding or expressing feelings and thoughts through speech, written language, or bodily gestures. It is caused by brain injury, usually to the left hemisphere of the brain (85% of the time).

- **Dysnomia.** Difficulty in remembering or retrieving names, words, a date, telephone numbers, passwords, or information during speaking or writing.

- **Dyscalculia.** Difficulty in understanding and doing mathematics such as multiplication, division, fractions, and algebra.

- **Dysgraphia.** Difficulty in writing letters legibly or written at an age-appropriate level.

- **Dyslexia.** Difficulty in interpreting or reading written language. Difficulties in spelling, writing, and listening are associated with dyslexia.

- **Dyspraxia.** Difficulty in performing purposeful novel motor tasks in the proper sequence such as in dressing, driving a car, playing tennis, or brushing one's teeth.

- **Perceptual Disability.** Dysfunction in discriminating, organizing, and processing visual, auditory, tactile, and kinesthetic information such as in reading or writing letters (i.e., b and d), differentiating in saying *seer* and *sear*, feeling metal or plastic, and throwing a ball.

- **Sensory Integrative Dysfunction.** Developmental disorder in which deficits in processing and integrating sensory input are hypothesized to result in problems in learning and behavior disorders in children.
- **Sensory Modulation Disorder.** Individual overresponds, underresponds, or fluctuates in response to sensory input in a manner disproportional to that input (i.e., <u>Tactile defensiveness</u>, gravitational insecurity). Examples include the following:
  - ○ **Tactile Defensiveness.** Defensive or fearful reaction to being touched or handled. The individual may complain or pull away from being touched and avoid activities that are messy and in engaging in body contact sports.
  - ○ **Gravitational Insecurity.** An emotional or fear reaction that is out of proportion to the actual danger of the vestibular-proprioceptive stimuli or position of the body in space (especially when the feet are off the ground).

Specific Interventions

- **Accommodations.** Computer software programs such as spelling and grammar checks and allowing more time to complete assignments.
- <u>Cognitive behavioral therapy</u> techniques
- <u>Role playing</u>
- <u>Behavioral rehearsal</u>
- <u>Relaxation therapy</u>
- <u>Stress management</u>
- **Assistive Technology.** Equipment such as computers, audio and video recorders, and communication devices.
- **Environmental Adaptation.** Adjusting heights of tables and chairs, providing adapted equipment, and providing a learning environment free of distractions, all of which enable the individual to learn.
- **Metacognitive Teaching.** Emphasizing the conscious learning of information through systematic practice, trial and error, rehearsal, and selection of the most effective ways to learn material such as through tape recorders or rewriting notes.
- **Multisensory Teaching.** Incorporates multiple sensory channels such as auditory, visual, tactile, and kinesthetic in learning (e.g., drawing a letter in sand while saying the letter).

- **Resource Program.** Classroom where the student has the opportunity for individual instruction and learning experiences outside the regular curriculum.

- **Sensory Integration Therapy.** Techniques that involve the use of enhanced, controlled sensory stimulation in the context of a meaningful, self-directed activity to elicit an adaptive behavior.

- **Special Education Techniques.** Specially designed instruction to fit the individual needs of a student with disabilities. Methods may include direct instruction in academic subjects and reading, writing, language, or arithmetic; adaptation of materials; or use of alternative methods. The interests of the student such as sports, fashion, popular music, automotive repair, or science fiction are incorporated into the learning exercises. The learning style of the student is considered, such as active/passive, field independent/dependent, reflective/impulsive, or verbal/auditory/tactile in structuring learning.

Leisure. A major occupation and performance area that relates to the individual's use of free time. It is related to Intrinsic motivation, quality of life, personal freedom, life satisfaction, relaxation, health, lifestyle, amusement, self-actualization, and pleasure. Leisure occupations include a wide range of activities such as gardening, sports, hobbies, social clubs, music, and traveling that are related to the specific interests of an individual. Cultural, psychological, social, developmental, family, and educational factors may influence leisure choices.

Level of Arousal. A cognitive construct that indicates an individual's alertness and responsiveness to environmental stimuli. An individual in early stages of a coma has little or no response when stimulated. As the individual progresses through coma stages, arousal increases. Similarly, in the conscious individual, levels of arousal vary throughout the day and in reaction to the occupation performed. For instance, sleeping is a low-arousal activity and playing baseball would be considered a rather high-arousal activity.

Limb Apraxia. Difficulty in motor planning of the limbs. See Apraxia.

Limb Synergies. A pattern of movement involving various muscle contractions that automatically occurs when one of the muscles (within the stereotypical movement) attempts to contract individually. These abnormal movement patterns are often present in persons who have hemiplegia. The upper and lower extremities can each demonstrate a Flexor and Extensor synergy. See Motor control problems for treatment methods.

Locomotion. The ability to move from one place to another.

Locus of Control. An individual's view that events can either be influenced by self (internal locus of control) or are predetermined or influenced by others (external locus of control). Persons with internal locus of control perceive themselves as having a fair amount of control over situational factors, whereas those with an external locus of control perceive themselves having very little influence on events.

Logical Positivism. A philosophical approach to verifying reality. Logical positivists assert that reality is a result of sensory data.

Lordosis. A convex curvature of the spine that may result from pathology or anterior pelvic tilt. See <u>Pelvic tilt</u>.

Low Back Pain (LBP). LBP is not a disease, but rather a condition affecting persons around the world, particularly in industrialized nations. The 2010 Global Burden of Disease study identified LBP as the highest in terms of disability and sixth in terms of burden, demonstrating the scope and impact of this condition (Hoy et al., 2014). In addition to major disability burden, LBP results in millions of dollars in workers' compensation annually and creates problems in performing <u>Self-care</u> and <u>Leisure</u> activities.

Multifactorial Causes

- Structural impairments of the spinal column
- Accident/trauma
- Overuse
- Prolonged static positions
- Incorrect continuous lifting
- Obesity
- Sedentary work
- Lack of exercise
- Stress also exacerbates the symptoms of LBP by creating tense and rigid muscles

Symptoms

- A common finding in LBP is the presence of a herniated intervertebral disk that impacts on the spinal nerves. The pain may radiate in the lower extremities through the sciatic nerve.

Specific Interventions

- **Psychoeducational Approach.** Teaching individuals to use:
  - Proper lifting techniques (e.g., lifting objects from the floor by bending the knees and keeping the object close to the body in a squat position)

- Preventative exercises in the morning, including stretching the back muscles by bringing the knees to the axilla, tilting the pelvis while in supine position, and modified sit-ups. The exercises are individualized.
- <u>Pain management</u>
- Ergonomics in performing <u>Self-care</u> activities, such as toileting, bed making, cooking, and laundering that reduce stress on the low back
- <u>Prescriptive exercises</u> such as walking and bicycling that stretch back muscles while increasing muscle strength. Vary movements and plan short stretch breaks at work and at home.
- <u>Stress management</u> techniques

- **Work Hardening**
  - Simulating bending, lifting, carrying, standing, and sitting positions
  - Setting up graduated activities with goal of the worker performing at 100% efficiency
  - Using Baltimore Therapeutic Equipment or other functional evaluation to determine client's capacities

- **Home Adaptation**
  - Recommending alterations in the client's home environment such as positioning of cabinets and appliances, hand rails in the bathroom, and the use of stools in raising legs while seated

- **Expand Leisure Activities**
  - Assisting the client to engage in occupations that are purposeful, meaningful, and increase <u>Muscle strength</u> and range of motion in back joints
  - Consider gross motor activities, such as woodworking, pottery, bowling, swimming, gardening, and bicycling. See <u>Coordination</u> and <u>Range of motion (ROM)</u> for treatment methods.

Contraindications/Precautions

- Discontinue exercise if client experiences pain.
- Observe for signs of <u>Depression</u> in a client that frequently accompany LBP.
- Rule out malingering syndrome, especially if the client is receiving workers' compensation.
- Monitor for muscle and joint substitutions in compensating for pain.

Low Vision. Typically, low vision is defined as a corrected eye vision of less than 20/70, yet some criteria include a best corrected acuity of 20/40 or less (National Eye Institute, n.d.). The definition may be expanded on to include not only loss of acuity, but also decreased vision in the visual fields. Smallfield, Clem, and Myers (2013) conducted a systematic review and found evidence for the use of occupational therapy vision rehabilitation to improve reading in older adults. A number of conditions may cause low vision, including <u>Macular degeneration</u>, cataracts, glaucoma, diabetic retinopathy, and other conditions secondary to illness and congenital deficits. Interventions include the use of visual strategies (e.g., turning head/scanning), contrast enhancement, lighting, magnification, sensory substitutions (e.g., use of key covers, auditory strategies), magnification, <u>Activities of daily living (ADLs)</u> and <u>Instrumental activities of daily living (IADLs)</u> adaptations, and caregiver training (Meibeyer, 2015). See <u>Blindness</u> for additional strategies.

Lower Motor Neuron Disorders. Lesions of the central nervous system may cause a loss of ventral horn cells or axons of the lower motor neurons, which are the cranial, spinal, or peripheral nerves that innervate muscles. These are referred to as *lower motor neuron lesions*, and they result in decreased muscle tone or flaccidity, decreased <u>Deep tendon reflexes</u> or areflexia, and fasciculations (a twitching-like contraction of the muscle under the skin) of the muscle as well as atrophy. Disorders and diseases that may result in a lower motor lesion include poliomyelitis, <u>Post-polio syndrome</u>, <u>Guillain-Barré syndrome</u>, radiculopathies, <u>Myasthenia gravis</u>, <u>Amyotrophic lateral sclerosis (ALS)</u>, and botulism.

Lymphedema. Impaired flow of the lymph resulting in swelling of the extremities. Causes include surgery, radiation, and, in developing countries, it may be a result of a parasitic infection. Therapists use individualized interventions and education to maximize occupational performance.

M

Macular Degeneration. A condition that results in degeneration of the macula of the retina, which is the location of the highest concentration of rods and cones for vision. Degeneration begins at the macula and proceeds outward; this may result in total blindness. See <u>Blindness</u> for further discussion of treatment.

Manual Contacts. Specific placement of the therapist's hands on the client to help facilitate movement and provide sensory cues during treatment within the framework of proprioceptive neuromuscular facilitation. The therapist should place his or her hands on the client to help reinforce the desired movement (e.g., if D2 flexion is desired, then the therapist should place his or her hands on the client's scapula to facilitate scapula elevation, rotation, and adduction). See <u>Motor control</u> problems and <u>Proprioceptive neuromuscular facilitation (PNF)</u> for treatment and techniques.

Manual Muscle Test (MMT). A technique used to evaluate the function of individual muscles and muscle groups (McGraw-Hill Global Education, 2018). The therapist usually tests a group of muscles together, which are responsible for the same action; these are called <u>Prime movers</u>. Grades are then given for the action rather than for each individual muscle. During this test, the only tool used by the therapist is his or her hands. Because there is no objective measurement tool for this test, the same therapist should retest his or her clients to provide more reliability to the strength grades. This tool should not be used with a person who demonstrates spasticity since the muscle contraction is not voluntary.

Stein, F., & Haertl, K.
Pocket Guide to Intervention in Occupational Therapy, Second Edition (pp 151-183).
© 2019 Taylor & Francis Group.

General Procedures

- The client's joints should first be passively moved through their full available range of motion (ROM).
- The procedure should be explained to the client, followed by demonstration if needed.
- The client should be allowed to rest for 2 minutes between tests if the same muscle is used to avoid inaccurate results from fatigue of the muscle.
- The client should then be positioned so that movement is against gravity.
- The therapist should stabilize the stationary/proximal part of the joint without placing his or her hands over the contracting muscles since stabilization helps isolate the proper movement and hinders substitutions.
- The client is then asked to actively move the extremity through full ROM while the therapist palpates the muscle bellies or tendons of the prime movers to check that no substitution is occurring. If the client actively moves through full ROM, the client is asked to hold near the end position of the range. After the client is allowed to give maximal effort, the therapist resists the motion by pushing against the distal end of the moving bone toward the opposite motion (e.g., if testing elbow flexion, the therapist pushes the forearm toward elbow extension). The therapist then grades the muscle strength.
- If the client is unable to actively move the joint through its available ROM, the client should be placed in a gravity-eliminated position. The client is asked to complete <u>Active range of motion (AROM)</u>, and the muscle strength is graded by observing the motion the client is able to accomplish. Maximum resistance should not be given if the client requires a gravity-eliminated position to complete motion. This specific type of MMT is called the *break test*.
- The *make test* can also be used. In this type of test, the therapist provides resistance to the moving part of the joint as it moves through its range.

Muscle Grading Scales

The following numerical or letter-grading scales are explained together since the systems are both widely used by therapists.

5	Normal	N	The part moves through full ROM against gravity and maximum resistance.
4	Good	G	The part moves through full ROM against gravity and moderate resistance.
3+	Fair plus	F+	The part moves through full ROM against gravity and minimal resistance.
3	Fair	F	The part moves through full ROM against gravity but with no resistance.
3–	Fair minus	F–	The part moves through partial (more than 50%) ROM against gravity.
2+	Poor plus	P+	The part moves through partial (less than 50%) ROM against gravity, or through full ROM in a gravity-eliminated position against minimal resistance.
2	Poor	P	The part moves through full ROM in a gravity-eliminated position with no resistance.
2–	Poor minus	P–	The part moves through partial ROM in a gravity-eliminated position.
1	Trace	T	No motion is observed, but an increase in tone can be palpated.
0	Zero	0	No motion is observed and no tone can be palpated.

Functional Muscle Testing

This technique, which condenses the full MMT, may be completed in the interest of time rather than the full MMT. If this is the case, treatment should focus on strengthening groups of muscles that complete actions rather than individual muscles. This technique may also be used as a screening tool or if weakness is not the client's primary symptom.

- **Procedure**
  - The client sits upright in a chair or wheelchair.
  - The therapist asks the client to complete a specific motion, while the therapist stabilizes the joint to isolate movement and check for substitutions.

- ○ If the client is able to complete full AROM, the therapist applies resistance near the end of the range after asking the client to hold the contraction.

- ○ If the client is not able to complete full AROM, the client should be placed in a gravity-eliminated position, or the appropriate grade below 3 should be assigned to the motion.

- ○ A therapist should use this form of muscle testing only after the therapist knows and understands the full MMT.

Contraindications/Precautions

- Muscle strength should not be measured in the presence of the following conditions: myositis ossificans, joint dislocation, surgery or repair to musculoskeletal structures at the site being tested, fractures that have not completely healed, inflammation, or pain.

- Precautions should be used if the client has osteoporosis, a subluxation, joint laxity, hemophilia, abdominal surgery or hernia, or a cardiovascular condition; takes muscle relaxants or pain medication; or has a condition that can be exacerbated by muscle fatigue.

Massage. Manipulation, methodical pressure, friction, and kneading of the body to reduce stress, increase relaxation, and reduce muscle tension. Massage is applied with firm pressure in a circular motion. This treatment method is often used over scars for Desensitization, as well as to help loosen scar tissue, which may be attaching to underlying structures and inhibiting movement.

Maximal Resistance. This term, when used within the framework of proprioceptive neuromuscular facilitation, refers to the greatest amount of resistance that can be given during an Isometric contraction without breaking the contraction, or during an Isotonic contraction without disrupting the movement of the body part. It does not refer to the greatest amount of resistance that the therapist can apply during movement. See Motor control problems and Proprioceptive neuromuscular facilitation (PNF) for further techniques.

MCP. Acronym for metacarpophalangeal.

Medial. Toward the midline of the body. See Anatomical position.

Medial Rotation. Turning toward the midline of the body. See Anatomical position.

Median Plane. Divides the body into right and left halves. See Anatomical position.

Medicaid. Federally mandated entitlement program that provides medical care for individuals who are indigent.

Medical Model. The traditional approach to diagnosing, preventing, and treating diseases. It is based on the scientific method of <u>Hypothesis</u> testing and experimental design. In the medical model, the physician focuses on detecting disease and treating it primarily through drugs and surgery. The physician is seen as the expert in treating the client. A client-centered approach, behavioral medicine, or <u>Alternative medicine</u> and <u>Holistic medicine</u> are contrasted with the traditional medical model, which has been attacked as being reductionistic.

Medicare. Federally mandated entitlement program that reimburses hospitals, physicians, and health care workers in providing services to individuals 65 years and older.

Meditation. Relaxation activity where the individual takes a comfortable position in a quiet environment, regulates breathing, and has a physically relaxed and mentally calm attitude while focusing on a mental image or word.

Memory. Cognitive ability to retrieve or recall information after either short or long periods of time. Memory is a component of information processing that involves learning information, storing it, and then recalling it. Memory deficits such as short-term recall are major symptoms in individuals with <u>Alzheimer's disease</u>. Therapists can use purposeful activities such as with cards or puzzles to stimulate memory. See <u>Cognitive-perceptual deficits</u> for further discussion and treatment.

Ménière's Disease. A condition that results in <u>Vertigo</u>, nausea, and vomiting, and may lead to total deafness.

Mental Retardation. This is a term formally used in the DSM-IV-TR (American Psychiatric Association [APA], 1994) and prior editions to indicate IQ and functional levels of persons with a developmental disability who had an accompanying intellectual disability characterized by subnormal intellectual aptitude potential with an IQ below 70, as well as significant limitations in adaptive behavior skills in at least two of the following areas: communication, <u>Self-care</u>, home and community living, <u>Social skills</u>, health and safety, <u>Leisure</u> activities, <u>Work</u>, and functional academics. The current DSM-5 (APA, 2013) no longer uses the term *mental retardation*; diagnostic criteria are now under "intellectual disabilities." See <u>Developmental disabilities</u> and <u>Intellectual disabilities</u>.

Metabolic Equivalent Levels (MET). A measure of the oxygen used by a person's body while completing activities and maintaining the body's metabolic processes such as respiration, body temperature, etc. The energy required by a person who is resting in a semi-reclined chair is equal to 1 MET.

Equivalencies

- 1.5 to 2 MET = Standing, driving, typing, or walking at 1 mph
- 2 to 3 MET = Playing piano, level bicycling, or walking at 2 mph
- 3 to 4 MET = Pushing a light mower, golfing with a pull cart, or walking at 3 mph
- 4 to 5 MET = Raking leaves, hoeing, ballroom dancing, or walking at 3.5 mph
- 5 to 6 MET = Skating, canoeing, or walking at 4 mph
- 6 to 7 MET = Water skiing, light downhill skiing, singles tennis, snow shoveling, or walking at 5 mph
- 7 to 8 MET = Vigorous downhill skiing, basketball, ice hockey, or jogging
- 8 to 9 MET = Fencing, vigorous basketball, or running
- 10+ MET = Handball or running

Most Self-care activities require fewer than 3 MET, with the exclusion of bathing/showering, washing hair, and toileting

Principles of Energy Conservation

- Plan ahead to use the most direct or easiest method for completion and reduce wasted motion.
- Sit while working, when possible.
- Avoid unnecessary tasks.
- To eliminate trips during a task, gather all the necessary tools prior to starting.
- Items that are used often should be lightweight and kept within easy reach.
- Combine tasks when possible (e.g., take one trip to the kitchen and complete all tasks there to reduce the number of trips between rooms).
- Use power tools, such as an electric can opener or mixer, to do the work when possible.
- Allow gravity to assist work rather than oppose it.
- Schedule rest breaks before becoming fatigued.
- Avoid stressful positions or situations such as the following: a hot, humid environment or quick temperature changes; reaching above the head; bending at the waist to reach to the floor or lower

extremities; standing for prolonged periods; <u>Isometric contractions</u>, such as pulling or pushing, which can cause a person to hold one's breath; exertion following meals since the distended stomach places pressure against the diaphragm; excessive bilateral extremity use; and overexertion.

Examples

- Spread tasks out over the day or week. Alternate between heavy and light tasks.
- Complete tasks often to keep the amount of work small. If dishes are left until the end of the week, a large amount of energy will be needed for the task. Doing a few dishes each day requires only a little energy.
- Organize trips to eliminate backtracking.
- Delegate tasks to family members or friends when possible.
- Soak dirty dishes before washing them, and then allow them to air-dry.
- Use fitted sheets.
- Schedule essential tasks, which require more energy, during peak hours of the day when the person has the most energy.
- Divide lengthy tasks into smaller tasks (e.g., iron for a short period and at different intervals during the day or week).
- Schedule frequent rest breaks, which last 10 to 15 minutes, especially following a heavy task.
- Do not start tasks, such as carrying a heavy item for a long distance, that do not allow a person to stop and rest.
- Avoid rushing.
- Avoid unnecessary stairs, bending, reaching, stretching, carrying, lifting, and holding.
- Use a utility cart on wheels for transporting items.
- Use the foot to close a low cabinet door rather than bending over.
- Slide a pan along the countertop from the sink to the stove.
- Use <u>Assistive technology</u> to make tasks easier. A nonskid mat will help stabilize pans or dishes. Long-handled reachers or dressing sticks will help a person don socks or pants.
- Maintain normal body weight.

- Use good <u>Body mechanics</u> during activities. Good posture can help prevent fatigue. Wear comfortable, supportive shoes, which will assist with proper posture.
- Remember that emotions also expend energy.

See <u>Work simplification</u> for more techniques to make activities easier and more manageable.

Metacognition. Often referred to as "thinking about thinking," metacognition involves an awareness of one's own thoughts and learning process. Metacognition involves self-reflection and may be used to enhance a client's ability to learn new information, leading to improved occupational performance.

Microcurrent Electrical Neuromuscular Stimulation (MENS). A physical agent modality that uses electrical current to help reduce acute or chronic pain; reduce inflammation; reduce spasm; and promote healing of bones, nerves, or connective tissue. The efficacy of this modality is controversial. See <u>Physical agent modalities (PAMs)</u> for further discussion and treatment.

MMT. Acronym for <u>Manual muscle test</u>.

Mobile Arm Support. An assistive device to assist a client who has weakness or decreased range of motion with feeding or other functional activities. This device may also be referred to as a *balanced forearm orthosis*. It attaches to the frame of the wheelchair along the edge of the seat back to assist the client with activities. Persons with the following diagnoses may benefit from this device: spinal cord injury, <u>Guillain-Barré syndrome</u>, muscular dystrophy, <u>Amyotrophic lateral sclerosis (ALS)</u>, and poliomyelitis. To benefit from the device and increase function, a client should have muscle strength at the elbow and shoulder that has been assessed with a <u>Manual muscle test (MMT)</u> at a level 1 to 3. See <u>Assistive devices</u> for a further discussion of adaptive equipment.

Model of Human Occupation (MOHO). Occupational therapy frame of reference that is based on the theory of general systems. Role acquisition, environmental and temporal adaptation, and skill development are emphasized in treatment. Volition, <u>Habituation</u>, and performance are key concepts (Taylor, 2017). See <u>Frame of reference</u>.

Modeling Behavior. A technique used in <u>Behavior therapy</u> to help the client acquire social skills by observing and then imitating behavior.

Mood Disorders. Disturbances of affect such as <u>Depression</u>, mania, and <u>Bipolar disorder</u>.

Moral Treatment. A movement during the 19th century that developed as a reaction to the inhumane care of the mentally ill who, up until that time, were abused and poorly treated. Arts and crafts, farming, and creative activities were emphasized in moral treatment.

Morbidity Rate. Relates to the frequency/rate of disease and illness within a population. Large health entities such as the Centers for Disease Control monitor morbidity rates and impact on the health of persons in the United States.

Moro Reflex. Infantile reflexive response when an infant feels a sudden loss of support. See <u>Reflexes and reactions</u>.

Mortality Statistics. Number of deaths in a target population during a specified period. For example, the mortality rate for stroke indicates around 140,000 people in the United States die from stroke (1/20 deaths) each year (Centers for Disease Control and Prevention, 2017b).

Motor Control. The ability to use the body in purposeful and versatile activities such as in learning how to dance, riding a bicycle, engaging in a sport, or doing intricate hand work in knitting, and also the identification of the underlying mechanisms that lead to the development of movement abilities. Newer treatment techniques such as constraint-induced motor training, mirror therapy, and task-oriented approaches to motor learning have been introduced in the last 10 years and compete with the traditional theories.

Specific Interventions

The following traditional theories of motor control outline interventions for persons not able to control voluntary movement, such as in <u>Stroke</u>, <u>Cerebral palsy (CP)</u>, and <u>Parkinson's disease</u>. These historical approaches share the following common assumptions: sensation is an important precursor to producing voluntary movement; motor control recurs approximately in a developmental sequence like that which occurs when a child grows; and the central nervous system is resilient and demonstrates plasticity and the potential to be reorganized. Some of the contemporary theories on motor control question these assumptions and dispute some of the traditional approaches. There have been a few studies recently to check the validity of these approaches, yet some of the techniques and ideas supported in the past may still benefit patients with movement difficulties. Newer interventions such as mirror therapy (Thieme, Mehrholz, Pohl, Behrens, & Dohle, 2013) can help improve motor function after stroke. Constraint-induced movement therapy (Corbetta, Sirtori, Castellini, Moja, & Gatti, 2015) for upper extremities in people with stroke and task-oriented approaches (Almhdawi, Mathiowetz, White, & delMas, 2016) in upper extremity post-stroke rehabilitation have shown efficacy and clinical utility and challenge some of these traditional approaches. This book still includes traditional approaches given their widespread use, yet continued research is needed to fully support or refute the approaches.

Traditional Approaches

The four motor control theories presented (Rood, Brunnstrom [movement therapy], proprioceptive neuromuscular approach, and Bobath [Neurodevelopmental treatment (NDT)]) are based on the following concepts (Pendleton & Schultz-Krohn, 2012):

1. Sensory stimulation is used to evoke a motor response.
2. Reflexive movement is used as a precursor for volitional movement.
3. Treatment is directed toward influencing muscle tone.
4. Developmental patterns/sequences are used for the development of motor skills.

Rood Approach

Margaret Rood, a scientist, clinician, and educator, had training as both an occupational and physical therapist. She applied a neurophysiological approach to individuals with brain injury such as in stroke and CP. The basic assumption is that sensation is able to produce motor responses (see Katusić, Alimovic, and Mejaski-Bosnjak, 2013 for more information).

General Principles

- Muscle tone can be normalized and motor responses can be evoked with appropriate sensory stimuli.
- Treatment occurs sequentially from the patient's current developmental level to higher levels of motor control.
- Purposeful activity or movement automatically programs the nervous system to facilitate the correct muscles involved in an activity; therefore, the patient can focus on a functional goal rather than a movement.
- Motor learning occurs through repetition of a movement.

Interventions

- Sensory input
- Facilitation
  - Fast Brushing over the skin of a muscle with a soft brush (avoid the face, head, and ear)

- ○ Light moving touch or <u>Stroking</u> with a fingertip, soft brush, or cotton swab (suggested frequency is three to five strokes with 30 seconds between)

- ○ <u>Icing</u> (suggested frequency is three quick strokes). Avoid icing the face, neck, ear, and midline of the body. Icing the midline of the body of a patient with a C4–C5 spinal cord injury can elicit <u>Autonomic dysreflexia</u> and cause seizures. Also avoid icing with patients who have cardiac problems as icing the region of the left shoulder can cause angina.

- ○ Heavy <u>Joint compression</u> can facilitate <u>Co-contraction</u> at a joint.

- ○ Quick <u>Stretch</u>, such as quickly bending the elbow to stretch the triceps

- ○ Intrinsic stretch, usually through pressure applied by a cone or handle, which can promote co-contraction at the shoulder (see Holmes et al., 2011). Forced steadiness during a co-contraction task can be improved with practice, but only by young adults and not by middle-aged or older adults.

- ○ Stretch pressure (which should last a suggested duration of 3 seconds) by placing firm pressure while pulling both hands apart, while stretching a superficial muscle with the fingertips of both thumbs and the first two digits

- ○ Resistance used in an isotonic manner so that the muscle contracts in a shortened length

- ○ <u>Tapping</u> a muscle or its tendon before or during a contraction (suggested frequency is three to five taps)

- ○ Vestibular stimulation mainly in the form of fast rocking. Slow, rhythmic rocking can have the opposite effect of inhibition.

- ○ Inversion, mainly to facilitate neck, trunk, and selected limb muscles

- ○ <u>Vibration</u> applied with light pressure over a muscle belly, parallel with the muscle fibers (suggested duration is not more than 2 minutes)

- ○ Osteopressure over a bony prominence; however, this should be preceded by light moving touch.

- • <u>Inhibition</u>

  - ○ <u>Neutral warmth</u>, such as wrapping the patient's body in a blanket for 5 to 10 minutes, may decrease muscle tone.

- ○ Gentle rocking while applying traction and/or compression to the joint being moved, as in the case with the patient's head, shoulder girdle, pelvis, or lower extremities

- ○ Slow stroking along both sides of the spinous processes of the patient's vertebrae, beginning at the occiput and continuing to the coccyx and alternating hands so that as the left hand reaches the coccyx, the right hand is beginning at the occiput

- ○ Slow "log" <u>Rolling</u> of a patient from a side-lying position into a prone position and back into side-lying so that the patient's shoulders and hips roll simultaneously. Some segmental rolling can be completed as well to separate the hips from the trunk so that the patient is able to turn his or her trunk independently from turning his or her hips.

- ○ Light joint compression less than body weight usually applied through two joints (e.g., approximating the head of the humerus into the glenohumeral joint by holding onto the proximal forearm while the patient's elbow is comfortably flexed and the humerus is slightly abducted). Once the tone begins to decrease, small circular movements can reduce pain in the shoulder and allow for greater range of motion (ROM; this can also be completed through the elbow and wrist with the elbow flexed comfortably and the wrist held in extension).

- Deep pressure to the tendinous insertion of a muscle
- Maintained stretch of a muscle for 1 to 2 minutes at its greatest length to lessen the effect of tone on a muscle during movement

Levels of Motor Control

Treatment should proceed in this developmental order:

- Shortening and lengthening of muscles to produce <u>Mobility</u> at a distal joint (e.g., a baby shaking a rattle)
- Co-contraction of muscles around a proximal joint to produce <u>Stability</u> (e.g., a baby learning to sit up)
- Mobility of proximal segments upon the stability of distal segments (e.g., a baby rocking back and forth in <u>Quadruped</u> position)
- Skilled and controlled mobility of distal segments on stability of proximal segments (e.g., walking or reaching)

Eight Functional Motor Patterns

This theory believes that a patient will develop the noted levels of motor control as he or she is progressed through the following sequence of patterns:

1. Supine withdrawal: The patient lies on his or her back with back flexed, hips flexed and abducted, shoulders adducted, and elbows flexed with extended hands toward his or her face.

2. Roll over: The patient's upper and lower extremity flex as the patient rolls toward the opposite side (e.g., the right arm and leg flex as the patient rolls to the left).

3. Pivot prone: The patient lies prone with the shoulders abducted, extended, and externally rotated; lower extremities extended; and neck and head extended so that only the area of the patient's trunk around the T10 level is touching the ground.

4. Neck co-contraction: The patient lies prone and is able to extend the neck and head against gravity.

5. Supporting self on elbows: The patient again lies prone with the neck/head extended and is able to flex the elbows and place weight on the elbows/forearms.

6. All-fours movement pattern: The patient bears weight on both knees and hands with the elbows extended, shoulder flexed, hips flexed, and neck/head extended.

7. Standing: The patient bears weight on both feet with upper and lower extremities extended.

8. Walking: The patient is able to stand, push off the floor with one foot, swing through with that same foot, strike the floor with that same heel, and repeat the process with the other foot.

Movement Therapy of Brunnstrom

This theory is particularly concerned with the rehabilitation of patients who have suffered a stroke (Brunnstrom, 1970, 1996; Burke, 2007; Houglum & Bertoti, 2012). It is based strongly on both the reflex and hierarchic models of motor control (see Pendleton & Schultz-Krohn, 2012).

Assumptions

- Normal development involves the reorganization of spinal cord and brainstem Reflexes and reactions into purposeful movement; therefore, reflexes can assist the recovery of normal movement following stroke.

- Sensory stimuli can elicit motion.

- The recovery of movement progresses from synergies, which are movement patterns that involve the entire involved limb, to normal voluntary movements.
- Learning through practice of the new voluntary movements, most effectively done through the incorporation of the movements into daily or purposeful activities, must be completed.

General Principles

- Treatment should progress according to normal motor development: reflexes, to voluntary, to functional movement.
- Reflexes, associated reactions, proprioceptive facilitation, and/or exteroceptive facilitation should be used to elicit movement when no motion is present.
- When the patient begins to demonstrate voluntary movement, he or she should be asked to complete an <u>Isometric contraction</u> (holding). After the patient has demonstrated success with this, an <u>Eccentric contraction</u> (lengthening) should be performed, with a <u>Concentric contraction</u> (shortening) being the final learned movement.
- Reversal of movement should also be stressed each treatment (e.g., after practicing flexion, the patient should also be asked to complete extension).
- Facilitation methods such as reflexes or exteroceptive stimuli should be removed from treatment as soon as the patient demonstrates voluntary control of movement.
- The patient's decision for voluntary movement is stressed to help overcome the patterns of movement or synergies so that the patient is able to move one part of the extremity without the others automatically responding.
- Practice, practice, practice while including functional activities to decrease the synergistic patterns and increase the patient's purposeful movement.
- Stages of recovery in the arm of a patient who has experienced a stroke:
  - <u>Flaccidity</u>: No voluntary movement noted
  - <u>Spasticity</u>: Starting to develop and synergies developing with flexion usually developing prior to extension
  - Increased spasticity but some voluntary movement beginning during synergies

- Spasticity is decreasing and some voluntary movement apart from synergy, usually (a) hand behind body, (b) arm to forward-horizontal position, and (c) pronation/supination with elbow flexed to 90 degrees

- Spasticity continues decreasing and more movement occurs that is independent from synergies, usually (a) arm to side-horizontal position, (b) arm forward and overhead, and (c) pronation-supination with elbow fully extended.

- Spasticity is minimal and joint movements are completed with nearly normal movement patterns.

• Stages of recovery in the hand of a patient who has experienced a stroke:

- Flaccidity: No voluntary movement noted

- Slight finger flexion possible

- <u>Hook</u> or mass grasp with no voluntary release

- Slight finger extension and <u>Lateral prehension</u> with release completed by thumb movement

- <u>Palmar prehension</u>, gross <u>Cylindrical</u> or <u>Spherical grasp</u>, and increased finger extension with the fingers acting together as a unit

- Full and voluntary finger extension and separate voluntary finger movements with increased ability to complete all prehension patterns

Interventions

Rehabilitation of Trunk Control

The patient is pushed in a direction so that trunk muscle contraction is facilitated to help restore the patient to an upright position. The patient should be encouraged to return to the upright position actively; however, the patient will most likely need assistance with this until the muscles have strengthened. Also, the patient should be guarded when he or she is pushed off balance to protect the patient from being hurt if he or she responds poorly to these activities at first.

1. The first step is facilitating contraction of the trunk muscles on the noninvolved side by gently pushing the patient toward the involved side. Once the person has acquired this skill, the therapist proceeds to step 2.

2. Next, the muscles on the involved side are facilitated by pushing the patient toward the noninvolved side.

3. Trunk flexion is practiced while the patient supports the involved arm with the noninvolved arm while sitting. The patient is assisted with forward flexion by the therapist. As the patient slowly bends forward, the therapist helps support the patient's upper extremities so that some shoulder flexion occurs while the patient is focusing on trunk control. The patient actively extends back to the upright position.

4. Trunk extension is practiced with the patient sitting in a chair without a back support. The patient is assisted with backward extension while supporting the involved arm as described earlier and encouraged to actively flex back to the upright position.

5. Trunk rotation is the final motion that is facilitated. Again, the involved arm is supported in the previously described manner while the therapist assists the patient in rotating his or her arm and trunk in one direction while rotating the patient's head in the opposite direction. This method uses the tonic neck and <u>Tonic lumbar reflexes</u> as a means of beginning the shoulder movements of the upper extremity synergies.

Rehabilitation of Upper Extremity Control

As the upper extremity recovers, the hand may return at a different rate of recovery than the shoulder; therefore, the stages and steps of regaining control are divided into proximal upper extremity and wrist/hand.

1. Proximal Upper Extremity Control. Treatment proceeds according to the stage of recovery of the patient's upper extremity.

   a. During stages 1 and 2 when the patient's arm is mostly flaccid, the goal is to elicit muscle tone and <u>Limb synergies</u> through the use of reflexes and associated reactions. The flexor synergy, usually the first to develop, may be produced through resistance to the noninvolved upper extremity during shoulder elevation or elbow flexion. Tapping the upper and middle trapezius, rhomboids, and biceps can facilitate it. Elbow flexion, which is the strongest component of the flexion synergy, usually develops first.

   b. The next goal is to have the patient begin to develop voluntary control of the synergy. Upper extremity control begins with scapular elevation. The therapist places the patient's involved arm on a table so that the shoulder is abducted and the elbow is flexed. Next, the therapist places his or her hands on the patient's upper trapezius area and on the lateral side of the head to provide resistance as the patient is asked to hold the head still and resist having the head laterally flexed toward the noninvolved side. This motion is the beginning of lateral neck flexion toward the involved side, which may help initiate scapular elevation since the upper trapezius performs both motions. When contraction begins in the trapezius on the involved side, the patient continues to work against the therapist's resistance while concentrating on attempting to laterally flex the head to the involved side and elevating the affected shoulder. As the contraction strengthens and motion is detected, the therapist should use an associated reaction to help produce movement by placing a hand on the noninvolved shoulder/scapula and asking the patient to elevate the noninvolved shoulder. If an associated reaction occurs, the involved shoulder will also elevate during this activity. The next step is to provide resistance against shoulder/scapula elevation on the involved side, as well as on the noninvolved side, while the patient is asked to hold the contraction. Individual elevation of the involved scapula is practiced next while using facilitatory techniques such as tapping or stroking if needed. The therapist helps the patient elevate the scapula who is then told to hold the contraction. The patient practices eccentric contraction of the shoulder when releasing the contraction slowly and lowering the shoulder back into place. Next, a concentric contraction is attempted by asking the patient to raise the involved shoulder toward his or her ear. Care should be taken to assist the patient with the remainder of the upper extremity as <u>Subluxation</u> may have occurred and can cause the patient pain during the activity. The head of the humerus should be approximated and the arm abducted so that proper <u>Scapulohumeral rhythm</u> can occur. The next motions to practice, which are the other components of the flexor synergy, are shoulder abduction, external rotation, and forearm supination.

c. Reversal of the flexor synergy movements, which are usually completed from the beginning of the earlier protocol, help develop voluntary control of the <u>Extensor synergy</u>. Again, associated reactions may help the involved arm complete the correct contraction. The extensor synergy may be produced through resistance to the noninvolved upper extremity during horizontal adduction. Horizontal adduction is facilitated by resisting the noninvolved arm while holding the involved arm midway between horizontal adduction and abduction and asking the patient to bring his or her arms together. Elbow extension is elicited through a technique named <u>Rowing</u>. The therapist sits facing the patient with his or her arms crossed at the wrists and grasps the patient's hands so that the therapist's right hand is holding the patient's right hand and left hand is to left hand. The patient sits with his or her arms supinated and flexed at the elbows. The therapist places his or her hands in the patient's palms so that the therapist is in pronation. The patient is asked to actively extend the noninvolved elbow while the therapist assists the involved arm to extend. As the patient extends, the patient's hands are guided so that the patient begins to pronate and cross the arms toward the opposite knees while the therapist supinates and uncrosses his or her arms. Once a contraction is felt in the involved arm, the therapist asks the patient to hold the contraction in near full extension while the therapist provides resistance. The therapist guides the patient's arms back into an uncrossed, supinated, and flexed elbow position while the therapist again pronates and crosses his or her arms. Again, the therapist resists elbow extension in the noninvolved upper extremity to help evoke an associated reaction in the involved arm. Resistance is then given against the involved extremity's action once a contraction has been produced in the affected arm. Once the extensor synergy has developed, voluntary movement is reinforced through resistance against near-full elbow extension. When active control of the extensor synergy is noted, bilateral <u>Weightbearing</u> on extended arms may begin. One method for weightbearing is to have the patient place his or her arms on a low stool in front of him or her while seated and support weight on both arms. Extension may be facilitated through stroking or tapping the affected arm's triceps during the activity. The patient then progresses to unilateral weightbearing on the involved extremity only. Any activity in which the patient supports an object with the involved extremity while working on it with the noninvolved extremity can fulfill this requirement. Once the involved triceps produces active extension, resistance is given while completing the motion. Further facilitation methods include the use of reflexes such as the <u>Asymmetrical tonic neck reflex (ATNR)</u> (watching the involved extremity during motion), the <u>Tonic labyrinthine reflex</u> (placing the patient in supine position), or having the patient work on extension with the forearm in pronation, which facilitates the extensor synergy.

d. Next, the extremity is facilitated to produce movement apart from the synergy. This begins by breaking up the motions that combine to form a synergy (e.g., in the extensor synergy, the patient is encouraged to extend the involved elbow while the therapist guides the patient's extremity into shoulder abduction or supination, which challenges the synergy's pattern of shoulder adduction and pronation).

e. Voluntary movement is encouraged, which combines aspects of both synergies in increasingly complex variations so that the effect of the synergies on movement decreases and willed movement increases. During this stage of rehabilitation, the therapist no longer uses associated reactions or reflexes to produce movement. Instead, the therapist isolates movement so that muscle groups can begin working independently of one another. Three specific movements deviating from synergy are listed as follows:

- Hand behind body may be easier for the patient to complete while standing if the patient demonstrates good balance. The patient combines shoulder abduction with elbow extension and forearm pronation in order to stroke the dorsal surface of the hand against the patient's back. This part of the activity provides sensory input and gives the voluntary movement a goal or direction. A swinging motion of the arm combined with trunk rotation can help assist the patient in getting the arm behind the back, or the therapist can actively assist the motion so that the patient completes the activity of stroking the back. The action should be practiced so that the therapist needs less help until the patient can complete the activity independently. Functional activities that use this motion include donning a belt or tucking a shirttail into pants.

- Shoulder flexion to a forward-horizontal position while extending the elbow is the second motion deviating from synergy. Again, the therapist may passively assist the patient if he or she is unable to complete the activity; however, facilitation should be used for the movements. Then <u>Place-and-hold</u> activities can be completed, with active motion being the final goal. Functional activities that use this motion include any vertically mounted game or sponge painting.

- Pronation and supination while flexing the elbow to 90 degrees is the final motion during stage 4 of upper extremity recovery. Supination should not be a problem since it is normally combined with elbow flexion in the flexor synergy. The therapist can begin by resisting pronation while the elbow is extended, and the therapist can then gradually bring the elbow into flexion while practicing pronation. Functional activities that use this motion include opening a door with a doorknob, using a screwdriver, or turning dials.

f. Movement in stage 5 of recovery involves increasingly complex movement, which is getting further away from synergy but does not require excess force. Again, three specific movements are noted:

- Arm raised to side-horizontal is the first movement to prove disassociation of the synergies. This motion combines full shoulder abduction with elbow extension. Proof that the synergies are still influencing movement include elbow flexion while abduction occurs or a drifting of the extremity toward horizontal adduction while the elbow is extended. The motion should be practiced until the patient can successfully demonstrate this motion. Functional activities that use this motion include placing objects on a strategically placed table, playing table tennis, and driving golf balls.

- Arm forward and overhead requires upward scapular rotation, so passive mobilization should be completed if the patient has spastic retractors or a weak serratus anterior. Retraining of the serratus anterior involves the patient placing the extremity in shoulder flexion and horizontal adduction and then trying to reach forward. Facilitation can be given through quick stretches into scapular retraction and then asking the patient to hold the scapula in that position. Next, the patient is asked to hold while the serratus is contracted and the scapula is protracted. As the serratus increases in strength, the shoulder is flexed in increasing increments until the arm is in the overhead position. Functional activities that use this motion include sanding on an incline, shooting baskets, or painting a wall.

- Supination and pronation with the elbow extended is the final motion during this stage of recovery. Brunnstrom (1970, 1996) gave no special treatment recommendations to help disassociate supination from elbow extension. One activity that could be used is performing ball-handling skills. The patient would grasp a ball with both hands and arms outstretched while rotating it so that first the affected arm was on top of the ball (pronating) and the unaffected arm was under the ball (supinating), and then the ball could be rotated so that the arms did the opposite motion of pronation/supination.

g. The final stage of recovery is willed movement; however, many patients with hemiplegia do not reach this stage.

2. Rehabilitation of the Hand and Wrist

a. Rehabilitation begins during stage 1 when the patient's hand is flaccid. If the patient cannot initiate finger flexion, then the therapist should give a quick stretch to the scapula adductors on the patient's affected side, which causes the fingers to slightly flex due to a traction response.

b. Once <u>Grasp</u> begins, the patient's wrist has a tendency to flex also. Treatment should focus on stabilizing the wrist during finger movement. This should first be attempted with the elbow in full extension, which helps facilitate wrist extension, and with the therapist supporting the patient's wrist. The therapist asks the patient to squeeze or strongly flex the fingers while the therapist facilitates contraction of the wrist extensor muscles. Once a contraction is felt in the wrist extensors, the therapist should discontinue support of the wrist during the "squeezing" or finger flexing and ask the patient to hold the contraction. Again, wrist extension can be facilitated, if necessary, through tapping. When the patient is able to grasp without flexing the wrist during full elbow extension, practice should occur while the elbow is slowly moved into a flexed position.

c. Next, finger flexion is inhibited and extension is facilitated through various techniques. One technique is placing the thumb in abduction/extension and then slowly pronating and supinating the patient's forearm, but especially emphasizing supination and holding the thumb more firmly during supination. Stroking or tapping can be done on the dorsal surface of the wrist and hand to help the flexion relax. Light tapping can also be done to the dorsal surfaces to the patient's fingers while holding the patient's forearm in supination so that the fingers slightly flex toward the palm, which gives a quick stretch to the extensors of the fingers. Following relaxation of the flexion, the patient's arm should be pronated and raised above horizontal (Souques' phenomenon) to assist with extension. Care should be taken to avoid maximum effort, as this can again increase flexor tension. Once the patient is able to extend the hand above the head, practice should occur as the arm is slowly lowered. Any functional grasp and release activity can help the patient practice extension.

d. Lateral prehension release is practiced next. The therapist can help facilitate the patient's lifting the thumb from the side of the index finger by stroking over the abductor pollicis longus tendon. Once the patient is able to release lateral prehension, then the patient is encouraged to practice using and holding lateral prehension. Functional activities to practice this motion include using a key or holding and then releasing a book.

e. After the patient is able to extend the fingers and successfully release objects, more complex prehensile patterns can be practiced such as palmar prehension, spherical grasp, or cylindrical grasp.

f. The final stage is individual finger movements. Functional activities such as typing, using an adding machine, or playing piano can be used; however, the patient should be warned that he or she may not recover completely.

Proprioceptive Neuromuscular Facilitation

This approach to motor learning originated in the mid-1940s by Herman Kabat, MD and was later developed by physical therapists Margaret Knott and Dorothy Voss in the 1960s (Knott & Voss, 1968).

[Proprioceptive neuromuscular facilitation (PNF)] is used as an intervention technique for numerous conditions, including Parkinson's disease, spinal cord injuries, arthritis, stroke, head injuries and hand injuries. It has been effectively combined with neuromobilization techniques to reduce sensory deficits in individuals who have sustained a CVA. (Pendleton & Schultz-Krohn, 2012, p. 805)

This approach is based on overall muscle movement patterns rather than individual muscle contractions.

General Principles

- All persons have potential that has not been fully developed (Voss, 1967). Therefore, all persons have the ability to make progress and further develop from their current state. This philosophy also pertains to therapy so that a patient can use a strong or able part to help a weaker part become further developed (e.g., a patient with a flaccid upper extremity can use his or her strong upper extremity to help increase movement in the affected arm).

- Normal development proceeds in a cervicocaudal and proximodistal direction (Voss, 1967). Treatment should adhere to this model so that treatment begins with motion in the head, neck, and trunk and should then branch into the extremities. This also supports the theory that stability must first be achieved proximally before fine motor skills can be practiced distally.

- Early motor behavior is dominated by reflex activity. Mature motor behavior is supported or reinforced by postural reflexes (Voss, 1967). Reflexes that exist in the newborn and help a child develop eventually become integrated so that reflex behavior is not visible or evident. When voluntary movement is not possible, a person's nervous system can recall those reflexes to help achieve movement.

- Voluntary movement must involve the reversal of a particular action or movement (Voss, 1967). In order to have motor control, both directions of movement must be practiced. For instance, a patient needs to be retrained on both how to dress and undress him- or herself. Likewise, a patient who is practicing standing must also practice sitting.

- The growth of motor behavior has cyclic trends, as evidenced by shifts between flexor and extensor dominance (Voss, 1967). Balance must be achieved between antagonist muscle groups (e.g., if a patient who has had a stroke demonstrates strong flexion, then extension should be emphasized during treatment).

- Developing motor behavior is expressed in an orderly sequence of total patterns of movement and posture. Treatment should incorporate a sequence of developmental positions (like that which infants go through during normal development: rolling, crawling, creeping, standing, and walking), which can facilitate movement. For instance, dressing can first be attempted while rolling,

Bridging, and going from supine to sitting rather than beginning in a less stable sitting or standing position.

- Normal development usually follows in an orderly sequence; however, overlapping occurs (Voss, 1967). A child does not wait until he or she has mastered one activity before beginning another such as sitting up and crawling before walking. Some children do not crawl before standing and walking. Likewise, during treatment, a patient does not wait to begin standing until he or she is able to sit perfectly.

- Movement depends on the balance and interaction between antagonists (Voss, 1967). This is one of the main objectives of this approach and again reiterates the importance of strengthening the weaker motion of an extremity or the trunk. Voluntary movement will be difficult if one motion such as flexion dominates. If spasticity is demonstrated, then it will need to be inhibited prior to the facilitation of antagonist muscles.

- Improvement in motor ability depends on motor learning (Voss, 1967). The therapist should provide as many sensory inputs as possible such as verbal, tactile, and visual cues to help the patient relearn a task.

- Frequency of stimulation and repetitive activity are used to promote and retain motor learning, and for the development of strength and endurance (Voss, 1967). The patient must practice for motor learning to occur and for the action to become automatic.

- Goal-directed activities coupled with techniques of facilitation are used to hasten learning of total patterns of walking and Self-care activities (Voss, 1967). Facilitation should not occur independent of a purposeful task, but neither should a functional activity be practiced with any facilitation of normal movements or motions.

Techniques Used During Proprioceptive Neuromuscular Facilitation

PNF superimposes these techniques on movement and posture (Voss, 1967; Voss, Iota, & Myers, 1985):

- Verbal cues can help reinforce movement.
- Visual cues help the patient identify the goal of the motion.
- Manual contacts refers to the therapist strategically placing his or her hands on the patient to provide pressure and sensory cues for facilitation. Contact should be given to reinforce the movement of the appropriate muscles completing the motion.

- Stretch is another facilitation method to help strengthen voluntary movement. Brazier's (1968) principle states that a stretch to a muscle sends excitatory messages to the stretched muscle while sending inhibitory messages to the antagonistic muscle. During PNF treatment, the muscle to be facilitated should be stretched during a movement pattern when it is in its lengthened range of the pattern.

- <u>Traction</u> promotes movement by sending messages to the joint receptors while the joint surfaces are separated. Traction can specifically facilitate increased ROM in painful joints.

- <u>Approximation</u> promotes stability by sending messages to the joint receptors while the joint surfaces are compressed. This technique can be applied during weightbearing activities.

- <u>Maximal resistance</u> is the greatest amount of resistance that can be given while a muscle contracts and/or completes its full ROM without disrupting the movement or breaking an isometric contraction. The theory again is based on Brazier's (1968) principle of irradiation, which states that stronger muscles can reinforce weaker ones. Resistance helps increase the patient's strength during the movement because the movement requires the patient's maximal effort.

- Repeated contractions, which are directed to the agonist, increase a patient's strength and endurance, as well as provide the practice necessary for motor learning.

- Rhythmic initiation, also directed to the agonist, provides sensory cues so that the patient feels a pattern before attempting to complete it. The therapist should first have the patient relax and passively complete the pattern. Then, the patient should be asked to assist with the movement until he or she can actively complete it unassisted. Finally, the motion can be resisted to help strengthen the contraction.

- <u>Reversal of antagonists</u> may increase pain and spasticity, so these techniques may be contraindicated for some patients:
  - Slow reversal begins with an <u>Isotonic contraction</u> of the antagonist against resistance followed by an isotonic contraction of the agonist against resistance. An isometric contraction at the end of the range following this sequence is a technique called *slow reversal-hold*.
  - Rhythmic stabilization may be contraindicated for cardiac patients due to the tendency for the patient to hold his or her breath during this technique. Repeating isometric contractions

increases stability. Resistance is placed against both agonist and antagonist muscles. The patient is asked to hold a contraction while resistance is given to the antagonist group. Then, the patient is asked to continue holding while resistance is switched to the agonist muscle group. Switching from one group to another continues for three to four repetitions without allowing the patient to rest.

- Relaxation techniques can help increase ROM.
    - Contact-relax begins with an isotonic contraction against maximal resistance during the antagonistic pattern, allowing movement during only the rotational component of the pattern. Next, the patient relaxes while the therapist passively completes the agonistic part of the pattern. This is commonly used when no active motion is present during the agonistic part of the pattern.
    - Hold-relax is similar to the previous technique; however, an isometric contraction is completed during the antagonistic pattern, followed by relaxation and active movement during the agonistic pattern. This technique may be beneficial for a patient with <u>Reflex sympathetic dystrophy (RSD) syndrome</u>.
- Slow-reversal-hold-relax starts with an isotonic contraction. Next, the patient completes an isometric contraction, followed by relaxation of the antagonistic pattern. Finally, the patient actively moves through the agonistic pattern.
- Rhythmic rotation occurs while the therapist passively moves a part through a pattern. Whenever resistance or tone is felt against the movement, the part should be rotated slowly in one direction and then the other until relaxation occurs. Recent research on the effectiveness of PNF includes Sato and Maruyama (2009); Hindle, Whitcomb, Briggs, and Hong (2012); and Lee, Park, and Na (2013).

Neurodevelopmental Treatment: The Bobath Approach

This intervention was specifically developed for patients with hemiplegia or CP, and the main goal is to train or retrain normal movement using a problem-solving approach. In the case of the patient with hemiplegia, the patient's muscles are reeducated both as single units and as groups. A recent study of the Bobath approach found that the method was effective in improving walking in individuals who had a stroke (García, Arratibel, & Azpiroz, 2015).

General Principles

- Movements that either increase abnormal muscle tone or facilitate abnormal movement patterns should be avoided.

- The goal is to produce normal movement or posture; however, treatment does not proceed in a developmental sequence. Rather, treatment should focus on movement that assists the patient with completing his or her functional activities.

- The patient's weak side should be included in all treatment so that functional use of the weak side becomes natural and so that symmetry between the patient's extremities can be reestablished.

- Treatment should demonstrate an improvement in the normal movement patterns and functional use of the patient's involved side.

  Problem Areas in the Patient With Hemiplegia

- Normal movement patterns cannot be produced when abnormal tone exists. Normal <u>Muscle tone</u> exists when the muscle has enough strength to move a body part against gravity but does not change the speed of a normal movement or restrict the movement in any way. Flaccidity occurs when a patient has very low muscle tone and is not able to lift the body part against gravity. Low muscle tone usually occurs during the acute stage of the stroke and immediately following. As tone redevelops in the body part, spasticity or very high tone may occur so that the patient cannot voluntarily move a body part against a very strong contraction in the <u>Antagonist</u> of the movement being attempted.

- A loss of postural control also inhibits normal movement. When completing activities, muscles automatically activate so that balance and equilibrium as well as stability at proximal joints occurs. The patient with hemiplegia can no longer rely on this automatic reaction of postural and stabilizing muscles, so he or she uses adaptive equipment such as a walker to compensate for this loss.

- Coordinated movements become difficult. When completing a motion, the patient's muscles may activate at the wrong time. Also, not all muscles required for a motion may have returned since the stroke; therefore, only a few muscles may be trying to substitute and compensate in order to complete a task.

- All of these deficits combine so that functional activities cannot be completed normally. The patient has difficulty coordinating the involved side with the noninvolved side while completing tasks.

Interventions

- Weightbearing on the affected extremity can have many positive effects. It can help normalize abnormal tone by either facilitating low tone or inhibiting high tone. It also provides the patient with sensory input and increases the patient's awareness of the affected extremity.

- The patient can be positioned in bed so that he or she is lying on the affected side.

- The patient should be encouraged to bear weight equally on both hips when sitting or on both feet when standing to complete activities.

- The therapist can help position the affected upper extremity in a weightbearing position during reaching activities, which is especially helpful for those patients who demonstrate flexor synergy. Prior to weightbearing, the therapist should complete scapular mobilization to ensure that the scapula is gliding well. Also, the head of the humerus should be repositioned into the glenoid fossa if subluxation has occurred.

  ○ The patient's affected hand should be placed on a chair or bench alongside the patient but far enough from the patient's hip so that the wrist is not hyperextended. The arm should be externally rotated (the hand is nearly perpendicular to the patient's trunk) and the elbow held in extension by the therapist. The elbow may be allowed to slightly flex; however, the therapist should not allow the elbow to flex too much, or the patient will not benefit from weightbearing through the shoulder. The patient should shift weight over the affected arm rather than "propping" him- or herself on the arm for extended periods, which could produce stress in the joints.

  ○ *Contraindications*: The patient should not complete this activity if there is extreme pain or edema in the affected arm.

  ○ The patient can also complete weightbearing activities on the affected forearm, which should be forward (0 degrees of rotation) with the elbow flexed and the wrist in neutral.

<u>Handling</u> occurs when the therapist directly facilitates or inhibits the patient's movements by placing his or her hands on the patient to provide normal alignment, complete normal movement patterns, or change abnormal tone. As the patient increases active movement, the therapist should lessen the amount of handling used.

The Bobaths (1990) suggested that handling was the method that should be used in rehabilitation. The use of <u>Key points of control</u> and reflex-inhibiting patterns would lead to normalization of tone and integration of reflexes. This would automatically lead to normal movement. All of the other techniques have been added on to NDT by different instructors who adapted them from Rood, Brunnstrom, PNF, and motor learning (functional task-oriented approaches). Modern NDT has become an eclectic approach that still is taught differently depending on the instructor teaching the course. The issue in the basic beliefs today is to emphasize function (previous criticism), use motor learning (include more up to date evidence), and emphasize the plasticity of the nervous system (when the original theory was produced, they believed in a hardwired developmental system, which is incongruent with plasticity; personal communication from James McPherson, October 24, 2017).

- Key points of control are the areas of the patient's body where the therapist can most effectively facilitate/inhibit movement, and they include the spine/ribcage, pelvis, shoulder, hand, and foot.

- Hand placement depends on the type of movement completed, as well as the amount of tone present. Firm pressure helps inhibit spasticity and abnormal patterns, while light pressure facilitates active movement and steers the patient in the correct pattern of movement.

- <u>Inhibition techniques</u> are used with patients who demonstrate spasticity or associated reactions. They include weightbearing, trunk rotation, and the lengthening of tight muscles (i.e., scapula mobilization, see later).

- <u>Facilitation techniques</u> are used with patients who demonstrate either spasticity or flaccidity. They include the therapist guiding the patient through normal movement patterns so that learning can occur and the patient can begin to actively assist with normal movement. If flaccidity is present, then <u>Stimulation techniques</u>, such as tapping or vibration, are used along with the facilitation techniques to help increase low tone.

Multidisciplinary Team. Professionals from various disciplines who assess and treat clients autonomously and meet regularly to coordinate treatment.

Multi-Infarct Dementia. A condition that results in impaired cognition from multiple sites of damage due to vascular disease. This form of organic brain disease can cause a rapid decline in mental ability.

Multiple Personality Disorder. The previous term used to denote <u>Dissociation</u> marked by the presence of two or more personalities that are distinct and can alternate in certain situations. Each personality is usually not aware of the other personalities. Interventions focus on skill training, <u>Coping skills</u>, <u>Stress management</u>, and expressive therapy. <u>Creative arts</u>, <u>Dialectical behavioral therapy (DBT)</u>, and insight-oriented interventions are often effective. See <u>Dissociative identity disorder</u>.

Multiple Sclerosis (MS). A disease of the nervous system that results in demyelination of nerve fibers in the white matter of the spinal cord and brain. After demyelination occurs, sclerotic patches form to create lesions. This disorder occurs in exacerbations and remissions, which cause a fluctuation in a client's function. The cause is unknown; however, some possible causes include decreased blood flow, vitamin deficiency, autoimmune reaction, a slow-acting virus, allergies, and trauma. Onset occurs in persons between 20 and 40 years of age, and women are 50% more likely to incur this disease.

Specific Interventions

- Complete resistive strengthening activities, but do not cause fatigue.
- Maintain coordination and reduce tremors by using weighted objects for activities or placing light weights on the wrists.
- Improve the client's endurance through exercise and rest, which are alternated to prevent fatigue.
- Fabricate splints or provide stretch to tight muscles to prevent deformity.
- Instruct the client on the importance of skin inspection to prevent pressure sores if the client demonstrates <u>Sensory deficits</u>.
- Increase the client's ability to use tactile or other sensory cues if vision is failing.
- Educate the client on energy conservation and work simplification techniques.
- Address safety and memory concerns by establishing reminders such as routines or tools like notebooks, signs, etc.

- Teach the client <u>Stress management</u> and <u>Relaxation therapy</u> techniques.
- Encourage the client to join a support group for socialization.
- Assist the client with adjustment to the disease by setting realistic goals.
- Recommend assistive devices to increase independence with self-care activities and equipment to increase safety and mobility in home.
- Explore leisure and job interests as needed, or help retrain skills to allow return to previous leisure and work activities.

Contraindications/Precautions

- Expect some loss of function following an exacerbation; a remission does not mean that all function will return exactly like it was prior to the exacerbation (see Yu & Mathiowitz, 2014 for a systematic review of MS interventions).

Muscle Strength. Neuromusculoskeletal ability that indicates the degree of muscle power when lifting objects, resisting force, or maintaining posture. Muscle weakness can occur in <u>Multiple sclerosis (MS)</u>, <u>Parkinson's disease</u>, <u>Muscular dystrophy</u>, <u>Stroke</u>, and other neuromuscular diseases. Treatment to increase muscle strength includes <u>Graded activities</u>, isotonic exercises, and isometric exercises such as weight lifting. It is important to consider occupational engagement in strengthening and to follow precautions and the physician's advice pertaining to the specific condition or reason for loss of strength. See <u>Appendix E</u>.

Muscle Tone. Neuromusculoskeletal component that indicates a muscle's degree of tension at rest or resistance in response to stretch. <u>Hypertonicity</u> or spasticity indicates high abnormal tone, while <u>Hypotonicity</u> or flaccidity indicates low muscular tone or tension. Abnormal muscle tone is one of the symptoms in children with <u>Cerebral palsy (CP)</u>; <u>Neurodevelopmental treatment (NDT)</u> is applied to reduce spasticity. It is assessed by measuring the amount of tension in the fibers of a muscle, or the amount of resistance in the muscle when it is stretched. Slight resistance can be felt in a muscle with normal tone when it is stretched. <u>Facilitation</u> and <u>Inhibition techniques</u> can be used to help increase or decrease muscle tone.

Music Therapy. Use of music for therapeutic purposes, including increased relaxation by creating an emotional climate, increasing movements in the client, or instruction on how to play a musical instrument (e.g., psychological goals can be used to increase self-esteem or decrease depressive thoughts). Music therapy sessions include singing, rhythmic movement where the client moves to the music, listening to music that can be relaxing or stimulating to the client, or playing a musical instrument. The goals for music therapy are individualized. Although music therapy is an established profession, many occupational therapists incorporate a music program in treatment. Research suggests benefits of music therapy for children with <u>Autism</u> (LaGasse, 2014), children and adolescents with psychopathology (Gold, Voracek, & Wigram, 2004), and for pregnant women (Chang, Chen, & Huang, 2008).

Mutism. Inability to speak. It is sometimes associated with social <u>Anxiety</u>.

Myasthenia Gravis. A chronic and progressive disorder that results in weakness of the voluntary muscles. Weakness is characterized by exacerbations and remissions. This disorder most likely occurs from an autoimmune cause, and onset is more prevalent in women if the person is between 20 and 30 years of age. When comparing the incidence after 40 years of age, this disorder occurs equally in men and women.

Specific Interventions

- Complete nonresistive activities to maintain range of motion, strength, and endurance.
- Apply equipment such as <u>Suspension slings</u> or mobile arm supports to assist with weak voluntary movement.
- Assist the client in establishing a time management program so that activity is spread throughout the day and completed when the client has the most energy.
- Instruct the client on energy conservation and work simplification principles.
- Teach safe transfer methods using equipment as needed.
- Educate the client on <u>Stress management</u> and <u>Relaxation therapy</u> techniques.
- Encourage socialization, but remind the client of the importance of frequent rest breaks to avoid fatigue.
- Demonstrate assistive devices that can increase the client's independence with <u>Self-care</u> activities.
- Recommend techniques and diet consistency to increase the client's ability to chew and swallow.
- Provide recommendations concerning the modification of home or the work site to increase the client's productivity and safety.
- Explore new leisure interests as needed.

Contraindications/Precautions

- Avoid overexertion and fatigue.
- Monitor respiration.
- Do not complete resistive activities.
- Avoid the use of materials or activities that can exacerbate difficulty with breathing (e.g., certain cleaning chemicals or sawdust from sanding wood should be avoided).

Myofascial Release. A method for treating myofascial pain that considers both the origin of the pain and the resulting dysfunction. The three aspects of this approach include manual therapy, movement and exercise, and client education. A whole-body "hands-on" approach is used to release soft tissue (muscle) from the abnormal grip of tight fascia (connective tissue).

N

Narcissistic Personality Disorder. An individual who shows signs of grandiosity toward self, fantasies of power over others, omniscience, self-importance, vanity, and a strong need for admiration by others and opportunities for exhibiting self. Sometimes, the individual shows a lack of empathy and understanding toward others. Group therapy may be effective to help the individual gain consensual validation of behavior and to develop compassion for others. Reality therapy has also been successful.

Naturopathy. Based on a therapeutic system that does not advocate the use of drugs. The naturopath employs natural forces such as light, heat, air, water, massage, herbs, healthy food, and vitamins in treating individuals with a dysfunction.

Neck Righting. See Reflexes and reactions.

Negative Symptoms. Losses or lessening of personal characteristics that should be present in everyday social interactions but are now lacking. Symptoms include loss of motivation, withdrawal from social interactions, apathy, flattening of affect, loss of words to say, and loss of critical thinking or problem-solving ability such as in making decisions. Negative symptoms are associated with Schizophrenia.

Nerves. A bundle of nerve fibers that utilizes chemical and electrical impulses to relay information and promote function throughout the body. Nerves have sensory, motor, and mixed functions.

Nervous System. Network of nerves that detects and relays information. The brain and spinal column make up the central nervous system. The cranial nerves and spinal nerves make up the peripheral nervous system. The autonomic system controls unconscious processes and is composed of the sympathetic nervous system that governs functions such as increases in activity and output of the muscles, heart, and sweat glands. The

Stein, F., & Haertl, K.
Pocket Guide to Intervention in Occupational Therapy, Second Edition (pp 185-186).
© 2019 Taylor & Francis Group.

parasympathetic nervous system conserves energy, such as in the slowing of the cardiovascular process.

Neuralgia. Severe pain that is caused by nerve irritation, damage, or impingement on a nerve such as in sciatic pain or shingles.

Neurodevelopmental Treatment (NDT). NDT (Bobath, 1990) is a traditional approach to the treatment of persons with motor control problems, specifically clients with hemiplegia or Cerebral palsy (CP). This approach states that treatment should focus on the goal of movement and increasing the client's ability to complete his or her functional activities. Other basic principles are that motor control redevelops in a proximal-to-distal sequence, and reflexes should not be used to assist the client with active movement. For more information, consult Vaughn-Graham, Cott, and Wright (2015). See Motor control problems and Neurodevelopmental treatment (NDT) for further discussion of treatment.

Neuroma. A mass of nerve fibers that forms alongside a nerve, often near a laceration site.

Neuromuscular Electrical Stimulation (NMES). A physical agent modality that uses electrical current to help reeducate and/or strengthen muscles, gain range of motion, and reduce spasticity through the stimulation of antagonist muscles (DeVahl, 1992; Knutson, Fu, Sheffler, & Chae, 2015). See Physical agent modalities (PAMs) for further discussion and treatment.

Neuropathy. Disease of the nerves such as sensory loss, motor weakness, impaired reflexes, and optic nerve Blindness.

Neurosis. A term that was first defined in the DSM-I (American Psychiatric Association [APA], 1952) as psychoneurotic and referred to behaviors in individuals marked by Anxiety, avoidance, feelings of inadequacy, phobias, unhappiness, excessive guilt, and obsessive behavior. Currently in the DSM-5 (APA, 2013), these behaviors are indicative of personality disorders.

Neutral Warmth. A technique used to inhibit high Muscle tone. The client is wrapped in a blanket for 10 to 20 minutes until the heat reaches the temperature center of the hypothalamus, which helps the client relax. See Motor control problems and Rood approach for further discussion of Inhibition techniques.

Nystagmus. Involuntary eye movement, which can occur in a horizontal or vertical direction, that can cause balance problems and difficulty with postural alignment. Lesions of the vestibular system, brainstem, or cerebellum may result in involuntary nystagmus.

Obesity. A rising problem in the United States based on the body mass index (BMI), which is calculated by weight and height (e.g., a male weighing 146 pounds with a height of 5 feet, 6 inches will have a BMI of 23.6, which is within normal range). BMI charts are readily available on the internet.

Categories
- Underweight = less than 18.5
- Normal weight = 18.5 to 24.9
- Overweight = 25 to 29.9
- Obese = 30 or greater

A position paper from the American Occupational Therapy Association (2007) on obesity emphasizes the role of occupational therapy in promoting healthy lifestyles to facilitate quality of life and healthy weight. Interventions include health promotion, community programs, and lifestyle redesign.

Object Permanence. A cognitive process in which infants (approximately 9 months) develop the concept that objects exist even if they are not in the child's line of vision.

Object Relations. A psychoanalytic term that refers to emotional attachment to persons or objects. Object relations is also associated with the psychoanalytic frame of reference. See <u>Frame of reference</u>.

Objective Psychological Test. A standardized test that contains comparative norms for interpreting individual raw scores.

Obsessive Compulsive Disorder/Obsessive Compulsive Personality Disorder. Obsessive compulsive disorder (OCD) was previously categorized under <u>Anxiety disorders</u>, but in the DSM-5 (American Psychiatric Association, 2013), it now stands on its own. Persons often confuse OCD

Stein, F., & Haertl, K.
Pocket Guide to Intervention in Occupational Therapy, Second Edition (pp 187-193).
© 2019 Taylor & Francis Group.

with obsessive compulsive personality disorder (OCPD). Typically, the personality disorder denotes an individual who has a morbid concern with neatness, orderliness, perfection, and ritualistic or repetitive behavior. Symptoms include extreme preoccupation with details that interferes with task completion, excessive time at work at the expense of leisure, over-conscientiousness regarding ethical or legal standards, lack of flexibility in decision making, a miserly spending attitude, and the hoarding of objects. OCD is often marked by excessive obsessions and compulsions that interfere with daily function. Intervention for both conditions often includes <u>Relaxation therapy</u>, <u>Stress management</u>, <u>Cognitive behavioral therapy</u>, <u>Dialectical behavioral therapy (DBT)</u>, creative expression, and <u>Paradoxical intention</u>, where the client learns how to control the behavior through self-regulation. Therapy also includes focus on strategies to maintain occupational performance in <u>Activities of daily living (ADLs)</u>, <u>Instrumental activities of daily living (IADLs)</u>, and <u>Work</u> due to the fact that obsessions and compulsions may interfere with daily routines (e.g., if an individual is washing his or her hands 50 times per day, it interferes with other activities). Reduction of the general <u>Anxiety</u> accompanying the behavior will often reduce the obsession or compulsiveness. Bringing humor into a client's life is also important to some clients who categorize their behavior or thoughts as catastrophic.

Occupational Performance. The Occupational Performance Model (Australia; 2014) defines occupational performance as "the ability to perceive, desire, recall, plan and carry out roles, routines, tasks, and sub-tasks for the purpose of self-maintenance, productivity, leisure and rest in response to the internal and/or external environment." Such performance relates to everyday activities such as <u>Work</u>, play, <u>Activities of daily living (ADLs)</u>, and <u>Instrumental activities of daily living (IADLs)</u>.

Occupational Profile. "The occupational profile is a summary of a client's occupational history and experiences, patterns of daily living, interests, values, and needs" (American Occupational Therapy Association, 2014, p. S13).

Occupational Science. An academic discipline providing the foundation for occupational therapy, occupational science is the study of human occupation and activity. Current research societies in occupational science are focused not only on individual occupations, but also how human engagement can advance global health and well-being.

Occupational Stress. The sum of the factors in the work environment that negatively affect the individual's psycho-physiological adjustment, or <u>Homeostasis</u>.

Occupational Therapy. As defined by the American Occupational Therapy Association (2014, p. S1) "the therapeutic use of everyday life activities (occupations) with individuals or groups for the purpose of enhancing or enabling participation in roles, habits, and routines in home, school, workplace, community, and other settings." This application of purposeful activities is aimed to prevent disability and injury in individuals who are at risk and to develop independence and restore functions in individuals who are disabled. Functional activities include the ability to Work, to be independent in Self-care, to engage in Leisure activities, and to be effective in social interactions. The effectiveness of occupational therapy depends on the therapist's ability to establish a therapeutic relationship and to select purposeful activities that are meaningful to the client in producing a desired outcome.

Occupational Therapy Practice Framework. The *Occupational Therapy Practice Framework: Domain and Process* (3rd ed.) is the official document of the American Occupational Therapy Association (2014) that provides an overview of the occupational therapy process, specific definitions, and a framework for practice. The document outlines aspects of the occupational therapy process to include occupations, client factors, performance skills, performance patterns, and contexts and environments. Within the framework, evaluation consists of creating an occupational profile and analyzing occupational performance. Based on the evaluation, intervention includes development of an intervention plan, implementation of the intervention, and review of the effectiveness of intervention as compared to targeted outcomes. Outcomes are seen as the evidence of success of the intervention plan.

Occupations. The culturally and personally meaningful and purposeful activities that humans engage in during their everyday lives. According to the *Occupational Therapy Practice Framework, Third Edition* (American Occupational Therapy Association, 2014), the term *occupation* refers to "client directed daily life activities that match and support or address identified participation goals" (p. S29). Examples of occupations include Work, Leisure, play, Self-care, rest, sleep, and social interactions.

Oculomotor. Relating to movement of the eyes. See Oculomotor function.

Oculomotor Control. The movement and position of the eyes. Six muscles around each eye work together in a coordinated manner to control eye movements.

Oculomotor Function. Movement of the eyeball, which is caused by the muscles attached to the eye. See Appendix E for specific muscles. The four parts of oculomotor function include range of motion, pursuits, convergence, and alignment.

- **Range of motion.** A test should be completed to check that all six extraocular muscles of the eye are able to contract and move the eye through its full available range. This is tested by holding a pencil in front of the client and moving the pencil in a large "H" pattern. The client should follow the pencil with eye movements without moving his or her head.

- **Pursuits.** The ability to track objects, or scan, is another component of oculomotor function, which is tested. The therapist should move a pencil while asking the client to follow the movement with his or her eyes.

- **Convergence.** A test should also be completed to check the ability of the eyes to focus on an object in close proximity. Measurement should be taken at the closest point of vision with both eyes. The therapist should slowly move a pencil toward the client's nose and take note of the point of convergence, which is normally 6 to 8 inches from the person's nose. The eyes will track the pencil together to the closest point of focus, but then one eye will drift while the other eye continues to track the object.

- **Alignment.** The final test of oculomotor function checks that both eyes are being used when viewing an object. The therapist should use the corneal light reflex by asking the client to look at a penlight held 12 inches in front of the client's eyes. The therapist should observe a reflection in the same location on the cornea of both eyes.

- Oculomotor function, <u>Visual acuity</u>, and <u>Visual fields</u> comprise the <u>Visual foundation skills</u>, which may decrease perception or negatively affect a test of perception. See <u>Cognitive-perceptual deficits</u> for further discussion and treatment of perceptual problems.

Olfactory Sensation. Receiving, distinguishing, localizing, and interpreting odors and smells through the nose. Damage to the olfactory mechanism will affect taste.

On-the-Job Evaluations. Situations in which the client is evaluated while employed.

Open Reduction. The act of correcting a fracture through surgical intervention. During surgery, hardware such as rods and screws are attached to the bone to help maintain alignment while the bone heals. The hardware is internal, which is referred to as an *internal fixator*. A client who has undergone this procedure has a diagnosis of open reduction internal fixator.

Operant Conditioning. <u>Behavior therapy</u> in which an individual's positive behavior is reinforced and negative behavior is not reinforced. Behavior is shaped by reinforcing sequential steps in a hierarchical manner.

Opioid Epidemic in the United States. Epidemic that became a health crisis in the first two decades of the 2000s. According to the U.S. Department of Health and Human Services (2017), in 2015, 12.5 million people in the United States misused prescriptions of opioids, and 33,091 died from overdosing on opioids. The economic costs were estimated at $80 billion. In addition to medical intervention from the health care team, occupational therapists often use <u>Cognitive behavioral therapy</u> and other common interventions used in <u>Addictions</u>.

Opposition. A motion that combines thumb flexion and abduction with medial rotation of the carpometacarpal joints and flexion of the metacarpophalangeal (MCP) joint in order to bring the palmar surfaces of the distal phalanxes of the thumb and each finger into contact. It should be noted that the tip of the thumb and each finger can achieve contact without having to perform opposition.

Optical Righting. Reflex that uses visual cues to help restore head righting and posture. See <u>Reflexes and reactions</u>.

Oral-Motor Control. The ability to coordinate the musculature around the mouth, tongue, lips, and palate in performing activities such as eating, speaking, singing, sucking through a straw, or playing a musical instrument such as the oboe. See also <u>Feeding/eating</u>.

Orientation. A component of cognition that refers to an individual's awareness and understanding of person, place, time, and situation. An item in an orientation test will ask the client to state who he or she is, where one is, the year it is, and why the individual is in a hospital or care center. See <u>Cognitive-perceptual deficits</u> for further discussion and treatment.

Orthomolecular Medicine. The study of the relationship between vitamins in the body and the onset of diseases, such as the relationship between B-complex vitamins and psychiatric disorders. Orthomolecular practitioners recommend megadoses of vitamins in treating specific psychiatric disorders.

Orthosis. An external device that is attached to a client's body for the purpose of restoring function. Orthoses may be used to (a) decrease the effect of abnormal muscle tone, (b) support a weak extremity, (c) immobilize an extremity following surgery or trauma, or (d) correct deformity. Orthoses that are applied to the hands are often referred to as <u>Splints</u>; however, with current terminology, fabricated devices should be referred to as *orthoses*.

Orthoses may be further subdivided into static and dynamic splints/ orthoses. *Static orthoses* have no moving parts and are used for support and stability, often to immobilize a joint or prevent contractures and deformity. *Dynamic orthoses* have moving parts that are used to assist the proper alignment of fractures, substitute for muscles that have undergone surgical repair, increase range of motion, and decrease contractures or control movement. The therapist fabricates a dynamic splint to increase mobility at a joint. Additional types of orthoses include *cervical collars* to prevent neck flexion; *back braces* to prevent curvature of the spine or to support weak musculature; *arm slings* to support the shoulder joint; *braces* to support the foot, which are often referred to as *ankle-foot orthoses*; *hinge splints/orthoses*, which are artificially powered to provide movement; and Suspension slings or *mobile arm supports* to assist if muscle contraction is difficult. For more information, see Coppard and Lohman (2015) and Appendix D.

Orthostatic Hypotension. A condition of dizziness, nausea, or loss of consciousness from rapidly changing positions. This most often occurs when a person has been lying down or sitting for an extended period, which can allow blood to pool in the lower extremities or abdomen. When the client then stands, blood pressure decreases rapidly and causes the mentioned symptoms. A client may be placed in a reclined position until the symptoms diminish. Some medications place a client at higher risk for hypotension.

Osteoarthritis. A disorder characterized by a loss of hyaline cartilage or changes in subchondral bone, which can affect one or many joints. This disorder is also referred to as *degenerative joint disease*. Osteoarthritis may be classified as primary or secondary. *Primary osteoarthritis* usually occurs due to genetic factors, whereas *secondary osteoarthritis* may occur from trauma, inflammation, endocrine and metabolic diseases, congenital or developmental defects, or prolonged Occupational stress. Onset can begin as early as 20 to 30 years of age; however, most people suffer from this disorder by 70 years of age.

Specific Interventions

- Apply paraffin or other thermal modalities prior to range of motion activities to help increase range.
- Fabricate Splints/orthoses to prevent deformity and increase functional use of the hands. Splints that may be useful include the wrist cock-up splint, resting hand splint, thumb spica splint, or finger gutter splint.

- Complete activities to increase strength of muscles surrounding the affected joints.
- Teach joint protection principles and remind the client to use these techniques during activities.
- Instruct the client on <u>Pain management</u> techniques.
- Educate the client on energy conservation and work simplification techniques.
- Help the client organize the home to make items more accessible and reduce barriers to mobility and function.
- Encourage the client to join a support group for socialization.
- Retrain <u>Self-care</u> activities by using techniques and devices that can reduce the stress on joints.
- Complete a home evaluation and modify equipment to make tasks simpler (e.g., elevate a chair or the bed for easier transfers).
- Suggest that the client purchase and wear clothing that is easy to don and doff (e.g., a female client can purchase a more elastic sports bra and don it overhead if she is unable to hook a brassiere).
- Encourage the continuation of job and leisure activities, but with utilization of new methods to decrease stress on joints.

Contraindications/Precautions

- Avoid overexertion.
- Monitor the skin for redness if splints are being used.
- Ask the client to avoid positions in bed that can lead to deformity, such as a prone position or the use of many pillows.

For more information, Aebischer, Elsig, and Taeymans (2016) provide a meta-analysis of interventions for those with trapeziometacarpal osteoarthritis.

Outcome. The result of a treatment intervention. Outcomes research is the investigation of treatment methods in producing desired outcomes, such as the decrease of negative symptoms in individuals with <u>Schizophrenia</u>.

Outcome Measure. A specific test, procedure, or tool that is used to measure the results of a treatment intervention (e.g., an outcome measure for pain is the *Assessment of Pain and Occupational Performance* [Perneros & Tropp, 2009]).

P

Paget's Disease. A condition that results in increased reabsorption and formation of bone, which causes softening and thickening of bones.

Pain. Physical or mental discomfort.

Pain Management. A holistic approach to treating chronic pain that takes into account the physiological, psychological, and cultural and spiritual aspects of the client. <u>Physical agent modalities (PAMs)</u>, <u>Stress management</u>, counseling and <u>Psychotherapy</u>, <u>Support groups</u>, and <u>Biofeedback</u> are used.

Pain Measurement. Pain, which is a subjective symptom, is measured, often by a visual analog. A wide range of scales is available for practice and research (Reips & Funke, 2008). Over time, progress may be measured by consistent changes in score.

Pain Response. A perceptual process that enables an individual to identify and localize tissue damage, physiological changes such as extreme temperature, and psychological or emotional stress. Acute pain is usually a warning sign of sudden change, such as a torn ligament or headache from emotional stress. Chronic pain that is continuous may have systemic symptoms affecting sleep, movement, the gastrointestinal tract, and personality. Occupational therapists can treat pain through <u>Stress management</u>, <u>Biofeedback</u>, <u>Splints/orthoses</u>, <u>Physical agent modalities (PAMs)</u>, arts and crafts, <u>Relaxation therapy</u>, and <u>Support groups</u>.

Palmar Grasp Reflex. Flexion of fingers in response to stimulation to palm in infants. See <u>Reflexes and reactions</u>.

Palmar Prehension. Also referred to as the <u>Three-jaw chuck pinch</u>, this pattern combines opposition and rotation of the thumb with flexion of the index and long fingers for pad-to-pad contact of the fingers and thumb. This pattern is used when tying shoelaces or picking small objects up off of a flat surface.

Stein, F., & Haertl, K.
Pocket Guide to Intervention in Occupational Therapy, Second Edition (pp 195-227).
© 2019 Taylor & Francis Group.

Palpation. The therapist uses the pads of his or her fingers (usually the index and long fingers) to feel bony landmarks, muscle contractions, or tone. This technique is important when finding landmarks for goniometer placement during measurement of range of motion and is essential in detecting a muscle contraction when the muscle is not strong enough to produce movement. Also, it is important to palpate a muscle while it contracts to ensure there is no substitution being made to complete a motion. See <u>Appendix H</u> for common substitutions for motions.

Panic Disorder. An <u>Anxiety disorder</u> characterized by panic attacks and accompanied by acute anxiety, terror or fright, hyperventilation, sweating, chest pain, dizziness, and a feeling of losing control of self. Panic attacks can occur suddenly and last for minutes with a sense of imminent danger or impending disaster. A panic disorder can lead to agoraphobia (fear of being in public and being alone). Treatment of this disorder includes <u>Cognitive behavioral therapy</u> techniques in which the individual learns how to self-regulate symptoms. Specific techniques include <u>Paradoxical intention</u>, <u>Desensitization</u>, and <u>Relaxation therapy</u>.

Paradigm. A conceptual model that becomes universally accepted. For example, during the age of <u>Institutionalization</u> (1920–1950) in the United States (Grob, 1991), the paradigm for treating mental illness was through hospitalization. In the 1960s, a shift in the paradigm occurred through efforts of the community mental health movement.

Paradoxical Intention. A <u>Behavior therapy</u> technique based on the theory that individuals develop fears and tensions because of anticipatory <u>Anxiety</u>. In using this technique, the individual is told to think of something he or she fears most or to create a negative emotion such as anxiety. By creating a negative feeling, the individual begins to cognitively control the symptom. It has been used as a successful technique with those who stutter, whom consciously produce stuttering and, by doing so, control the speech (Frankl, 1967).

Paraffin. A physical agent modality that uses conduction to transfer heat to superficial physiological tissue. See <u>Physical agent modalities (PAMs)</u> for further discussion and treatment.

Paraffin Therapy. The application of hot wax, usually to the hand and fingers, to relieve pain such as in <u>Rheumatoid arthritis</u> or <u>Osteoarthritis</u>. Precautions should be noted when there are any skin infections.

Paralysis. Loss of sensation and purposeful motor function. This can be the result of a spinal cord or brain injury.

Paranoid Personality Disorder. Marked by extreme suspiciousness and distrust of others. An individual with this disorder attributes hidden motives and agendas of hostility directed by others toward self. The individual is easily offended, tends to misread and distort verbal and nonverbal communications, and is hypervigilant. Treatment is based on the assumption that the client is harboring much anger that needs to be channeled into socially acceptable behaviors. Anger management, expressive arts, Stress management, and Relaxation therapy have been shown to be effective.

Paranoid Schizophrenia. This term was a previous subcategory of Schizophrenia, characterized by Delusions, irrational beliefs, excessive suspicion, and feeling of persecutions by others. The new DSM-5 (American Psychiatric Association, 2013) no longer recognizes the subtypes of schizophrenia but acknowledges that associated symptoms such as paranoia may accompany schizophrenia.

Paraplegia. Paralysis of both lower extremities, usually due to a spinal injury.

Parataxic Distortion. The "uncommunicative, unintelligible, and misleading statements in allegedly communicative interpersonal contexts" (Sullivan, 1963, p. 23).

Paresthesia. The condition of feeling a "burning" or "pins and needles" sensation.

Parkinson's Disease. A degenerative disorder of the central nervous system, specifically the basal ganglia. It results in the degeneration of dopaminergic neurons in the substantia nigra of the midbrain and the development of neuronal Lewy bodies. Symptoms include Cogwheel rigidity, Bradykinesia, Akinesia, and impaired posture. Onset most commonly occurs after 40 years of age, and the cause is unknown. It is the second most common progressive neurodegenerative disorder affecting older American adults. Foster, Bedeker, and Tickle-Degnen (2014) identified rehabilitation for Parkinson's to fall under three areas: physical activity/exercise, environmental cues, and self-management and Cognitive behavioral therapy strategies.

Specific Interventions

- Complete activities to maintain range of motion, especially extension.
- Provide stretch to tight muscles to prevent contractures.
- Use repetitive tasks to improve dexterity and coordination.
- Remind the client to continue reciprocal arm movements, moderate-sized steps, and initiation of ambulation.

- Use music, singing, and dancing to assist with initiation of movement.
- Treat motor planning and movement, especially trunk rotation, through the application of <u>Proprioceptive neuromuscular facilitation (PNF)</u> patterns.
- Cue the client to check balance and posture and use self-correcting techniques when possible.
- Complete a home evaluation and remove barriers to mobility.
- Provide beat or rhythm through the use of a metronome or music while teaching balance and posture skills.
- Instruct the client on energy conservation and work simplification techniques.
- Educate the client on the disease process and expectations for therapy.
- Teach the client to use <u>Inhibition techniques</u> to help normalize increased muscle tone.
- Train the client to use relaxation techniques as a means for also decreasing high tone.
- Encourage the client and family to join a support group.
- Ask the client to verbalize often during treatment to help maintain volume of the voice.
- Teach the client compensatory techniques to help maintain independence with <u>Self-care</u> activities; if the client demonstrates tremors, positioning the arms close to the body may help with stability during feeding, or stabilizing the arms on a table surface or the lap can help control tremors.
- Explore job and leisure interests as needed.
- Utilize current research on the effective use of physical activity for functional movement.

Contraindications/Precautions

- Stand near the client when the client is standing or walking, as there is an increased risk for loss of balance, which can result in falls.
- Observe the client for symptoms that may result as side effects from medication.
- Monitor the client for signs of <u>Depression</u>.

Partial Hospitalization. Includes day, evening, night, and weekend day treatment programs for individuals who need a supportive environment during a period of crisis but are able to avoid hospitalization and stay in the community.

Passive-Aggressive Personality Disorder. Characterized in previous versions of the *Diagnostic and Statistical Manual* system (American Psychiatric Association, 1952, 1994, 2013) by stubbornness, procrastination, indecisiveness, envy, and resistance to requests and demands from others. An individual with this disorder tends not to be overtly hostile, but through indecision and defiance, creates negative confrontations with others. A Psychodynamic approach using expressive and creative media is effective in helping the client resolve feelings.

Passive Range of Motion (PROM). The amount of movement at a joint when the joint is moved through its range by an outside force rather than by the muscles that act on that joint. A therapist often passively moves body parts through a range to help prevent stiffness and contractures when the muscles are too weak. If only one extremity demonstrates limited ROM, then the therapist should compare to the unaffected extremity to determine the amount of impairment. If this is not possible, the therapist should refer to a table of average ranges, which can be found in Appendix F. For *contraindications/precautions* to ROM/measurement and specifics on measurement, see Range of motion (ROM).

Pelvic Tilt. A term used to refer to the position of the pelvis and its relationship to the spine. A client's pelvis can demonstrate a posterior or anterior pelvic tilt. A client who demonstrates *posterior pelvic tilt* appears to sit on the lower part of the sacrum, which makes the person look like he or she may slide out of the chair. The pelvis is tipped backward with the anterior superior iliac spines and the posterior superior iliac spines tilted more posteriorly than normal. Flexion of the spine results to help the client keep the head upright, which may result in a concave curvature of the spine known as Kyphosis. A client who demonstrates *anterior pelvic tilt* has the pelvis tipped forward with the anterior superior iliac spines down and the posterior superior iliac spines tilted more anteriorly than normal. Hyperextension of the spine allows the client to remain upright, but this may result in a convex curvature of the spine known as Lordosis.

Perception. The ability to gather sensory information and apply it within a meaningful framework of knowledge to help assign meaning to the sensory input (e.g., a client with intact spatial relations is able to feel his or her body position but then applies that to his or her existing knowledge of directions such as over, under, above, and so on to determine body position). See Cognitive-perceptual deficits for further discussion and treatment.

Perceptual Deficits. See Cognitive-perceptual deficits for discussion and treatment.

Performance Areas of the Uniform Terminology. In the historical document *Uniform Terminology* (American Occupational Therapy Association, 1994), occupational performance areas included <u>Activities of daily living (ADLs)</u>, <u>Work</u> and productivity, and play or <u>Leisure</u>.

Performance Components of the Uniform Terminology. In the historical document *Uniform Terminology* (American Occupational Therapy Association, 1994), performance components underlying the <u>Performance areas</u> included <u>Sensorimotor</u>, cognitive integration, and <u>Psychosocial skills and psychological components</u>.

Performance Contexts. The *Occupational Therapy Practice Framework* (3rd ed.; AOTA, 2014) performance contexts include cultural, personal, physical, social, temporal, and virtual.

Performance Test. A measure of an individual's skill or capacity such as grip strength, <u>Range of motion (ROM)</u>, manual dexterity, or driving skills.

Peripheral. Relating to the outside surface. See <u>Anatomical position</u>.

Peripheral Nerve Injuries. Different nerve injuries result in different deformities. An ulnar nerve injury or palsy may cause the client to have a <u>Claw hand</u>. A radial nerve injury or palsy can result in wrist drop.

Specific Interventions

- Depending on which branches are injured, either or both sensory and motor reeducation may be necessary to the affected area.

- <u>Sensory reeducation</u> should be started as soon as possible. The client can rub various textures over the affected area or immerse the affected part into containers of different-textured materials. For a more complete description of this treatment technique, see <u>Sensory deficits</u> and <u>Treatment protocol</u>.

- The affected part may need to be immobilized for 3 to 5 weeks to allow some healing of the nerve, depending on the severity of the injury. Motor reeducation may begin following immobilization in the form of gentle active and passive range of motion to decrease stiffness.

- A <u>Splint/orthosis</u> may be necessary to help oppose the agonist muscles since nerve damage can result in paralysis of antagonist muscles (e.g., a client with a radial nerve injury could get a contracture in wrist flexion, since the wrist extension muscles are not able to oppose the strong wrist flexors).

- <u>Neuromuscular electrical stimulation (NMES)</u> is used in some cases to assist the client with the paralyzed or weak motion and to help prevent atrophy of muscles.

Personality. The complex of characteristics, behavioral traits, and attitudes that distinguish an individual from others.

Personality Disorders. Identified by the DSM-5 (American Psychiatric Association, 2013) as an enduring pattern of experience and behavior differing markedly from an individual's culture. Several types of personality disorders are identified, including paranoid, schizoid, schizotypal, antisocial, borderline, histrionic, narcissistic, avoidant, dependent, obsessive compulsive, and other subtypes. The disorder usually begins during childhood or adolescence and continues into adulthood. Many times, the disorder leads to self-defeating behaviors that interfere with the individual's ability to adapt to changes in the environment and to meet societal expectations.

Pet Therapy. The therapeutic use of pets or service animals to create an animal–human bond, which may improve a client's physical and emotional health.

Phantom Pain. The sensation of pain along the nerve root of an amputated body part. Many times, it interferes with use of a prosthetic.

Phenomenological. The subjective experiences and feelings of an individual. Depressed feelings and <u>Delusions</u> in an individual with mental illness can be considered phenomenological symptoms.

Phobia. An abnormal fear or irrational dread of a specific object (e.g., spiders), activity, (e.g., flying), or situation (e.g., being in an open plain).

Phonophoresis. The application of ultrasound in conveying medication into a tissue, such as in <u>Pain management</u>. See <u>Physical agent modalities (PAMs)</u> for further discussion and treatment.

Physical Agent Modalities (PAMs). "Techniques that produce a response in soft tissue through the use of light, water, temperature, sound, or electricity. These techniques are used as adjunctive methods in conjunction with, or in immediate preparation for, occupational therapy services" (California Board of Occupational Therapy, n.d.).

PAMs use physical energy to promote physiological change in body tissue for the purpose of reducing symptoms and enhancing function (Bracciano, 2008). In using PAMs, the therapist applies electrical current, sound waves, light waves, and hot or cold temperatures to enhance therapeutic effects. Modalities are applied to enhance circulation, connective tissue extensibility and healing, pain control, muscle facilitation, relaxation, or retraining. Examples are <u>Transcutaneous electrical nerve stimulation (TENS)</u>, <u>Paraffin therapy</u>, <u>Hydrotherapy</u>, <u>Phonophoresis</u>, <u>Cryotherapy</u>, <u>Biofeedback</u>, and <u>Ultrasound</u>. Therapists using PAMs should have specialized training and/or certification in the use of the modality, and the applications may be limited based on state laws and practice acts. The American Occupational Therapy Association recommends that an occupational therapist may use PAMs prior to or during treatment provided that the main focus of treatment is functional activities. The therapist must also demonstrate knowledge of the theory, purpose, and technical skills required by the modality being used. PAMs are also classified into two major categories: thermal modalities and electrical modalities.

- **Heat.** Heat modalities increase blood flow, which can reduce pain, decrease spasticity, and reduce muscle spasm. Heat also increases the metabolic rate, facilitating healing of connective tissue. Gradual elevation of tissue temperature increases connective tissues' extensibility and the viscosity of synovium. Heat modalities may be applied via conduction, convection, or conversion. An example of conduction is direct surface-to-surface contact via hot pack. Convection is via moving particles such as fluidotherapy and whirlpool. An example of conversion is ultrasound that produces heat effects through cellular interactions. The therapeutic temperature for heat application varies by modality but in general is 105°F to 113°F. Precautions must be taken with heat application to prevent tissue damage.

- **Cold.** Cold causes vasoconstriction, which initially decreases blood flow and metabolic rate, slowing inflammation; the pain threshold is elevated through free nerve endings. Cold can be transferred through conduction, as in cold packs, such as coolant gels. Cold is used to help decrease acute pain and muscle spasm, maintain muscle length, reduce spasticity and <u>Clonus</u>, and decrease inflammation and edema. The therapist should closely monitor the use of cold with clients since cold can cause skin burn. Cold can be transferred through conduction and evaporation.

- **Conduction.** This method of heat transfer occurs from one object to another through direct physical contact.
    - ○ **Paraffin Bath.** Paraffin baths are heat units that store a mixture of seven parts paraffin wax and some mineral oil maintained at a therapeutic temperature between 125°F and 130°F. Paraffin baths are useful when the therapist is attempting to apply superficial heat to an area that is hard to reach, such as the fingers of a client who has <u>Rheumatoid arthritis</u> or <u>Osteoarthritis</u>.
        - ▪ **General Procedure.** Before the client puts an extremity into paraffin, the client should wash thoroughly to prevent

contamination. The client then dips the hand into the tub 6 to 12 times, or as tolerated, while being sure to lift the hand completely out of the tub between dips. The therapist should then wrap the hand in a plastic bag and towel or other insulated fabric mitt/cover with the paraffin applied for 10 to 20 minutes. It is also good practice to elevate the client's hand on an inclined surface, stack of towels, or pillow to help prevent edema and to position the treated part on stretch to provide prolonged gentle stretch during treatment. The client should hold the hand still since movement of the hand would break the paraffin seal and allow the heating benefit to escape.

- **Contraindications.** A client who has open wounds should not apply paraffin. Paraffin is a type of heat that may cause vasodilation, so a client with severe or moderate edema should also not use this modality. Other conditions that are contraindicated for paraffin treatment include fever, active bleeding, site of malignancy, peripheral vascular disease, and cardiac or arterial insufficiency. Caution should be used when applying heat to a client who has <u>Sensory deficits</u>, slight <u>Edema</u>, or confusion.

○ **Hot Packs.** Packs that contain silicate gel are heated and stored in a hydrocollator, or unit which contains water that is heated to 158°F to 176°F. The pack is generally able to retain heat for 30 minutes.

- **General Procedure.** Since the packs are heated to a level that can burn and cause tissue damage, hot packs are applied to the client with towels or other insulated fabric pieces placed between the skin and the packs. Clothing and jewelry should be removed from the area being treated. It is generally recommend that six to eight layers of fabric between the packs and the client's skin. The therapist should check the client's skin for redness or blotching after the packs have been applied for 5 minutes. If the client complains of too much heat or the skin is red, more layers of insulation should be added between the packs and the skin. Treatment should last for 15 to 30 minutes. Hot packs may be applied to a client who has open wounds.

- **Contraindications.** Heat is contraindicated with a client who has moderate to severe edema, fever, active bleeding, site of malignancy, peripheral vascular disease, and cardiac and arterial insufficiency. Caution should be used when applying heat to a client who has sensory deficits, slight edema, or confusion. This modality serves as an alternative to paraffin for the client who has an open wound since hot packs may be used on open wounds unless otherwise indicated by the physician.

- **Convection.** Heat transfer may occur through the motion of fluid surrounding tissues.
  - ○ **Hydrotherapy.** The physical properties of water can benefit affected body parts during immersion in many ways. Thermal effects occur similarly to the application of superficial thermal agents; however, the client's body may respond systemically since more body surface area is generally affected during hydrotherapy. Warm temperatures will initially increase blood pressure and heart rate, but vasodilation will occur and decrease blood pressure. Cold temperatures will cause vasoconstriction, which will increase blood pressure and decrease heart rate. Water creates buoyancy of the body near the surface of the water, which can assist the client with movement. If body parts are immersed below the surface of the water, water creates resistance to movement for strengthening benefits. The density of water helps support the affected body part, which can decrease stress on the joints. The pressure of water helps promote circulation. Mechanical devices can agitate the water, which helps with wound <u>Debridement</u> and pain relief.
  - ○ **Whirlpool.** The most common form of hydrotherapy. The various benefits of whirlpool treatment include debridement of wounds from water agitation, massage of the affected tissues, and buoyancy and resistance of water against movement, which can promote active movement and exercise during whirlpool.
    - ■ **General Procedure.** When using whirlpool as a thermal modality, the water should be heated to 100°F to 105°F for upper limbs and 100°F to 102°F for lower limbs. If necessary, the water can be heated to 110°F, but full-body immersion should occur in water that is 100°F or below. Treatment may be completed for 10 to 20 minutes as tolerated by the client. If using the whirlpool for wound care, a sterilizing agent must be added during treatment. Care should be taken to sanitize and drain the whirlpool

following every treatment. It should be noted that some clinics have removed the use of whirlpools due to risk of infections.

- **Contraindications.** See general hydrotherapy contraindications later.

o **Pool Therapy.** May be used with clients for relaxation, increased circulation, increased motion, strengthening, stress reduction to joints, and leisure. Clients with the following diagnoses may benefit from aquatic therapy: mild spastic <u>Cerebral palsy (CP)</u>, orthopedic and musculoskeletal conditions, neurologic disorders, and rheumatoid arthritis. See <u>Aquatic therapy</u> for further discussion of treatment and specific contraindications.

o **Contrast Bath.** Used to help decrease edema or <u>Hypersensitivity</u>. Clients with the following diagnoses may benefit from this modality: rheumatoid arthritis, joint sprains, muscle strains, <u>Reflex sympathetic dystrophy (RSD) syndrome</u> (complex regional pain syndrome), or mild peripheral vascular diseases. See edema for further discussion of treatment and specific contraindications.

o **Contraindications.** Hydrotherapy is contraindicated for clients with the following diagnoses/conditions: fever, infections, sensory deficits, trauma or hemorrhage, sites of malignancy, bleeding disorders, cardiac instability, inability to communicate pain, atrophic skin, acute edema (except with contrast baths), ischemic areas, poor thermal regulation, and immature scar tissue.

- **Fluidotherapy.** A limb can be placed in a fluidotherapy machine, which circulates finely ground corn husks in warm air (102°F to 118°F). This heating mechanism has proven to be an excellent modality for raising the temperature of tissue in hands and feet. Benefits include heat as well as <u>Desensitization</u>, massage, and slight resistance while providing an environment conducive to active motion/exercise.

o **General Procedure.** The machine should be started prior to treatment so that the particles are warm when treatment begins. The temperature ranges from 102°F to 125°F, and this should be set according to the client's tolerance. The client then places the limb in the machine, and the therapist should tightly fasten the band around the client's limb to avoid particles from exiting the machine. Treatment lasts 20 to 30 minutes.

○ **Contraindications.** Clients who have open wounds or edema should not use fluidotherapy unless the wound is covered with a plastic bag. Care should be taken with clients who have sensory deficits. See <u>Paraffin</u> or <u>Hot packs</u> for general contraindications/precautions when using heat.

- **Conversion.** The final method of heat transfer occurs when a modality creates internal friction to generate heat.

  ○ **Ultrasound.** This machine produces inaudible sound waves, which can penetrate tissue to create thermal and nonthermal effects. Thermal effects are the results of sound wave compression and decompression of cellular molecules, resulting in heat from friction. Nonthermal effects in some fractures, wound healing, and reduction in inflammation occur through increasing cellular permeability. Ultrasound is helpful with the management of clients with the following diagnoses/conditions: scar tissue/keloids, tendinitis, bursitis, joint contractures, myositis ossificans, pain, and muscle spasm.

    - **General Procedure.** A small transducer head transmits sound waves through a gel that is applied to the client's skin. Ultrasound produces deep heat, which penetrates deeper than the previously mentioned modalities, usually to a depth of 1 to 3 cm, depending on the size of the head and sound wave frequency. Sound waves can be set to cycle at a frequency of 1 or 3 MHz When cycling at 1 MHz, tissue penetration depth is increased; tissue can be heated more superficially through use of the 3-MHz setting. Sound absorption varies depending on the fluid content of the tissue. The strength of ultrasound is also set by programming the intensity of the sound waves, which are measured in watts per square centimeter. Intensity can range between 0.25 and 3 W/cm^2 during treatment; however, most treatment occurs between 1 and 2 W/cm^2. If applying ultrasound for thermal benefit, then *continuous wave* should be used. If mechanical benefit is the goal, then *pulsed wave* should be used. When placing the transducer on the client's skin, small circular motions should be used to help avoid overheating a specific spot, and the therapist should maintain even contact between the transducer with the treatment site. Also, the intensity of the waves should be reduced when using ultrasound over bony prominences.

Once the ultrasound has been started, the head of the transducer should immediately be applied to the client's skin. Sound waves cannot be transmitted through air, so the crystal of the transducer may shatter or depolarize if not permitted to transmit its waves. Ultrasound is applied to the affected area for a duration of 8 to 10 minutes. A client has this modality applied for 6 to 12 treatment sessions. Ultrasound may be applied with tissue on stretch, with therapeutic activities immediately following treatment.

Ultrasound may also be used as a nonthermal agent to help drive topical medication into deeper tissue, which is called *phonophoresis*. The medications most commonly used include local anesthetics and corticosteroids. This modality may be once per day for up to 10 days. The transducer may be set at a frequency of 1 or 2 MHz and an intensity of 1 to 3 W/cm^2 for a duration of 5 to 7 minutes per site. The efficacy of this use of the modality is controversial; therefore, therapists should consult recent research. Clients with the following diagnoses/conditions may benefit from phonophoresis: epicondylitis, tendinitis, tenosynovitis, bursitis, capsulitis, fasciitis, strains, contractures, osteoarthritis, impingement of shoulder, scar tissue, adhesions, and <u>Neuromas</u>.

- **Contraindications.** Ultrasound should not be used over the following areas: heart, pacemakers, brain, eyes, laminectomized spine, testes, carotid sinus, cervical ganglia, acute joint pathologies, active bleeding, thrombophlebitic sites, growth plates, infected bone or other sites of infection, sites of malignancy, and fluid-filled cavities. Care should be taken to avoid overheating specific sites when using ultrasound over metal implants/hardware.

- **Cryotherapy.** Cold is used in treatment to help decrease edema, inflammation, and pain, as well as reduce spasticity and clonus. The application of cold results in vasoconstriction, decrease of peripheral nerve conduction velocity, decrease in cellular metabolic rate, and increased stiffness due to decreased elasticity of tissue.

  - **Cold Packs.** These silicone gel packs are stored in a freezer at 23°F to 45°F. When applied to a client's skin, a moist towel should be placed between the pack and the client's skin to prevent tissue damage. Cold packs should be applied for 15 to 30 minutes.

- o **Ice Packs.** Plastic bags can be filled with ice and used for cooling if cold packs are not available. Ice packs are actually colder on the skin than cold packs. The therapist again places a moist towel between the pack and the client's skin. Ice packs should be applied for 10 to 20 minutes. After completing a home program, the client can complete this cooling at home with ice in a plastic bag or a bag of frozen vegetables.

- o **Ice Massage.** Water can be frozen in Styrofoam (The Dow Chemical Company), plastic, or paper cups. Following exercise, the therapist can retrieve a cup from the freezer, tear the bottom from the cup, and use the top half of the cup to hold the ice. The therapist should massage over the affected area for 5 to 10 minutes until the skin becomes numb.

- o **Vapocoolant Sprays.** The most commonly used spray for superficial cooling is fluorimethane. The therapist should spray two or three times across an area of the skin where the client complains of pain during stretch of a limb. Care should be taken so the skin is not frosted. After the skin has been sprayed, the therapist should stretch the limb and attempt to increase the range of motion. Coolant sprays can also assist in maintaining gains in muscle length through cooling of tissues in stretch position. This superficial cooling does not have the same stiffening effect as ice that is applied for a longer duration.

- o **Cold Baths.** Body parts can also be immersed into a container filled with ice and water. The water temperature should range between 55°F and 65°F. The client should place the affected part in the water 10 to 20 minutes or as tolerated. If a client is unable to tolerate the ice bath, the therapist can strain the ice out of the water immediately before the client inserts his or her limb, which will allow the water to slightly heat back toward room temperature quicker.

- o **Contraindications.** Clients with the following diagnoses/conditions should not have cryotherapy applied: Raynaud's phenomenon; extreme hypersensitivity; compromised circulation; peripheral vascular disease; cardiac or respiratory involvement; initial stage of wound, fracture, or tendon healing; an inability to communicate pain; severe hypertension; replantations; and crush injuries. Caution should be taken when applying cryo-therapy to a client who has sensory deficits, as well as with the elderly or very young clients.

- **Electrical Modalities.** Various forms of direct and alternating electrical current in small increments can help excite nerve or muscle tissue to help promote the restoration of lost function. The biophysiological effects of current are thermal, chemical, neural, and physiological. Thermal effects are reduced by pulsing the current; care must be taken to monitor the current density at electrode sites to reduce skin reaction. The primary use of electrical modalities is neural stimulation and physiological healing of wounds and fractures. The flow of electrons is able to transfer to the flow of ions within biological tissues through the application of electrodes to the client's skin. The flow of ions in biological tissue is then able to produce an action potential within a nerve. Larger cutaneous nerves, which are closer to the surface of the skin, are the first nerves to be stimulated. A client may report a "tingling" sensation, which results from the firing of the cutaneous nerves. If the amplitude is increased, the deeper motor nerves can be stimulated, resulting in muscle contraction. Research has shown that the application of electrical modalities can also increase local blood flow, stimulate soft tissue regeneration, increase levels of endorphins in the blood, and increase the absorption of fluid (edema) from the affected site. The treatment of pain is also based on the gate-control theory, which posits that electrical current can close the gates that allow the pain impulses to reach the brain. Electrical modalities can help decrease pain, promote healing, increase movement/strength, decrease edema, and reeducate muscles.

  - **Contraindications.** Clients with the following diagnoses/conditions should not receive electrotherapy treatment: cardiac problems and/or pacemakers, active cancer/malignancy, local infections (except if use is for wound healing), decreased cutaneous sensation, pregnancy, <u>Seizure disorders</u>, thrombotic blood vessels, fresh fractures, fusion, sutured nerves or tendons, edema, active hemorrhage, site of the carotid sinus, and on the anterior chest wall. Care should be taken when using electrical current with a client who has high blood pressure, circulatory problems, peripheral vascular disease, problems communicating pain, or small body mass.

- **Iontophoresis.** This modality utilizes continuous low-voltage current that flows in one direction (DC current), otherwise known as *galvanic current*. Current of this type helps to promote wound and fracture healing. When ions are applied to the client's skin, this current helps drive the ions into underlying tissue. This process is called *iontophoresis*. Different topical medications that contain ions can be applied to help facilitate various processes such as the following: reduce edema with corticosteroids, reduce pain with local anesthetics, relax muscles with magnesium sulfate, reduce calcium deposits with acetic acid, treat infections with copper sulfate, heal wounds with zinc oxide, or soften scars and adhesions with sodium chloride. Iontophoresis uses a current ranging from microamperes up to 30 mA. One smaller active electrode is used with a larger dispersive electrode. The electrical unit should be set so that its polarity is the same as the medication being used. This will cause the current to repel the ions and drive them into the treatment site. The active electrode should be applied to the treatment site, while the dispersive electrode is applied ipsilaterally on the same general body area. It is important to note that premanufactured IontoPatches (Travanti Medical) of varying sizes and doses are now available commercially, replacing most clinical iontophoresis units. The IontoPatch or unit uses an active electrode and a dispersive electrode set for polarity of the medication used.
  - **Contraindications.** Clients who have decreased sensation should not have DC current applied as DC current can burn the skin. Clients should also not have medications applied that cause the client to have an allergic reaction. In addition, take care not to apply over open wounds or rashes.
- **Microcurrent Electrical Neuromuscular Stimulation (MENS).** Use of low-frequency and low-intensity current so that the current is not sensed by the client. This type of modality may be used to help reduce acute or chronic pain; reduce inflammation; reduce spasm; and promote healing of bones, nerves, or connective tissue. Some evidence supports its use to enhance tissue healing.
- **Transcutaneous Electrical Nerve Stimulation (TENS).** This modality helps decrease pain based on the endorphin release principle and on the gate-control theory principle. Both acute and chronic pain may be relieved by TENS (Zeng et al., 2015). The application of this device may help a client with acute or chronic pain. An example is a client who needs to begin movement following

surgery, such as capsulotomy or <u>Tenolysis</u>, but complains of pain. TENS may be set at a short pulse duration, a frequency of 50 to 100 Hz, and an amplitude of 10 to 30 mA (or within limits of perception). This setting brings relief that may last 1 to 3 hours within 1 to 20 minutes of application; however, relief may also end immediately following application. This setting is based on the gate-control theory. TENS may also be set at a long pulse duration, a frequency of 1 to 4 Hz, and an amplitude of 30 to 80 mA (or until a slight motor response occurs). This setting brings relief within 20 to 30 minutes of application but lasts from 2 to 6 hours following treatment. This setting is based on the endorphin release theory. When using conventional mode TENS (50 to 100 Hz), the electrodes may be placed at the local site of pain. If using low-frequency TENS (1 to 4 Hz), the electrodes should be placed in the segmental myotome that is related to the involved area. Electrodes may also be placed on motor, trigger, or <u>Acupuncture</u> points. Once educated, the client can apply TENS daily as needed for pain.

- **Neuromuscular Electrical Stimulation (NMES).** NMES uses an alternating current; it is used with innervated muscle tissue. This modality helps reeducate and/or strengthen muscles, reduce atrophy, gain range of motion, and reduce spasticity through the stimulation of antagonist muscles. NMES uses an interrupted current to allow the muscle to relax between contractions. The electrodes should be placed on motor points of the muscles being stimulated in line with the muscle fiber stimulated. The current is increased slowly until a motor response is demonstrated. If the therapist uses unipolar motor point stimulation, one electrode is small and the other is large. The same amount of current passes through both electrodes; however, the current is more concentrated under the small electrode. The small electrode is the active one and should be placed on the motor point. When finding the motor point, refer to a motor point chart, if possible. If no references are available, the motor point tends to be in the middle of the muscle belly. In general, a greater distance between electrodes increases current depth; a shorter distance will result in a more superficial flow of current. Lightly place the active electrode on the approximate motor point. While the unit delivers current, slowly slide the active electrode around on the skin until the strongest contraction is demonstrated. The active electrode can then be firmly attached to the motor point site. The larger, dispersive electrode is often placed distally over the tendinous portion of the muscle. Unipolar stimulation may be applied to a client with <u>Peripheral nerve injury</u> or tendon transplant. Bipolar stimulation utilizes two equally sized electrodes with equal strength of current. The electrodes may both be placed on the muscle being stimulated; however, the distance between the electrodes should at least be the length of the diameter of one electrode to prevent short-circuiting. The unit can produce a contraction near a frequency of 30 pps. A ratio of one unit of "on time" to five units of "off time" is a good starting point if using NMES with a client who has hemiplegia. Orthopedic clients benefit from a 1:3 ratio, while a client who needs to increase muscle strength will benefit from a 1:1 ratio of "on time" to "off time." The electrical unit should always be turned back to 0 following treatment. Duration of treatment can range between 10 and 45 minutes depending on the goal of treatment and the client's tolerance. NMES can also be referred to as <u>Functional electrical stimulation (FES)</u> if applied while asking the client to complete functional activities.

- **High-Voltage Galvanic Stimulation (HVGS).** HVGS is direct current usually used for denervated muscle tissue primarily to treat muscle atrophy. Direct current is also used for tissue repair (electrical stimulation for tissue repair). This modality may also be referred to as *high-voltage pulsed current* to treat pain and edema and heal wounds. The active electrode should be placed over the involved site, while the dispersive electrode is placed on the body at a good distance from the treatment site. Some dispersive electrodes are so large that they must be placed on the back or abdomen. This electrical unit differs from low-voltage units in that the current has a higher voltage (up to 500 volts) and waves that are unidirectional and close together. This modality may treat various conditions using different settings.

- **Interferential Electrical Stimulation.** This modality is sometimes referred to as <u>Interference current (IFC)</u>. It is used to treat chronic pain and edema. The electrical unit has two equal currents delivered to the affected tissue at two different frequencies. This causes a summation of current (70 to 100 mA), which is greater than the current provided to the tissue by TENS, and this current is then able to stimulate both sensory and motor nerve fibers. Stimulation results in muscle contraction of deeper, larger muscles, which may be pain-relieving. The IFC electrical unit may be set at the maximal output that the client is able to tolerate.

Pilates. A method of physical movement, exercise, and stabilization developed by Joseph Pilates, a German fitness instructor, who originally designed his exercises to rehabilitate soldiers returning from the war. The exercises may be done with or without the special Pilates equipment.

Pinch. Usually referred to when testing a client's finger strength. A pinch meter is used for measuring a client's palmar, lateral, and tip pinch in pounds of pressure. See Prehension.

PIP. Acronym for proximal interphalangeal.

Place and Hold. Activities completed with the therapist's assistance by persons who demonstrate weakness or the inability to control movement. The therapist assists the client with movement, such as flexing the shoulder to 90 degrees, and then asks the client to attempt to hold the extremity in that position. The therapist should decrease the amount of assistance being given to hold the affected extremity in place, but not withdraw assistance completely at the beginning of place-and-hold activities. As the client increases voluntary muscle contraction, the therapist should decrease assistance until the client is able to both place and hold the extremity in the desired position independently. See Motor control problems.

Placebo Effect. A placebo is a treatment or substance with no known active ingredient. The placebo effect occurs when the individual's belief in the actual treatment causes beneficial results that cannot otherwise be explained by the treatment itself.

Placing Reflex or Placing Reaction. Reflex present in infants. See Reflexes and reactions.

Plantar Grasp Reflex. Reflex where the toes flex when the sole is stroked. See Reflexes and reactions.

Plantarflexion. A joint motion at the ankle that results in the toes being pulled downward away from the knee. This is ankle joint flexion, which is often mislabeled as extension. See Appendix F for the normal range of this motion.

Poetry Therapy. Use of poetry to help clients express their feelings and innermost thoughts. The poetry is designed to convey a vivid and imaginative sense of experience. It can be insightful in discovering a person's fantasies, desires, and fears.

Position in Space. The ability to understand terms that define position, such as *over, under, above, beneath,* and so on, and then apply those to objects. See Cognitive-perceptual deficits for further discussion and treatment.

Positioning. Clients who are unable to move themselves or particular body parts must be positioned appropriately by the therapist. Incorrect positioning can result in contractures, foot drop, subluxation, <u>Decubitus ulcers</u>, pain, disfigurement, and decreased functional ability. A client must be positioned correctly while in bed as well as while in a wheelchair or dining room chair. Often, common items such as pillows can be used to promote proper alignment; however, special equipment should be fabricated or ordered as needed.

Bed Positioning

Recommended positioning for clients with hemiplegia: For all lying down positions, the bed should be flat. In general, avoid the half-lying position. This position can worsen muscle tightness.

- When lying on your affected side, use one or two pillows for your head. Your affected shoulder should be positioned comfortably. Place your unaffected leg forward on one or two pillows. Place more pillows in front and behind you. This is an important position as it increases awareness of your affected side as you are lying on the bed. It also leaves your unaffected side available for tasks.

- When lying on your unaffected side, use one or two pillows for your head. Your affected shoulder should be forward with your arm supported on another pillow. Place your affected leg backward on one or two more pillows. Place a pillow behind you. This position can let you practice doing tasks with your affected side, if possible.

- When lying on your back, place three pillows supporting both your shoulders and your head. Place your affected arm on a fourth pillow. Keep your feet in a neutral position. You can also place another pillow beneath your affected hip. You do not need to stay in this position if you find it uncomfortable. See https://ahc.aurorahealth-care.org/fywb/x14042.pdf.

- This is the preferred position for clients who have hemiplegia. Lying on the affected side helps provide input through weightbearing. The client should be positioned with the head symmetrical; a pillow may be used if the head is not flexed too much. Next, the affected arm should be fully protracted and flexed at the shoulder to at least 90 degrees with the elbow flexed and the forearm supinated so that the affected hand is under the pillow. The elbow may also be extended with the wrist slightly off the bed to help encourage wrist extension. The affected leg should be extended at the hip and slightly flexed at the knee, while the unaffected leg is supported on a pillow in hip and knee flexion for comfort.

- Lying on the nonaffected side begins with the head positioned symmetrically on a pillow. Again, the affected shoulder is fully protracted and flexed to 90 degrees. The affected arm should be supported on a pillow so that the wrist is placed in neutral and not allowed to flex. The affected leg should also be supported by a pillow so that the hip and knee are flexed and the foot and ankle are supported so that the foot does not invert.

- Lying supine begins with the head symmetrical. A pillow should be placed under the affected shoulder so that it is symmetrical with the nonaffected shoulder; however, care should be taken so that it is not overly raised as this could result in anterior subluxation. The affected arm should be slightly flexed and abducted at the shoulder, extended at the elbow, and supinated or neutral at the forearm with the hand open and a pillow supporting the entire arm.

- If a client has sustained a brain injury, side-lying is the preferred position. The supine position may facilitate the <u>Tonic labyrinthine reflex</u>, which will govern the client's position. The client may lie on either side with a small pillow to support the head in alignment with the trunk. Both upper extremities should be protracted at the shoulders in slight shoulder flexion. A pillow may be placed between the arms to prevent horizontal adduction of the uppermost arm. The client's wrists should be extended, and cones may be placed in the client's hands to prevent contractures due to increased tone. The lower extremities should be slightly flexed at the knee and hip with a pillow to prevent hip adduction and internal rotation of the uppermost leg. Pillows may also be needed behind the client's back to help the client maintain a side-lying position. Padded boots may be applied to the feet to prevent pressure areas on the feet and to position the ankle near 90 degrees flexion to prevent foot drop. If the client does lie in supine, pillows should be used to protract the shoulders. The upper extremities should be abducted slightly and externally rotated. Cones may also be used in this position if a client demonstrates increased tone.

Wheelchair Positioning

- The first step of positioning is to produce correct placement and position of the client's pelvis. The client should be sitting on the pelvis symmetrically, rather than having more weight on one hip than the other. A wedge cushion may be used to support the side of the pelvis that is supporting more weight in order to redistribute the client's weight equally.

- The client's pelvis should be in neutral or slightly tilted anteriorly. A solid seat may need to be installed since a regular fabric seat encourages posterior <u>Pelvic tilt</u>, which will lead to poor posture, as well as internal rotation and adduction of the hips. A small lumbar roll also facilitates anterior pelvic tilt.

- When sitting, the client should have the hips at 90 degrees flexion. A wedge cushion can be used with the higher side of the wedge placed toward the front of the wheelchair seat, at the client's knees, to achieve proper hip position.

- A seat belt provides safety as well as good positioning. The belt should fasten along the lower pelvis area to help continue proper pelvic tilt and even weightbearing through the hips.

- Pads may be placed along the lateral aspect of the thighs to prevent the client from excessively abducting the hips.

- A pad or swing-away abductor may be placed between the client's thighs to prevent the client from excessively adducting the hips. An abductor that can be lowered under the chair as needed preserves the client's ability to transfer, while a pad that is permanently in the chair can increase the assistance needed for the client to transfer.

- If a client tends to slide forward in the wheelchair, the abductor or wedge cushion may be indicated. A larger wedge cushion, called an *anti-thrust cushion*, may be used to prevent the client from falling out of the chair. This cushion may cause hip flexion greater than 90 degrees; however, if the client is at risk of hurting him- or herself by falling, the cushion should be used.

- If the client is prone to skin breakdown from poor nutrition or incontinence, a gel cushion or other pressure-relieving device should be used in the seat. Clients with spinal cord injury are specifically at risk due to absent or decreased sensation and decreased ability to reposition oneself.

- The client's trunk should be aligned with the pelvis. A solid seat back may be required to prevent the client from leaning back too far into the existing fabric seat back. This back may be reclined 10 to 15 degrees to align the trunk and head with the pelvis. If trunk flexion is an extreme problem, the seat may be reclined farther to prevent the client from falling out of the wheelchair. Care should be taken during meals to return the client to a more upright position for safety in swallowing.

- If the client tends to lean to one side, lateral supports may be used to elongate the shortened side of the trunk.

- A client may have shoulder straps applied to the wheelchair to prevent falls from extreme trunk flexion. This may be viewed as a restraint, so the proper channels should be used to approve this positioning device.

- The client's knees and ankles should be flexed as close to 90 degrees as possible. The client's feet should be placed against the footrests in neutral with the entire foot supported; pronation/supination and inversion/eversion should be avoided at the ankle. Calf pads or straps behind the footrests can be used to help the client keep the feet on the footrests. Guards can be placed along the front of the footrests to prevent the client from extending the feet over the front edge of the footrest.

- The ideal upper extremity position is as follows: neutral scapular elevation/depression with slight protraction; slight shoulder flexion, abduction, and external rotation; comfortable elbow flexion supported by the armrests; forearm pronation; neutral wrist flexion/extension and ulnar/radial deviation; comfortable slight finger flexion; and thumb abduction. If the client has hemiplegia or weakness, the affected arm should be supported to prevent <u>Subluxation</u>. A lapboard may be used across the armrests of the wheelchair both as support for the upper extremities and as a surface for completing activities such as feeding or exercises. A special arm trough may be purchased or fabricated to prevent the affected arm from sliding off of the armrest. An inclined cushion may be used if the client demonstrates edema. If the client demonstrates flaccid or spastic hemiplegia, the affected hand may require a splint to prevent contractures and maintain skin integrity. See <u>Splints/orthoses</u>, <u>Cerebrovascular accident (CVA)</u>, and <u>Edema</u> for more specific instructions concerning these conditions.

- The client's head should be aligned with the trunk for safety in swallowing. The neck should be extended so that the head is upright with the chin slightly tucked. If the client is not able to hold the head upright, a headrest may be used to support the head from the back, side, or front. If a front support is needed during eating, it is beneficial if this device is detachable to make transfers easier.

Positive Behavior Support. Research-based strategies used to manage challenging behaviors and promote positive behavior. Focus includes providing a healthy supportive environment and supporting skill development.

Positive Symptoms. These symptoms are often present in a psychiatric illness such as <u>Schizophrenia</u>. Positive symptoms represent an excess or distortion of normal functions (e.g., normal suspicion becomes delusional thinking or illusions become <u>Hallucinations</u>). Other examples of positive symptoms include disorganized speech and thinking, bizarre dressing, and exaggerated postures or hand movements.

Post-Polio Syndrome. In 2006, the European Academy of Neurology came up with a common definition of post-polio syndrome, which is characterized by "new or increased muscular weakness atrophy, muscle pain and fatigue several years after acute polio" (Farbu et al., 2006, p. 975). The disorder may also result in cold intolerance and breathing difficulties. The recurrence of symptoms of polio may be linked to overuse or disuse of muscles as well as motor unit dysfunction.

Specific Interventions

- Complete aerobic exercise for strengthening, but avoid fatigue and pain.
- Train the client to use a new orthosis or power wheelchair if applicable.
- Teach the client energy conservation and work simplification techniques.
- Assist the client with establishing a diet to help lose weight and increase the client's energy level.
- Establish a time management program that alternates periods of activity with periods of rest.
- Instruct the client on <u>Stress management</u> and relaxation techniques.
- Encourage the client to join a support group for socialization and adjustment to the disease.
- Provide education on assistive devices and equipment that can increase or maintain the client's independence with <u>Self-care</u> activities.
- Modify work or leisure tasks as needed to allow the client to continue with previous responsibilities/tasks.

Contraindications/Precautions

- Avoid overexertion and fatigue since this could result in a loss of muscle strength for a duration of days.

Post-Traumatic Stress Disorder (PTSD). Mental health condition or <u>Anxiety disorder</u> as a result of an intense or terrifying experience such as war, physical/mental torture, criminal assault, rape, or natural disasters. The symptoms include recurring vivid memories of the past experience causing insomnia, recurrent nightmares, hypervigilance, and other symptoms related to anxiety. The disorder can last for many years. Interventions include <u>Stress management</u> techniques, relaxation therapies, and expressive media, which can be effective in helping the client, as well as <u>Cognitive behavioral therapy</u>, medications, and assisted animal therapy (Krause-Parello, Sarni, & Padden, 2016).

Posterior. Toward the back of the body. See <u>Anatomical position</u>.

Postrotary Nystagmus (PRN). A normal reaction of the eyes in reaction to the body being rotated in a swing. The eyeballs respond by constantly moving in a cyclical direction. PRN is assessed by therapists using sensory integrative therapy.

Postural Alignment. The coordination and integration of joints during movements to maintain neutral positions (e.g., in the wrist, elbow, shoulder, torso, and hip). When teaching correct biomechanical principles in standing, sitting, lifting, and transferring objects, consider postural alignment.

Postural Control. The ability to use righting and equilibrium adjustments to maintain balance during functional movements, such as returning to an upright position after bending down, prolonged standing in an awkward position such as in a job, or dancing. <u>Tai chi</u>, <u>Yoga</u>, and <u>Range of motion dance</u> can be modified to meet the individual's needs for improving postural control.

Postural Tone. The amount of <u>Muscle tone</u> necessary in the trunk muscles that is great enough to allow a person to remain upright against the force of gravity but low enough to permit movement such as bending, <u>Righting</u>, or <u>Equilibrium reactions</u>.

Practice Framework. See <u>Occupational Therapy Practice Framework</u>.

Prader-Willi Syndrome. A congenital condition that often results in <u>Intellectual disability</u>, short stature, inability of sexual organs to mature properly, and obesity.

Praxis. Ability to conceive and execute a motor act such as dressing, brushing one's teeth, or driving a car. The motor act is carried out in a sequential pattern of purposeful movements. A <u>Task analysis</u> can be useful in analyzing a motor activity into discrete actions, such as tying shoelaces. Individuals with brain damage such as in <u>Cerebrovascular accidents</u>

(CVA) can develop <u>Apraxia</u>. This skill may also be referred to as *motor planning*. A client who is not able to brush his or her hair even though the client's motor, sensory, and coordination abilities are intact demonstrates apraxia. See <u>Cognitive-perceptual deficits</u> for treatment and further discussion.

Preferred Provider Organizations (PPOs). Networks of health care professionals who provide services to a group health plan such as a <u>Health maintenance organization (HMO)</u>. PPOs are paid a capitation fee for each subscriber to the plan, and on that basis they provide comprehensive health care services.

Prehension. The act of bringing the thumb and fingers into contact in order to manipulate small objects.

Types of Prehension

- **Palmar Prehension.** Also referred to as the <u>Three-jaw chuck pinch</u>, this pattern combines opposition and rotation of the thumb with flexion of the index and long fingers for pad-to-pad contact of the fingers and thumb. This pattern is used when tying shoelaces or picking small objects up off of a flat surface.

- **Lateral Prehension.** This prehension pattern is composed of opposition of the thumb to the radial side of the index finger (either the middle or distal phalanx). This pattern is used when turning a key or holding a fork.

- **Tip Prehension.** This pattern combines opposition and flexion of the interphalangeal (IP) joint of the thumb with proximal interphalangeal (PIP) and distal interphalangeal (DIP) flexion of the index finger so that the tips of the distal phalanxes are touching. This pattern is used when picking up a very small object such as a hair pin or penny.

Prescriptive Exercise. Any physical activity that is planned, purposeful, and structured. It includes aerobic and anaerobic exercises, as well as isometric, isotonic, stretching, relaxation, and passive motions. In general, exercise is beneficial for almost every client and is used to meet the health needs of every individual. As part of an occupational therapy program, prescriptive exercise is goal directed; meaningful to the client; and provides sensorimotor, cognitive, and psychosocial stimulation (Wykoff, 1993). In designing a therapeutic exercise program for an individual, the therapist should consider the (a) type of exercise, such as walking, swimming, <u>Progressive relaxation</u>; (b) duration of time in doing the exercise; (c) intensity of the exercise, such as mild, moderate, or intense; (d) frequency such as daily, two to three times per week, or weekly; and (e) methods to increase compliance to the exercise schedule, such as daily monitoring and external reinforcement. To be successful, the therapist should consider the following:

- Select an exercise that is meaningful to the client.
- Incorporate the exercise into the client's everyday schedule.
- As a general target goal, have the client engage in moderate exercise for 30 to 35 minutes daily.
- Have the client keep a diary of exercise.
- Encourage the client to evaluate the effects of the exercise.
- Have the client incorporate an aerobic, relaxation, and stretching exercise in the morning or early evening.

Pressure. A technique that can be used for either facilitation or inhibition of Muscle tone. If facilitating tone, the pressure is applied with the thumb and first and second digits placed in close proximity to one another, while the therapist begins a stretch of the muscle fibers of a muscle belly. The stimulus should be applied for 3 seconds. As the Stretch occurs, the thumb will gradually move away from the first and second digits. Lotion may need to be applied to prevent heat friction. If inhibiting tone, the pressure is applied to the tendinous insertion of the muscle being inhibited (e.g., if inhibiting the biceps, then deep pressure should be applied to the inside of the elbow or the bicipital aponeurosis). A hard surface helps inhibit tone to a greater extent, which explains the technique of placing a cone in a client's hand or fabricating a hard Splint/orthosis. See Motor control problems and Rood approach for further discussion of Inhibition techniques.

Pressure Sores. Ulcers or decubiti. See Decubitus ulcer for interventions.

Prevention. Deterring a disease from occurring through lifestyle changes such as exercise, diet, Stress management, counseling, education, and social support. Primary prevention refers to the initial prevention of a disease, such as a vaccine to prevent polio. Secondary prevention refers to the recurrence of an illness, such as a second stroke. Tertiary prevention refers to secondary conditions, such as pressure sores that occur in individuals with spinal cord injuries who are confined to bed.

Prevocational Evaluation. Program to assess a client's ability to work (e.g., in a Sheltered workshop, competitive employment, or as a homemaker).

Primary Care. Initial assessment or intervention by a health care professional providing integrative and personal care using a <u>Biopsychosocial approach</u> and referring to specialists as needed.

Primary Prevention. Prevention of the initial onset of a disease (e.g., the prevention of polio with a vaccination).

Prime Mover. A muscle or group of muscles primarily responsible for a particular movement (e.g., the prime movers for elbow flexion are the biceps, brachialis, and brachioradialis).

Problem-Oriented Medical Record (POMR). Systematic method of recording progress notes in a client's chart that prioritizes the symptoms and problems and includes a plan to treat these problems. The initial notes are periodically evaluated and progress notes are recorded. <u>SOAP notes</u> are part of a problem-oriented record.

Problem Solving. Cognitive ability that entails recognizing and defining a problem, identifying alternative solutions, selecting the most feasible solution, devising a plan to implement the solution, evaluating the outcome, and readjusting the solution. Problem solving is an important task of the occupational therapist, such as in <u>Ergonomics</u> where the therapist devises a plan to prevent injury on the job, home health where the therapist helps the client to be independent in <u>Self-care</u> activities, and psychosocial rehabilitation where the client learns how to self-regulate stress. Problem solving by the client is encouraged through trial-and-error learning.

Procrustean Bed. Applying a treatment method such as a panacea to all clients, regardless of individual differences and needs (e.g., applying a treatment procedure to all clients with arthritis, as well as to all clients with cancer, without regard to the individual and specific needs of each client). In this method, the client is fitted to the treatment method rather than, in good treatment, being given the best and most effective treatment method.

Prodromal. The initial symptoms that can lead to precipitating an episode of a disease in a vulnerable individual.

Professional Standard Review Organization (PSRO). The PSROs are an outcome of the Social Security Amendment of 1972 (Public Law 92-603), which requires the setting up of PSROs to monitor health care services paid for, wholly or in part, under provisions of the Social Security Act. Each PSRO serves a specific geographic area and develops or selects its own norms of care, diagnosis, and treatment. The norms are based on typical patterns of practice in the area being served, including typical lengths of stay for institutional care by age and diagnosis.

Prognosis. Clinical forecast of the probable course of the illness and the eventual outcome of the disease or condition (e.g., the prognosis of an individual diagnosed with <u>Schizophrenia</u> will depend on the age of the initial onset, severity of symptoms, intelligence level, and environmental factors).

Progressive Relaxation. A treatment method developed by Edmund Jacobson (1929, 1978) based on systematically tensing and relaxing muscle groups in the body. The procedure involves identifying a local state of tension and relaxing it away by learning to control all of the skeletal musculature through systematic muscle tension and relaxation. In practicing progressive relaxation, the client should consider the following:

- Set aside a specific time during the day such as before dinner and about 15 to 20 minutes to practice.
- Block out distracting noises or interruptions.
- Use a firm mattress, tatami, or exercise mat.
- Have the client learn how to flex and relax individual muscles starting with the upper extremities, head and neck, and then lower extremities.
- Incorporate relaxing music into the exercise.
- As a precaution do not move muscles that are tender, strained, or produce pain. The purpose of the exercise is to gently flex and relax muscles in a progressive manner.
- Continuously have the client evaluate the benefits of the exercise.

PROM. Acronym for <u>Passive range of motion</u>.

Pronation. Rotation of hands or forearm downward or the foot/ankle inward. See <u>Anatomical position</u>.

Prone. A term that refers to the position of a client while the client lies on a horizontal surface with the stomach and front of the legs touching the supporting surface.

Proprioception. The ability to identify where body parts are in space. This is one of many components included in a sensory evaluation to test for deficits. See <u>Sensory deficits</u> for further discussion and treatment.

Proprioceptive Neuromuscular Facilitation (PNF). A traditional approach to the treatment of persons with <u>Motor control</u> problems, specifically clients who have <u>Parkinson's disease</u>, spinal cord injury, arthritis, stroke, head injury, and <u>Hand injuries</u>. This approach is based on overall muscle movement patterns rather than individual muscle contractions. Other important principles include the following: normal development proceeds in a cervicocaudal and proximodistal direction, a person's nervous system can recall reflexes to help achieve movement, and the client must practice for motor learning to occur (Kabat, 1961; Voss, 1967; Voss, Ionta, & Myers, 1985).

Proprioceptive Sensation. Receiving and interpreting stimuli originating primarily in the joints and muscles, which gives information about the position of bodily parts in space and in relation to each other (e.g., touching the nose with a forefinger with eyes closed).

Prosthesis. A device fabricated to substitute for a missing part of the body. Clients who have had parts of the body amputated may require a simple prosthesis for cosmetic reasons or a very complex, electrically powered prosthesis for completing work tasks. See Amputation for further discussion and treatment.

Protective Arm Extension. Reflexive motion where arms go out in response to a fall. See Reflexes and reactions.

Protective Reaction. A reaction of the extremities during an Equilibrium reaction. If equilibrium cannot be reestablished by the body, then the extremities will automatically abduct and/or extend to protect the body when falling. See Reflexes and reactions for further discussion.

Proximal. See Anatomical position.

Proximal Traction Response. Flexion of *all* flexor muscles of the upper extremity in response to a stretch of the flexor muscles at one joint of the upper extremity (e.g., if the elbow flexors are stretched, then all muscles of that extremity will flex, resulting in a flexor synergy). See Motor control problems and Movement therapy of Brunnstrom.

Psyche. A term that refers to the mind and its processes, such as conscious and unconscious aspects of the mind.

Psychedelic. A term popularized in the 1960s during the "hippie era" that referred to an altered state of consciousness and visual Hallucinations produced by drugs such as mescaline, psilocybin, or lysergic acid diethylamide (LSD).

Psychiatric Diagnostic Interview. An exploration of the client's symptoms and problems; past psychiatric treatments, hospitalizations, and medications; medical history of past diseases, allergies, and bodily injuries; family history of mental illness; psychosocial development, education, occupation, family relationships, friendships, and sexual experiences; mental status examination, including assessment of appearance, behavior, current mood, cognition, suicidal or homicidal thoughts; and reality testing.

Psychiatric Rehabilitation. Multidisciplinary approach with the goal of restoring function in social skills, <u>Self-care</u>, leisure, and work (Anthony, 1979). Psychiatric rehabilitation refers to restoring function in an individual with a psychiatric disability.

Psychoanalysis. A systematic method of <u>Psychotherapy</u> founded by Sigmund Freud that employs free association, dream analysis, analyses of transference, and other <u>Psychodynamic</u> techniques to help an individual understand the unconscious feelings and desires that shape his or her personality and behavior.

Psychodrama. A form of group <u>Psychotherapy</u> in which clients act out assigned roles. The therapeutic goals are to reduce emotional symptoms and encourage personal growth. The psychodrama includes a protagonist who is the center of the drama, alter egos who help the protagonist to think through identified issues, a director who sets the stage and scenes, and an audience who comment on the actions and give insight to the protagonist.

Psychodynamic. Refers to the understanding of the conscious and unconscious forces that motivate behavior, cause symptoms, and shape one's personality. Psychotherapists such as psychoanalysts use a psychodynamic approach in treating individuals with mental disorders.

Psychoeducational. In this approach, the therapist uses educational technology such as lecture, discussion, seminars, handouts, <u>Role playing</u>, and videotapes in teaching clients how to deal more effectively with their illness (e.g., the therapist using a <u>Group therapy</u> format can help clients with arthritis to learn energy conservation methods, ergonomics, mechanics of lifting, and methods to reduce stress). This approach has been effective with clients with <u>Depression</u>, <u>Low back pain (LBP)</u>, and stroke. The therapist designs the group by:

- Developing specific objectives for the clients, such as learn relaxation techniques
- Organizing a time schedule for group, such as nine sessions once per week for 1 hour
- Identifying course content, such as demonstrating and practice with heart rate <u>Biofeedback</u> to increase relaxation or providing a film on nutrition
- Setting up homework assignments for clients to practice skills or an exercise program
- Having the client keep a diary of symptoms and progress of improvement
- Having closure activity and follow-up recommendations

Psychomotor Agitation. Describes the state of a client who is in constant motion with severe restlessness, pacing, wringing of hands, and purposeless activity accompanied by a high level of <u>Anxiety</u>.

Psychoneuroimmunology. Study of the relationships and interactions between the mind, central nervous system, autonomic nervous system, and endocrine system. It represents the effects of psychological states on the immune system. It has been found in some studies that extreme <u>Stress reactions</u> can dampen the immune system and leave the individual vulnerable to disease.

Psychopathic. Antisocial behavior such as violence, criminal activity, physical or sexual abuse, or related behaviors that reflect a lack of moral and ethical standards. Synonymous terms are *sociopathic* and *antisocial reaction*.

Psychosis. A severe mental disorder characterized by <u>Delusions</u>, <u>Hallucinations</u>, thinking disturbances, and inability to perform <u>Activities of daily living (ADLs)</u> as occurs in <u>Schizophrenia</u>, extreme <u>Depression</u>, dementia, and chronic alcoholism.

Psychosocial Skills and Psychological Components. Terms used in the old <u>Uniform Terminology</u> to include individual's abilities and characteristics to engage and interact in society and to express and control emotions. These include psychological <u>Values</u>, <u>Interests</u>, and <u>Self-concept</u>; social <u>Role performance</u>, conduct, <u>Interpersonal skills</u>, <u>Self-expression</u>, and management of <u>Coping skills</u>; temporal planning; and <u>Self-control</u>.

Psychosomatic Medicine. The study of the relationship of psychological factors and the etiology of physical and psychiatric disorders. Current investigators in psychosomatic medicine examine both the physical and psychological factors as causes and effects and treat mind and body as one.

Psychotherapy. Method of treating individuals with mental illnesses through verbal means. It originated from Sigmund Freud's work on <u>Psychoanalysis</u> and was called the "talking cure." The various schools of psychotherapy include psychoanalytic, <u>Client-centered</u>, <u>Rational-emotive</u>, cognitive, <u>Cognitive behavioral</u>, Adlerian, Jungian, behavior modification, <u>Transactional analysis (TA)</u>, and <u>Psychodrama</u>. Within these models there are many more frames of reference in psychotherapy. As a treatment technique, it relies primarily on the verbal interactions between the therapist and client. The methods used in psychotherapy vary considerably depending on the theoretical model espoused by the therapist. In general, the phases in psychotherapy include:

- Establishing rapport and a therapeutic alliance with the client
- Understanding the client's problems and making a tentative diagnosis
- Helping the client to understand and gain insight into the causes of his or her problems
- Setting goals for treatment that are mutually acceptable by the therapist and client
- Implementing treatment where the client learns and tests out new behaviors
- Closure and discharge of the client

Ptosis. A condition in which the upper eyelid droops.

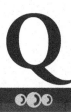

Quadriplegia. Paralysis of all four extremities.

Quadruped. The position referred to by Rood when a client is bearing weight on all four extremities with shoulders flexed with elbows extended and hips and knees flexed. See <u>Motor control</u> problems and <u>Rood approach</u> for further discussion and treatment.

Quality Assurance. A system to measure the effectiveness of a hospital or treatment facility to meet standards of care established by governmental agencies or hospital associations. A quality assurance program in a hospital includes an evaluation component to identify problems and an action component to improve client care.

Quality of Life. According to the Centers for Disease Control (2016), health-related quality of life for the individual includes personal perception of physical and mental health, including factors such as personal health (risks and conditions), functional status, social support, and socioeconomic status.

Stein, F., & Haertl, K.
Pocket Guide to Intervention in Occupational Therapy, Second Edition (p 229).
© 2019 Taylor & Francis Group.

R

Raimiste's Phenomenon. A term used for a specific associated reaction when resistance against hip abduction or adduction in the noninvolved lower extremity elicits the same motion in the involved extremity. See <u>Motor control</u> problems.

Range of Motion (ROM). The amount of movement available at a joint. A client must have a functional ROM in order to complete most functional activities; therefore, ROM may be included in a client's plan of treatment as an adjunctive treatment to help increase the client's independence with daily activities. The therapist should measure ROM if a client demonstrates impairment to help monitor and document progress during treatment. The therapist uses a goniometer to measure the number of degrees available at a joint.

Methods of Measurement

- When measuring the range of most joints, the 180-degree system is used. The starting point of the joint motion (which begins from <u>Anatomical position</u>) is 0 degrees, and the degrees increase toward 180 as the motion continues. When documenting measurements, the degrees for extension and flexion are written together as a range. If using the neutral-zero method when measuring an impaired joint, then the number of degrees for the joint range is written as "extension limitation: 15 to 140 degrees" or "flexion limitation: 0 to 100 degrees." If hyperextension occurs at the joint, past the expected starting point, then that range is written separately as "hyperextension: 0 to 20 degrees."

- Many therapists document the limitations using a different method. An impairment in extension is measured as the number of degrees the joint lacks from the starting position, or it could be written as

Stein, F., & Haertl, K.
Pocket Guide to Intervention in Occupational Therapy, Second Edition (pp 231-250).
© 2019 Taylor & Francis Group.

15 or as "-15 degrees." *Flexion* is written as the number of degrees from the starting position, or "100 degrees." *Hyperextension* may be measured and stated as the number of degrees the joint has in addition to the normal range, or "+20 degrees." Thus, a client who is able to hyperextend at the metacarpophalangeal joints (MCPs) may receive a range of "+20 to 90 degrees," which denotes the range's starting and ending points. A therapist should check his or her facility's requirements for documenting ROM, as methods can vary. Motion can be measured during active movement through the range, or while the therapist passively moves the joint through the range. When possible, the therapist should compare limited ROM in a joint to the corresponding joint of the unaffected extremity. If this is not possible, the therapist should refer to a chart of average ranges, which can be found in <u>Appendix F</u>.

Types

- **Active Range of Motion.** The amount of movement at a joint when the client actively contracts appropriate muscles acting on that joint. The acronym commonly used is AROM. When possible, the therapist should compare limited ROM in a joint to the corresponding joint of the unaffected extremity. If this is not possible, the therapist should refer to a chart of average ranges, which can be found in <u>Appendix F</u>.

- **Passive Range of Motion.** The amount of movement at a joint when the joint is moved through its range by an outside force, rather than by the muscles that act on that joint. The acronym commonly used is PROM. A therapist often passively moves body parts through the range to help prevent stiffness and contractures when the muscles are too weak.

General Procedures for Testing

- The client is seated comfortably. The joint to be measured is exposed so that bony landmarks and muscle contraction can be observed.

- The therapist should passively move the joint through its range to estimate the available ROM. The joint should be returned to its starting position.

- The therapist should place the goniometer with the stationary arm on the stationary part of the joint and the movable arm on the moving part. Bony landmarks should be identified and used to help find proper placement for the axis. The joint should be measured at the starting position, and the goniometer should then be removed from the joint. The client should actively move the joint as far as possible toward the ending point of motion, or the therapist should passively move the joint through its range, without force, toward the ending point. The goniometer should be placed again and the joint should be measured at the ending position.

- If the client is unable to reach the estimated ROM (PROM), then muscle weakness is limiting AROM. If AROM = PROM but PROM is not equal to the unaffected extremity or average ranges, then joint limitation exists and PROM should also be measured. In the interest of time, if limitations in PROM are observed during the beginning estimation of ROM (prior to AROM), measurements for PROM can be taken at that time. If PROM or AROM are comparable from one arm to the other or to average ranges, then ROM can be recorded "within normal limits," and measurements do not need to be taken.

Functional Range of Motion Testing

The therapist may use this abbreviated version of testing to screen the client. If the client demonstrates deficits, then the entire test should be given.

Procedure

The client should be seated upright while the therapist asks the client to complete the following motions. The therapist may demonstrate the motions if needed.

- Trunk flexion/extension: "Please reach down to your toes and then come back up."
- Trunk lateral flexion: "Please reach down to the floor to the left side of your chair with your left hand and to the right side of your chair with your right hand."
- Shoulder flexion: "Raise your arms up in front of you as high as you can."
- Shoulder external rotation: "Place your hands behind your head or neck."
- Shoulder internal rotation: "Place your hands behind your back."
- Shoulder abduction: "Raise your arms up and out to the side of you as high as you can."
- Supination/pronation: "Turn your palms up toward the ceiling and then down toward the floor."

- Elbow flexion/extension: "Bend your elbows to touch your shoulders and then straighten them."
- Wrist flexion/extension: "Bend your wrist up and down."
- Radial/ulnar deviation: "Bend your hands out toward your small finger and then in toward your thumb."
- Finger flexion/extension: "Make a tight fist with each hand and then straighten your fingers."
- Thumb opposition: "Touch the tip of each finger to the tip of your thumb."

The therapist should use this abbreviated test only if he or she knows and understands the full AROM test.

Contraindications/Precautions

- Joint motion should not be measured or completed in the presence of the following conditions: myositis ossificans, joint dislocation, surgery or repair to any soft tissue surrounding the joint, or fractures that are not completely healed.
- Precautions should be used if the client has osteoporosis, a Subluxation, inflammation at the joint, joint laxity, hemophilia, or hematoma, or if the client takes muscle relaxants or pain medication.
- When the therapist is unable to compare to the noninvolved extremity, refer to Appendix F for average ranges of motion.

Specific Interventions

- **Active Assistive Range of Motion.** This technique is used when a client does not have enough muscle strength to move a joint through its available ROM. The therapist should hold the affected extremity near the joint being moved, with one hand stabilizing the joint and the other holding the moving part. As the client actively attempts to move the body part, the therapist should only assist when needed. This technique is also referred to as *active-assisted range of motion*, and the acronym listed in the client's chart is A/AROM. Activities should emphasize meaningful occupation.
- ROM arc: The client slides rings up and over a large arc and moves toward meaningful occupational activities.
- Bean bag activities: The client slides the bags off a large table to either side or forward, or tosses the bags into a bucket placed at a distance. The activity can be progressed to a bean bag game.

- Clothespins: The client places clothespins as high as possible onto a vertical rod, which is taller than the client's highest reach, and works toward the ability to use a clothesline and other functional activities.

- ROM exercises/dowel or broomstick exercises: The client can complete motions unassisted and actively, or the client can use a dowel, broomstick, or towel to allow the unaffected extremity to assist the affected extremity through increased range in preparation for daily functional activities.

- Reaching for items above the head

- Playing catch

- Washing tables with a wet rag

- Wiping vertical surfaces such as mirrors or walls

- Skateboard: The client places the affected upper extremity on a skateboard to go from one side to the other or forward and back on the surface of a table.

- Pulleys: The unaffected upper extremity can assist the affected upper extremity in reaching full shoulder flexion; in the same manner, the upper extremity bicycle allows the unaffected upper extremity to assist the affected upper extremity with elbow flexion and extension.

- Ring tree: The client may use one or both extremities to retrieve one ring at a time from a horizontal rod on one side of the "tree" and move it to a horizontal rod on the other side of the "tree."

- Finger ladder: The client uses the fingers to inch up a small ladder on the wall (or can simply walk against the surface of the wall) to help assist shoulder flexion.

- Balloon volleyball

- Large tabletop board games like giant checkers

- <u>ROM dance</u> program

- Note: The emphasis for all ROM activities should be occupational and meaningful.

Range of Motion Dance (ROM Dance). A movement therapy described by Van Deusen and Harlowe (1987) composed of expressive dance and relaxation techniques. It incorporates joint motion in all ranges to help individuals with joint and muscle limitations. It is also an educational process that assists individuals in improving movement through hands-on patterning and verbal instruction.

Rational-Emotive Therapy (RET). A direct <u>Psychotherapy</u> technique originated by Albert Ellis (Ellis & Whiteley, 1979) that helps the client to problem solve by working through solutions and stating the options. The therapist frequently confronts the client with the consequences of his or her behavior and assigns homework problems for the client to try out new behaviors.

Reactive Attachment Disorder (RAD). The DSM-5 (American Psychiatric Association, 2013) involves criteria including (a) a pattern of emotionally withdrawn behavior toward adults/caregivers, (b) a persistent social/emotional/behavioral disturbance, (c) historical past of insufficient care by caregivers, which are presumed to cause the behavioral disturbance, (d) the criteria are not due to <u>Autism</u>, (e) the disturbance begins before 5 years of age, and (f) the child has a developmental age of at least 9 months. Early intervention for children with RAD often includes parental education; addressing any developmental, social, and behavioral difficulties; and occupational- and sensory-based interventions.

Reality Orientation. Treatment that assists confused clients in understanding the current situation. For example, during a treatment group, the therapist may have each client give his or her name, the date, or the situation that brought the client to the hospital. Discussion between the members of the group may help orient the client to reality in a less threatening manner than if the therapist completes orientation. If the client is being treated individually, the therapist may have a memory board posted that the client uses each day to recite the time and place. The therapist may then discuss the client's situation and other personal items of concern. See <u>Cognitive-perceptual deficits</u> for further discussion and treatment.

Reality Therapy. A <u>Psychotherapy</u> technique introduced by Glasser (1965) that focuses on helping the client take responsibility for his or her behavior and confront problems directly.

Rebound Phenomenon of Holmes. Inability to control movements so that a contraction can be stopped quickly in order to avoid hitting an object. A client who demonstrates this deficit will hit him- or herself in the face or arm if the client is flexing the elbow against the therapist's resistance and the resistance is quickly withdrawn without warning the client.

Recognition. The cognitive ability to identify familiar faces and objects. It is based on the individual's ability to retrieve memory. Activities to aid memory include cue cards, use of compensatory techniques, and <u>Assistive technology</u>.

Reductionism. Reducing complex situations, data, phenomena, and experiences to simple terms. An example is treating major <u>Depression</u>, a complex illness that affects an individual's ability to <u>Work</u>, socialize with others, engage in <u>Leisure</u> activities, and regulate one's <u>Self-care</u>, by taking a drug to relieve symptoms. A holistic approach is in contrast to reductionist treatment.

Reflex. An involuntary muscle response to sensory stimuli. Some reflexes occur during infancy and disappear later (e.g., the <u>Asymmetrical tonic neck reflex (ATNR)</u>, <u>Moro reflex</u>, <u>Neck righting</u>, rooting, stepping, and sucking). Other reflexes are purposeful in the adult, such as flexor withdrawal, postural proprioception, and pupillary.

Reflex Sympathetic Dystrophy (RSD)/Complex Regional Pain Syndrome (CRPS). Also known as *causalgia*, RSD/CRPS are denoted by a compilation of symptoms, including complex chronic pain that often starts in the hands, legs, or feet; tenderness; possible swelling; and other symptoms. The syndrome may occur following an injury to a nerve or tissue in the affected area. Rest and time may only make it worse.

Symptoms in the affected area are:
- Dramatic changes in skin temperature, color, or texture
- Intense burning pain
- Extreme skin sensitivity
- Swelling and stiffness in affected joints
- Decreased ability to move the affected body part

This disorder results in pain, edema, and sympathetic nervous system dysfunction that is much worse than expected from the client's original condition (such as nerve injury). The exact cause is unknown; however, the syndrome often occurs following trauma, nerve injury, or a central nervous system disorder. This disorder may be classified into the following types of RSD:
- Shoulder–hand syndrome
- Causalgia
- Neurovascular dystrophy
- Sudeck's atrophy
- Idiopathic peripheral autonomic <u>Neuropathy</u>
- Post-traumatic dystrophy
- Algodystrophy

Onset most often occurs between 45 and 65 years of age, and this disorder is more common in women. Intervention techniques often focus on education, stress loading (involving compression activities), scrubbing, <u>Graded motor imagery</u>, and working toward tolerance of normal occupational activities.

Reflexes and Reactions. As an infant, sensory stimulation can evoke automatic movements. As motor development occurs, these automatic movements become integrated by the central nervous system (CNS). CNS integration allows a person to move voluntarily rather than being governed by those automatic movements. However, if a person sustains a brain injury, the person may revert to automatic movements based on the location of brain insult. Mathiowitz and Bass-Haugen (1994) listed the following locations of integration for some of the reflexes and reactions.

Locations of Integration

- **Spinal Level.** <u>Extensor thrust</u>, flexor withdrawal, crossed extension, negative supporting reaction, <u>Grasp</u>, and cutaneous fusimotor reflexes
- **Brainstem Level.** <u>Tonic labyrinthine reflex</u>, tonic neck reflexes, <u>Tonic lumbar reflexes</u>, and associated reactions (Mathiowitz and Bass-Haugen [1994] also placed positive supporting reaction in this category)
- **Midbrain/Cortical Level.** <u>Body on body righting</u>, body and head righting, <u>Labyrinthine righting</u>, <u>Neck righting</u>, <u>Optical righting</u>, protective extension, and <u>Equilibrium reactions</u>
- **Cortical Level.** Higher-level voluntary movement

Following is a list of reflexes and reactions that can be observed as <u>Developmental milestones</u> in children, but some of them may also be demonstrated by a person who has had a stroke or other insult to the brain. The general time for integration is listed to help the therapist determine if a child is delayed in development. A diagnosis of delay should not be based solely on the integration of reflexes and reactions, but to measure a child's performance in order to determine the performance in comparison to norms.

Developmental Reflexes

- **Oral Reflexes**
  - ○ **Rooting.** When a child's skin is stroked at the corner of the mouth, the child turns his or her head toward the side being stimulated. This reflex begins at birth, and integration occurs between 2 and 3 months of age.

- ○ **Suck-Swallow.** When liquid is presented to a child, the child sucks and reflexively swallows. This reflex begins at birth, and integration occurs around 4 months of age.

- ○ **Bite.** When a child's gums are touched with an object, the child bites down on the object. This reflex begins near 4 months of age, and integration occurs around 7 months of age.

- ○ **Gag.** When pressure is applied on the middle to back of the child's tongue, the child grimaces, constricts the pharynx, and thrusts the tongue. This reflex begins at birth, and it exists throughout the lifespan. As a child, the reflex occurs more forward on the tongue and moves back as a person gets older.

- ○ **Palatal.** When the faucial arches are stroked, the arches constrict and the uvula elevates. This reflex begins at birth and exists throughout the lifespan. It helps protect a person's airway and produce swallowing.

- **Moro Reflex.** A child is held in supine and the child's head is allowed to suddenly drop backward 20 to 30 degrees. The head is then supported again. The response to the stimulus will first be abduction and extension of the child's arms, followed by flexion, adduction, and crossing of the arms across the body. This reflex begins at birth, and integration occurs around 5 to 6 months of age.

- **Palmar Grasp Reflex.** When an adult places a finger (or object) into a child's palm from the ulnar side, the fingers flex and grasp the adult's finger. This reflex begins at birth, and integration occurs around 2 months of age.

- **Plantar Grasp Reflex.** When an adult places pressure on the sole of a child's foot, the toes flex around the adult's hand (or object being used). This reflex begins at birth, and integration occurs around 12 months of age.

- **Positive Supporting Reaction.** When a child is positioned with the ball of the foot in contact with a surface, the leg will extend and bear some weight. This reflex begins at birth, and integration occurs around 6 months of age. If a client exhibits this reflex following a brain injury, he or she will have difficulty with ambulation and transfers since the affected leg will want to rigidly extend whenever it contacts a surface.

- **Automatic Stepping.** When a child is held in a slightly forward position so that the soles of both feet are in firm contact with a surface, the legs will make rhythmical and alternating stepping movements. This reflex begins at birth, and integration occurs around 2 months of age.

- **Placing Reflex or Placing Reaction.** When a child's palm comes into contact with a hard surface, the client will bear weight on that extremity. This reflex begins at birth, and integration occurs around 2 months of age.

- **Tonic Neck Reflex.** A brainstem-level reflex present early in life but may return due to a brain injury. A child or client demonstrates this reflex when the position of the person's neck affects the person's limbs. This reflex has been further subdivided into an asymmetrical tonic neck reflex and a symmetrical tonic neck reflex.

  ○ **Asymmetrical Tonic Neck Reflex.** When a child's head is turned 90 degrees to one side, he or she extends the upper extremity nearest the face and flexes the upper extremity nearest the back of the head. This reflex is present at birth, and integration occurs around 4 to 6 months of age. A client who has had a brain injury may also exhibit this reflex. When a client's head is turned 90 degrees to one side, he or she demonstrates an increase in extensor tone of the upper extremity nearest the face and an increase in flexor tone of the upper extremity nearest the back of the head. If a client exhibits this reflex, he or she will have difficulty moving the affected arm voluntarily since movement will be dependent on his or her head position.

  ○ **Symmetrical Tonic Neck Reflex.** When a child's head is flexed, the child demonstrates flexion of the arms and extension of the legs. Likewise, when the child's head is extended, the child demonstrates extension of the arms and flexion of the legs. This reflex is present at birth, and integration occurs around 4 to 6 months of age. If a client who has had a brain injury exhibits this reflex, he or she will have difficulty transferring from sitting to standing since his or her legs will extend when the head flexes.

- **Tonic Lumbar Reflex.** When a child's chest is rotated to the right, the child flexes the right upper extremity and extends the right lower extremity. Simultaneously, the left upper extremity extends and the left lower extremity flexes. This reflex is present at birth, and integration occurs at 4 to 6 months of age. A client who had a brain injury may have difficulty voluntarily controlling the affected extremities if this reflex is present.

- **Landau Reflex.** When a child is supported at the stomach while in prone, the hips, back, and neck extend. This reflex begins to form at birth but is not complete until 6 months of age. Integration occurs at 10 to 12 months of age.

- **Galant Reflex.** When the child is stroked along one side of the vertebrae, the spine will flex or curve toward the side being stimulated. This reflex begins at birth.

- **Crossed Extension.** When a child is in supine, one leg begins in extension while the other is in flexion. As the extended leg is flexed, the flexed leg will extend, adduct, and internally rotate. This reflex begins at birth, and integration occurs around 2 months of age. If a client exhibits this reflex, he or she will have difficulty with ambulation since abnormal extension will occur in the affected leg when the unaffected leg is flexing.

- **Flexor Withdrawal.** When the sole of a child's foot is tickled or pricked, the leg receiving the stimulus will flex to withdraw from the stimulus. This reflex begins at birth, and integration occurs around 2 months of age.

- **Extensor Thrust.** The child begins with one leg flexed. When the sole of the foot of the flexed leg is stroked, the leg extends. This reflex begins at birth, and integration occurs around 2 months of age.

- **Tonic Labyrinthine Reflexes.** This brainstem-level reflex is present early in life but may return due to a brain injury. A client demonstrates this reflex when the position of the client's trunk influences movement. This reflex can be subdivided into a *tonic labyrinthine supine reflex* and a *tonic labyrinthine prone reflex*. If a client exhibits this reflex, he or she will have difficulty going from supine to sitting. Extensor tone will make trunk flexion difficult at first. Then, as forward movement occurs, flexor tone will increase and put the client at risk for falling forward off the bed.

  - **Tonic Labyrinthine Supine Reflex.** When a child is placed in supine (the neck is usually flexed), both upper and lower extremities extend. This reflex begins at birth, and integration occurs around 4 months of age.

  - **Tonic Labyrinthine Prone Reflex.** When a child is placed prone (the neck is usually extended), both upper and lower extremities flex. This reflex begins at birth, and integration occurs around 4 months of age.

- **Grasp Reflex.** The application of deep pressure (of the therapist's hand) to the child's palm results in digit flexion and adduction, or a closing of the fist. This is also referred to as <u>Palmar grasp reflex</u> (see earlier). The client will not be able to open his or her hand, even if able to actively extend the fingers of the affected hand. This reflex is used to elicit movement when treating with the <u>Brunnstrom approach</u>. See <u>Motor control</u> problems.

- **Babkin Reflex.** When pressure is applied to a child's palms, the child's mouth opens. This reflex begins at birth, and integration occurs around 4 months of age.

- **Babinski Reflex.** A stimulus (such as a light stroke) is presented to the plantar surface of the foot, which results in <u>Dorsiflexion</u> of the great toe. This reflex occurs when the upper motor neuron tracts of the spinal cord are interrupted before reaching the lumbosacral reflex center. This reflex may be demonstrated by a client who has had a stroke, spinal cord injury, or <u>Multiple sclerosis (MS)</u>.

- **Finger Extension.** When the child's ulnar border of the hand is stroked, the fingers extend and the hand opens.

- **Deep Tendon Reflexes.** Reaction of the tendons of specific muscles to a tap resulting in a slight and quick jerk (e.g., the test for the quadriceps is completed by the physician tapping on the tendon distal to the patella, resulting in a knee jerk). Other commonly tested tendons include the biceps brachii, brachioradialis, triceps brachii, and gastrocnemius-soleus. Deep tendon reflexes are tested to help check for symptoms of <u>Upper motor neuron disorders</u>.

- **Associated Reactions.** When voluntary movement in a child's limb is resisted, the opposite limb moves involuntarily (e.g., if the therapist resists shoulder flexion with the left upper extremity, the right upper extremity will flex at the shoulder). This reflex begins at birth, and integration occurs between 8 and 9 years of age.

Developmental Reactions

- **Optical Righting.** When a child is tilted so that the body is no longer vertical, the head will right itself so that it remains vertical. This reaction begins around 2 months of age, and it continues throughout the lifespan.

- **Labyrinthine Righting.** When a child is tilted so that the body is no longer vertical, the head will right itself to the vertical position, even though the client's eyes are covered so that visual cues cannot be used to orient the head. This reaction begins around 2 months of age, and it continues throughout the lifespan.

- **Neck Righting.** When a child's head is turned to one side, the body rolls to that same side at the same time. The head and body cannot roll separately from one another, so the client "log-rolls." This reaction begins at birth, and integration occurs around 6 months of age.

- **Body Righting on Body.** When a child's head is turned to one side, the body is able to roll segmentally. The upper trunk rolls first, and the pelvis and lower extremities follow. This reflex may also be referred to as *body-on-body righting*. This reaction begins at 6 months of age, and integration occurs around 18 months of age.

- **Body Righting on Head.** When a part of the body is touching a supporting surface, the head adjusts to a vertical position. For example, when a child is lying prone, the neck flexes so that the head is lifted to between 45 and 90 degrees vertical. Likewise, when a child is lying supine, the neck extends to lift the head. This reaction begins at 1 to 2 months of age when the child is prone, and 5 to 6 months of age when the child is supine.

- **Protective Arm Extension.** A reaction of the extremities during an equilibrium reaction. If equilibrium cannot be reestablished by the body, then the extremities will automatically abduct and/or extend to protect the body when falling. Protective arm extension occurs in a forward direction, lateral direction, and backward direction. This reaction begins at 6 months of age for both forward and lateral extension, but it is not present in the backward direction until 9 months of age. It continues throughout the lifespan.

- **Equilibrium Reactions.** A reaction of the body to shift its center of gravity to maintain balance when a supporting surface is moved. During the equilibrium reaction, <u>Righting</u> of the head and upper trunk can be observed, as well as <u>Protective reactions</u> of extremities. A child learns to use equilibrium reactions while in prone, supine, <u>Quadruped</u>, sitting, and standing positions. These reactions begin between 6 and 21 months of age, and they continue throughout the lifespan.

Reflexology. The application of massage to reflex points on the feet and hands to encourage health and well-being.

Regression. Relapse or exacerbation of symptoms in which an individual's illness gets worse (e.g., an individual who is making improvement from an episode of <u>Depression</u> suddenly regresses with exaggerated feelings of suicide).

Rehabilitation. The restoration of function in an individual with an acquired disability. Function relates to competence in an individual's ability to work; to be independent in <u>Self-care</u>, <u>Work</u>, and <u>Leisure</u> activities; and to have the social skills for effective personal interactions.

Reinforcement Schedule. The method of reinforcing a client's behavior. This can be on a ratio or interval schedule to help a client to learn or maintain a task or behavior. In a ratio schedule, a client is reinforced for completion of a specific task (e.g., tying a shoelace or demonstrating positive interactions). In an interval schedule, the client is reinforced for appropriate behavior based on a time interval, such as every 15 or 30 minutes.

Relaxation Response. An intervention method created by Herbert Benson (1975) based originally on transcendental meditation. In this method, the client is taught to have a passive attitude and to recite a verbal phrase to him- or herself while in a comfortable position. The physiological reaction that is sought is produced by sitting serenely and alone in a quiet place with eyes closed and arms and hands relaxed, paying careful attention to breathing, and repeating a brief word or phrase at each respiratory cycle. The aim is to reach a tranquil mental state that refreshes the mind and body. It is recommended that the client practice the technique every day and to incorporate it into his or her schedule.

Relaxation Therapy. Techniques that help an individual to reduce bodily tension, <u>Anxiety</u>, heart rate, blood pressure, and overall sympathetic responses that occur when an individual is overaroused. In designing a relaxation program, the therapist should consider the following:

- The purposes of the program, such as reducing the individual's anxiety so that he or she will be better able to work, engage in leisure activities, or be independent in <u>Self-care</u>
- The context of the therapy, such as group or individual sessions, number and length of sessions, and environment where sessions will take place
- The specific therapies used, such as <u>Relaxation response</u>, <u>Progressive relaxation</u>, <u>Visualization</u>, or meditation
- The evaluation of the relaxation experience through client evaluation, standardized test, or physiological measure

Remission. The lessening of symptoms or complete recovery from an illness (e.g., in an individual diagnosed with <u>Schizophrenia</u>, the symptoms of <u>Hallucinations</u> and <u>Delusions</u> may disappear and the individual is able to work and engage in normal activities). Individuals may be in remission for weeks, months, or years.

Repetitive Strain/Repetitive Stress Injury. Refers to painful conditions of the muscles and tendons that may be caused by occupations that require repetitive tasks. Initial interventions include rest, ice, compression, and elevation of the affected joint. Taping and wraps may be helpful to align the joint. Adaptation of the job involving frequent rest breaks and job rotation may also help.

Resting Tremor. Tremor that occurs when the muscles are relaxed; it is often associated with <u>Parkinson's disease</u>. See <u>Tremor</u>.

Retrograde Massage. A technique used to help reduce and control edema. See <u>Edema</u> for further discussion and treatment method.

Rett Syndrome. A genetic developmental disorder usually in girls about 6 to 18 months of age that progresses from impaired hand function to <u>Ataxia</u>, autistic characteristics, intellectual disability, language problems, and dementia.

Reversal of Antagonists. A technique that was originally used by Voss (1967) during treatment within the framework of proprioceptive neuromuscular facilitation. The supporting theory states that a stronger antagonist can help facilitate a weaker agonist. Resistance is given to the antagonist to help promote contraction of the agonist. Three specific techniques include slow reversal, slow reversal-hold, and rhythmic stabilization. See <u>Motor control</u> problems and <u>Proprioceptive neuromuscular facilitation (PNF)</u> for more discussion of these techniques. Slow reversal techniques include an <u>Isotonic contraction</u> of the agonist followed by an isotonic contraction of the antagonist. The slow reversal-hold includes an isotonic contraction of the agonist followed by an <u>Isometric contraction</u>. All may employ a quick stretch to facilitate muscular activity.

Reye's Syndrome. A condition that occurs after a client has contracted a virus. Symptoms begin with vomiting and can proceed to cognitive impairments such as disorientation, lethargy, and possibly a coma. Death can also occur from edema of the brain that may cause cerebral herniation.

Rheumatoid Arthritis. A systemic and autoimmune disease that results in inflammation of the joints (especially the synovial lining) that can destroy surrounding joint structures. Rheumatoid arthritis occurs in remissions and exacerbations. Symptoms include pain, morning stiffness, fatigue, muscle wasting, anemia, and decreased movement of the affected joints. The cause is generally unknown but is probably due to genetic and environmental factors that make a person more vulnerable to developing the illness. Onset usually occurs between 25 and 50 years of age. Ekelman, Hooker, Davis, Newburn, and Ricchino (2014) appraised six systematic reviews and found evidence to support the use of patient education; therapeutic exercise; and splinting for pain, inflammation, and grip strength. The following are possible interventions.

Specific Interventions

- Complete activities to maintain range of motion, strength, and endurance.
- Fabricate splints to prevent deformity: a resting hand <u>Splint/orthosis</u> or a splint to prevent ulnar deviation is indicated for a person with this diagnosis.
- Recommend the use of knee extension splints at night.
- Instruct the client on <u>Pain management</u> techniques.
- Educate the client on the importance of avoiding fatigue or overexertion.
- Teach the client to use energy conservation, work simplification, and especially joint protection principles during activities.
- Encourage the client to join a support group to assist with emotional adjustment to the disease.
- Provide education on assistive devices to increase the client's independence with <u>Self-care</u> activities as needed.
- Complete a home evaluation and give recommendations to improve the client's mobility in the home, as well as ability to continue functional tasks such as laundry or cooking.
- Help the client modify <u>Leisure</u> activities as needed or explore new leisure interests.

Contraindications/Precautions

- Stress the importance of compliance with joint protection, energy conservation, and work simplification principles to prevent deformity.
- Monitor for skin breakdown from splints.
- Avoid overexertion.
- Monitor for symptoms of <u>Carpal tunnel syndrome</u>.

RHUMBA. An acronym for **R**elevant, **H**ow long, **U**nderstandable, **M**easurable, **B**ehavioral, and **A**chievable. It is used as a guide in writing operational occupational-based goals for clients. In order to achieve <u>Client-centered therapy</u>, it is important the client have input into the goal area.

Right/Left Discrimination. The perceptual process or ability to differentiate between the right and left sides of the body. Individuals with <u>Learning disabilities</u> can have difficulty with this skill. See <u>Cognitive-perceptual deficits</u> for further discussion and treatment.

Righting Reaction. A reaction of the body to gain normal alignment between the head and trunk or extremities, or to position the head in its normal upright position in space so that the head is vertical and the mouth is horizontal. For specific reactions, see <u>Reflexes and reactions</u>.

Rigidity. <u>Hypertonicity</u> of both agonist and antagonist muscles so that resistance to passive movement can be felt in any direction or at any point in the range of motion.

Types of Rigidity

- **Cogwheel Rigidity.** Characterized by a rhythmic relaxation and contraction of muscles during passive movement. When moving a body part with cogwheel rigidity, the part may be difficult to move at first, but then both agonist and antagonist muscles will relax so that movement is easier. However, the muscle <u>Co-contraction</u> will again occur, making movement difficult. This contracting and relaxing will occur many times while the therapist moves the part through its range of motion so that movement feels like it keeps "catching."

- **Lead Pipe Rigidity.** Characterized by *constant* resistance to movement in any direction with no relaxation of the agonist or antagonist muscles occurring. This hypertonicity is uniform so that the same resistance is felt at any point in the affected joint's range of motion.

Rocking. Rocking has multiple definitions, as it may be used in sensory strategies and/or a client may self-stimulate with rocking to provide vestibular input. Rocking is also referred to as a technique used to either facilitate or inhibit <u>Muscle tone</u>. If completed in a fast manner, rocking produces vestibular stimulation, which helps facilitate tone. If completed in a slow manner, rocking helps inhibit tone so that a spastic muscle relaxes through a wider range of motion. See <u>Motor control</u> problems and <u>Rood approach</u> for further discussion of <u>Facilitation</u> and <u>Inhibition techniques</u>. Rocking behavior is also noticeable in individuals with a diagnosis of <u>Autism</u> and may indicate vestibular seeking behavior.

Role Performance. Roles are socially constructed and relate to behavioral expectations within specific roles (Bonsaksen & Kvarsnes, 2016). Roles involve a social component that includes the individual's position in a family, job, culture, nation, or religion. These role functions may include family roles (e.g., husband/wife) vocational title or job (e.g., nurse), and societal roles such as friend or volunteer. Role functions are gained through education and social and family expectations. Role performance is key in the <u>Model of Human Occupation (MOHO)</u> frame of reference (Kielhofner, 2008). Throughout one's life, role functions are assumed and changed. Occupational therapists can help clients gain insight into their various role performances and develop new roles (e.g., volunteering, changing jobs, becoming a better parent). Use of role <u>Performance tests</u>, counseling, and <u>Role playing</u> are used to assist the client.

Role Playing. Simulation of family, work, social, interpersonal, or community situations. The client portrays roles in previous situations (e.g., conflicts) and in future situations (e.g., applying for a job). The therapist provides a supportive environment and coaching to help the client increase social skills. Can also be used in a <u>Group therapy</u> context where other clients can give feedback and consensual validation. The therapist can also use role reversal to help clients gain insight into roles.

Rolfing. The application of deep massage to the connective tissue, which is the wrapping that binds and connects muscles and bones (Rolf, 1977). The purpose of rolfing is to increase the range of motion of the joints and to enhance suppleness by stretching and unwinding the fascias, which become thickened and stuck together, causing pain and immobility in the client. The massage involves deep sliding movements to the neck, shoulder, torso, and lower extremities.

Rolling. A technique that can help decrease high muscle tone. The client assumes a side-lying position on the uninvolved side. The therapist sits behind the client and places his or her hands on the client's affected hip and shoulder/ribcage. The therapist slowly rolls the client from side-lying into prone and back to side-lying, with a slow rhythmic motion. A pillow under the client's head or between the knees may be necessary to preserve alignment during this activity. Rolling should be completed first with the client side-lying on the nonaffected side and then side-lying on the affected side. See <u>Motor control</u> problems and <u>Rood approach</u> for further discussion of <u>Inhibition techniques</u>.

Romberg Sign. A test that examines the proprioceptive function of the dorsal columns.

- The client is asked to stand with heels together while keeping the eyes open.

- The therapist should observe how much the client sways, and then ask the client to maintain balance while closing the eyes and keeping the feet together.
- If the client sways much more or even nearly falls when the eyes are shut, this is a positive Romberg sign that the dorsal columns, which are responsible for proprioception, are affected by injury or disease.
- A client who has cerebellar dysfunction will sway equally or more when the eyes are open.

Rood Approach. A traditional approach to the treatment of a person who has difficulty controlling movement. This treatment is based on the premise that sensory stimuli can normalize abnormal muscle tone, which helps elicit motor responses. Sensory stimuli can be used for the facilitation or inhibition of muscle tone. Other important principles include the following: motor control returns in a developmental sequence, and treatment should focus on the goal of a movement, rather than the movement itself, since the nervous system is able to automatically elicit the correct movement to reach a specific goal. See Motor control problems.

Rotator Cuff Muscles. The four muscles that attach around the shoulder joint and help form a musculotendinous cuff to help hold the head of the humerus in the glenoid fossa. These muscles include the supraspinatus, infraspinatus, teres minor, and subscapularis. See Appendix E for a table of the muscles of the body, including their origins, insertions, actions, and innervations.

Rowing. A technique used to facilitate elbow extension within Brunnstrom's (1970, 1996) framework of movement therapy to regain motor control.

- The therapist sits facing the client with his or her arms pronated, extended at the elbows, and crossed at the wrists.
- The client has his or her arms supinated and flexed at the elbows.
- The therapist places his or her hands in the client's palms.
- The therapist asks the client to help actively extend the elbows while the therapist assists.
- As the therapist flexes his or her elbows and supinates his or her forearms (which results in the therapist uncrossing his or her arms), the client extends his or her elbows while pronating and crossing his or her arms at the wrists.
- The therapist should resist the noninvolved arm as it moves into elbow extension to help produce an associated reaction in the involved arm. See Reflexes and reactions.

- The therapist should have the client relax as the therapist passively guides the client's arms back into flexion and supination, while the therapist returns to elbows extended and forearms pronated and crossed at the wrists.

See <u>Motor control</u> problems.

S

Saccades. Small, rapid, often jerky movements of the eyes that change the point of visual fixation. Occupational therapy often assesses saccadic movement as part of a comprehensive vision screen.

Sagittal Plane. Anteroposterior plane dividing the body (also referred to as the *medial plane*). See <u>Anatomical position</u>.

Scapula Abduction. Movement of the scapula away from the spine. This is the preferred term for <u>Scapula protraction</u> and occurs as the scapula moves laterally and anteriorly.

Scapula Adduction. Movement of the scapula toward the spine. Currently, this term is preferred over <u>Scapula retraction</u>.

Scapula Depression. A gliding movement of the scapula downward or away from the client's head.

Scapula Elevation. A gliding movement of the scapula upward or toward the client's head.

Scapula Protraction. The act of bringing the scapula forward around the ribcage, which naturally occurs when a person reaches forward. Bobath (1990) stressed the importance of the therapist passively completing this motion when a client demonstrates a flexor synergy. Treatment must begin proximally and move distally. <u>Scapula abduction</u> is currently the preferred term for this motion. See <u>Motor control</u> problems and <u>Neurodevelopmental treatment (NDT)</u> for more treatment techniques.

Scapula Retraction. See <u>Scapula adduction</u>.

Scapular Mobilization. A technique initially referred to by Bobath (1990) to help maintain the glide of the scapulothoracic joint and allow the extremity its full range of motion. This technique is often completed while the client is in supine, but it may also be completed in a side-lying or seated

Stein, F., & Haertl, K.
Pocket Guide to Intervention in Occupational
Therapy, Second Edition (pp 251-285).
© 2019 Taylor & Francis Group.

position. The therapist places one hand on the client's scapula and the other on the proximal humerus to help externally rotate the humerus. The therapist then elevates/depresses and abducts/adducts the scapula with the client's arm at 0 degrees flexion. If there is no resistance to gliding, the arm is flexed to near 90 degrees during the same motions. When the scapula demonstrates glide in all three positions, the therapist may proceed to passive range through full range. There are actually a few current strategies for scapular mobilization.

Scapulohumeral Rhythm. The coordination of the scapulothoracic, glenohumeral, acromioclavicular, and sternoclavicular joints to produce 60 degrees of scapulothoracic movement and 120 degrees of glenohumeral movement, which allows a full 180-degree range of motion at the shoulder. If one of these joints is disrupted, then the combined scapula–humerus motion will be inhibited and shoulder movement will be decreased. Scapular mobilization should be completed prior to range of motion activities, especially if the client has abnormal muscle tone, to make sure that the scapula is gliding along the ribcage and not inhibiting shoulder motion. Yang, Jan, Chang, and Lin (2012) found that the end-range mobilization/scapular mobilization approach was superior to standard therapy in certain subgroups of physical rehabilitation clients.

Schizoaffective Disorder. This disorder, as identified in the DSM-5 (American Psychiatric Association, 2013), combines symptoms of Criterion A for Schizophrenia (Delusions, Hallucinations, disorganized speech, etc.) along with a mood component such as mania or Depression.

Schizoid Personality Disorder. Symptomatic of individuals who are withdrawn, introspective, oversensitive, seclusive, and detached from initiating and maintaining close relationships. The individual with a schizoid personality disorder tends to prefer working alone and has difficulty in expressing feelings. Treatment includes Social skills training, Role playing, and creative expression.

Schizophrenia. A severe psychotic mental disorder affecting approximately 1% of the population. In the previous DSM classification, schizophrenia was classified into subtypes such as paranoid, catatonic, disorganized, undifferentiated, and residual. The current DSM-5 (American Psychiatric Association, 2013) no longer distinguishes subtypes of schizophrenia. In the DSM-5, persons with schizophrenia must have at least one of three major Positive symptoms, including Hallucinations, Delusions, and/or disorganized speech. An individual must also have at least two of the following: delusions, hallucinations, disorganized speech, negative symptoms, and catatonic or disorganized behavior (for a minimum of

6 months). The symptoms of schizophrenia interfere with the individual's ability to carry out the normal role functions in areas such as <u>Work</u>, <u>Leisure</u>, <u>Self-care</u>, and social interactions.

There are several theories to explain the cause or causes of schizophrenia:

- Genetic factors, which assumes that the individual has inherited a vulnerability or tendency toward introversion, social withdrawal, and a low threshold for coping with stress.

- Biochemical theories, which assume that individuals with schizophrenia have neurological impairments such as high levels of <u>Dopamine</u> in the brain, which leads to hyperarousal, or structural differences in the ventricles of the brain.

- Psychological theories based on developmental factors in the individual, such as family relationships where high <u>Expressed emotion</u> may cause the individual to have lowered self-esteem and ability to cope with everyday problems of living.

- Sociocultural theories relate to factors such as impoverishment, poverty, class prejudice, and social disorganization that lead to severe anxiety, inadequacy, passive dependence, and alienation.

- Eclectic theories assume that there is a multifactorial nature to schizophrenia where genetic, biochemical, psychological, and sociocultural factors interact to cause a schizophrenic illness.

- Currently, biopsychosocial theories are often favored and acknowledge the role stress may play in manifesting illnesses a person may otherwise be genetically predisposed to.

Symptoms of schizophrenia are characterized as either positive or negative. Positive symptoms include the addition or exaggerating of normal functions such as visual or auditory hallucinations, delusional thinking, or disorganized speech or behavior. Negative symptoms, on the other hand, reflect a loss of function such as social withdrawal, lack of affect, apathy, and low motivation

Course of Illness

The average onset of schizophrenia in males is late teens to mid-twenties; for females the onset is slightly later. About one-quarter of individuals with one episode of schizophrenia eventually recover completely; another one-third of individuals require continuous treatment and respond well to medication and combined interventions focused on <u>Activities of daily living (ADLs)</u>, <u>Instrumental activities of daily living (IADLs)</u>, self-management, and education; while another one-third seem to be resistant to treatment and require long-term support. A robust meta-analysis found that intervention methods utilizing cognitive remediation (involving a variety of cognitive techniques) were associated with improved cognitive performance, reduced symptoms, psychosocial functioning, and functional outcomes (McGurk, Twamley, McHugo, & Mueser, 2007).

Specific Interventions

- The holistic approach is usually the most effective (Stein & Cutler, 2002).
- Medication such as atypical neuroleptics (antipsychotics), which serve to reduce the positive symptoms, is paired with medication training by the occupational therapists.
- Training in ADL/IADL and self-management skills for living in the least restrictive environment possible
- Social skills training in attention and listening skills, ability to converse, being supportive, problem solving, and self-assessment
- Stress management training in developing Coping skills to manage the symptoms of stress and the situations that trigger stressful reactions
- Leisure skills training, identifying leisure activities that the individual enjoys and can gain gratification through incorporating into the everyday schedule
- Psychoeducation of the client and family on the illness, medication management, and prevention of relapse
- Exercise and healthy eating to increase general well-being of the individual and to control Depression
- Housing referral to help the individual to locate housing arrangements such as a Halfway house, a transitional apartment, or foster care that enables an individual to be maximally independent
- Support groups to give the individual an opportunity to express feelings and thoughts without critical judgments while developing reality testing
- Creative arts to give the individual opportunities to develop specialized skills and interests in music, art, poetry, literature, ceramics, weaving, computers, and jewelry making
- Counseling and Psychotherapy, including individual or group therapy, in which the mental health professional works in alliance with the individual in solving problems of everyday living, including family conflicts

- Vocational programming to help an individual gain vocational skills, experience in working, and placement in appropriate jobs
- Skill training
- Assessment of cognitive function and basic living skills with recommendation for discharge planning and supports needed
- <u>Family therapy</u> and conflict resolution into the individual's illness to help family members gain insight

Specific Occupational Therapy Guidelines

- Develop a therapeutic alliance with the individual based on mutual trust.
- Help the individual to incorporate activities, such as exercise, health, nutrition, medication, creative arts, leisure, and social skills into the daily schedule.
- Encourage the individual to monitor behavior and to ask for help when relapses may occur.
- Develop an individualized stress management program.
- Focus on the strengths of the individual.

Scoliosis. A lateral curvature of the spine that may be congenital or caused by trauma or acquired conditions. Interventions include <u>Traction</u>, braces, plaster casts, exercises, breathing techniques, and orthopedic surgery. Occupational therapists may be called upon to facilitate adaptive and compensatory techniques to maximize occupational performance.

Seasonal Affective Disorder (SAD). A mood disorder accompanied by symptoms of <u>Depression</u> such as fatigue, diminished concentration, sadness, sleep and eating disturbances, and a general malaise. It is thought to be caused by the diminishing of daytime sun in late fall and winter. Treatment includes light therapy, medication, <u>Stress management</u>, and exercise.

Secondary Prevention. Prevention of the recurrence of a disease (e.g., preventing a second stroke in an individual).

Seizure Disorder. A sudden convulsion or involuntary contraction caused by abnormal activity in the brain. Seizures may be generalized, focal, or due to unknown onset and may include motor and non-motor symptoms.

Self. The individual's typical characteristics or personality that constitutes his or her identity. It is composed of the affective, cognitive, and spiritual qualities that are distinctive.

Self-Care. Activities that are completed daily to maintain good hygiene and appearance; meet basic needs such as eating, grooming, and voiding; and for functional mobility from one necessary area (such as the kitchen) to another (the bathroom). These basic required activities can be grouped together in a category also referred to as <u>Activities of daily living (ADLs)</u>. Following are subcategories of activities included in this area. Each subcategory contains adaptive techniques helpful to clients who exhibit impairments with specific performance components. In addition, skill training and habilitative/rehabilitative approaches are often used in ADLs/<u>Instrumental activities of daily living (IADLs)</u>. Also refer to specific diagnoses/conditions within this guide for more treatment ideas. See <u>Assistive technology</u> for a list of devices that may assist clients with self-care activities.

Dressing

A self-care activity that includes the following: retrieving clothing appropriate for weather and time of year from storage areas; donning/doffing items in the proper sequence (socks before shoes); fastening all pieces of clothing, including shoes; and donning/doffing prostheses or orthoses.

- **Donning a Shirt.** Methods for approach will depend on the client's condition and current skill and functional level.
  - Method I (button-down shirt): For a client with <u>Hemiplegia</u>, he or she may grab the shirt by the collar and lay it across the lap so that it is inside out with the collar up by the stomach. The client first opens the armhole nearest the affected arm and places the affected arm in it. Then, the unaffected arm is placed in its armhole. Care should be taken to push the sleeve above the elbow on the affected arm. The client then gathers the shirt and grasps it by the collar. While ducking the head, the client uses the unaffected arm to pull the shirt over the head. The shirt is then pulled down in back and the buttons are fastened. To remove the shirt, the same steps are completed in reverse order. The shirt is first gathered up at the collar and pulled forward over the head. The final step is to remove the affected arm from the shirt.
  - Method II (button-down shirt): For a client with hemiplegia, the shirt is positioned on the lap as in Method I. The client places the affected arm into the shirt first. The client then grasps the shirt by the collar and pulls it around behind the back. The unaffected arm is then placed into the shirt, and the buttons are

fastened. Again, to remove the shirt, the steps are completed in reverse so that the unaffected arm is removed first. The final step is to remove the affected arm.

- ○ Method III (button-down shirt): The client can first button the shirt while it is lying on his or her lap, and then use Method IV for donning a pullover shirt. The shirt is also removed by reversing the pullover shirt method.

- ○ Method IV (pullover shirt): The client positions the shirt so that the bottom hem is nearest the client's stomach and the back side of the shirt is up. The client then places the affected arm in the shirt and uses the unaffected arm to pull the sleeve on up past the elbow. Next, the client places the unaffected arm in its armhole. The client then gathers the back of the shirt and grasps it at the collar while pulling it over the head. The final step is to adjust the shirt in the back. To remove a pullover shirt, the method is reversed so that the shirt is first gathered up to the collar and pulled forward over the head.

- **Donning a Brassiere**
  - ○ Method I (back fastener): The client can tuck one end of the brassiere into the pants' waistband while pulling the other end around the waist. The client should then hook the brassiere and pull the fastener around to the back. The affected arm is placed through the arm strap, and the strap is pulled up onto the shoulder. The unaffected arm is then placed through the strap and positioned correctly. The brassiere is removed in the reverse order. For clients with strength limitations, a simple fastener bra may be preferable to a one-piece bra that must be placed over the head.

  - ○ Method II (back fastener): The client can fasten the brassiere while it is lying on her lap and then don it over the head. After it has been fastened, the affected arm is placed through its strap. The unaffected arm is also placed through its strap, and then the back piece of the garment near the fastener is grasped and pulled overhead. The client must then pull the brassier down completely in front and back. The brassiere should be removed in the reverse order. If the brassiere is too tight to easily be pulled down, a bra extension can be sewn onto the garment to increase its elasticity around the client's middle.

○ Method III (sports bra): A bra can be purchased that is very elastic and has no fastener. This bra should be donned overhead, as was done in Method II.

○ Method IV (front fastener): The client should first place the affected arm through its strap and pull it completely onto the shoulder. Next, the client places the unaffected arm through its strap and pulls it onto the shoulder. The front of the bra should be positioned with the affected arm stabilizing that end of the garment. The client then uses the unaffected arm to fasten the brassiere. The garment is removed in the reverse order. Additional options may include use of alternative fasteners such as Velcro.

• **Donning Pants.** The approach to donning pants again is dependent on the condition of the client. In addition to positioning, the type of clothing (e.g., warm-up pants vs. formal pants with zipper) should be considered along with the type of fabric. Some pants have elastic, while others have fasteners; match the type of clothing to the client's preference and skills.

○ Method I: For those with an affected leg, the client positions the pants on the lap with the affected leghole in front of the affected leg and the unaffected leghole in front of the unaffected leg. The client then crosses the affected leg over the unaffected leg at the knee, with help of the unaffected arm if needed. If unable to cross at the knee, the client may cross the legs at the ankle. The client places the affected leg through the leghole and pulls the pants completely over the foot while pulling the waistband only up to the knee. This allows the client to place the unaffected leg into its leghole. The client then pulls the pants completely over the unaffected foot and pulls the waistband as close to the hips as possible. If the pants do not have an elastic waist, the client may place the pocket or belt loop in the affected hand to prevent the pants from falling to the floor while the client stands. The client then stands and pulls the pants to the waist. If the pants are large enough and the client demonstrates good balance, the client should fasten the button while standing. The client can then fasten the zipper after sitting again. When removing the pants, complete the previous steps in the reverse order.

○ Method II: The client uses the previous method to place the legs into the legholes. Instead of standing, the client extends the hips by pushing against the back of the chair and using the unaffected leg to push against the floor. While the hips are elevated from the seat, the client pulls the pants to the waist and fastens the button if possible. The client then fastens the zipper when sitting against the seat. The pants are removed in the reverse order.

- ○ Method III: The client completes this method while in bed. If possible, the head should be slightly elevated to assist the client in reaching the feet. The client first places the affected leg in the pants by crossing the leg over the unaffected leg or by bending the affected leg. The client then places the unaffected leg in the pants. The client uses the unaffected leg and arm to push against the bed and lift the bottom from the bed while pulling the pants to the waist. The client can then lie against the bed while fastening the pants. When removing the pants, complete these steps in reverse.

- **Donning Socks.** The client should cross the affected leg over the unaffected leg at the knee if possible. If the client is not able to do this, the legs can also be crossed at the ankles. The client then opens the end of the sock and pulls it onto the foot. The client can insert the unaffected hand and spread the fingers apart in order to get the toes into the sock. Once the toes are completely in the sock, the client can pull the sock over the heel and up into place. The client then dons the sock onto the unaffected foot in the same manner. When removing the socks, complete the steps in the reverse order. Adaptive equipment such as a sock aid may also be used.

- **Donning Shoes**
  - ○ Consider the type of shoe used (e.g., slip-on shoe, Velcro shoes, laces), along with the client's preference and functionality.
  - ○ The client can slip the toes on the affected foot into the shoe if the client can plantarflex enough to point the toes slightly. The client should then cross the affected leg over the unaffected leg (as long as it is not contraindicated per condition) to pull the shoe onto the heel. If the shoe needs to be fastened, this should also be completed while the legs are crossed. The client then dons the shoe onto the unaffected foot.
  - ○ If the client is unable to plantarflex, the client can don the shoe onto the affected toes while sitting and crossing the affected leg over the unaffected knee. Otherwise, the client can stand to help position the toes into the shoe.

- A client who demonstrates good balance may be able to bend over and use the finger to help push the heel into the shoe.

- **Donning an Ankle-Foot Orthosis (AFO)**
  - The leg of the pants should be lifted up past the area where the AFO will be applied. The client should lift the affected leg while plantarflexing or allowing gravity to point the toes. The toes are then placed into the AFO, which is placed in the shoe. The toes are slowly pushed into the shoe. The client may lift the back of the AFO upward to assist with pushing the heel into the AFO/shoe, or the client can push on the knee to help push the heel down. The client should then fasten the Velcro straps and lower the pant leg. If the client is unable to bend over to fasten the straps, the client can carefully cross the affected leg with the AFO over the knee of the unaffected leg to fasten the AFO.
  - A client with severe swelling in the foot will have difficulty placing the foot into the AFO while it is already in the shoe. This client can attempt to don the AFO first and then use the unaffected hand to help lift the leg to place the toes in the shoe. The client will require a long-handled shoehorn to help push the heel into the shoe.
  - Use adaptive equipment to assist with activities according to the client's needs. See <u>Assistive technology</u> and specific diagnoses/conditions for treatment ideas.

Grooming

A self-care activity that includes the following: retrieving items necessary for maintaining good hygiene; washing, combing, and styling the hair; removing unwanted hair (shaving); caring for the nails; brushing the teeth or completing other mouth care; cleaning the ears; applying deodorant; and caring for other skin.

- A client who demonstrates decreased endurance or back pain should sit to complete activities when possible.
- Assistance from another person may be needed to help a client wash and style the hair or apply cosmetics.
- Labels can be placed on items to help the client identify objects.
- Use adaptive equipment to assist with activities according to the client's needs. See <u>Assistive technology</u> and specific diagnoses/conditions for treatment ideas.

Feeding/Eating

A self-care activity that includes washing hands before the meal; opening containers or other items that will be necessary during the meal (i.e., milk carton); using appropriate utensils and dishes; transferring food from the dish to the mouth; chewing and swallowing the food; cleaning oneself following the meal as needed; and managing other means of nutrition if needed (tube feeding).

- The therapist should first check that the client is positioned properly while eating for safety in swallowing.

- For those with severe oral-motor and <u>Dysphagia</u> issues, be sure to use specialized techniques. Additional training may be needed.

- A coated spoon should be used if the client has a tendency to clench the teeth following oral stimulation.

- The therapist may also complete an oral stimulation program to assist the client with moving food around the mouth or desensitizing the client to textures that are uncomfortable.

- Use adaptive equipment to assist with activities according to the client's needs. See <u>Assistive technology</u> and specific diagnoses/conditions for treatment ideas.

- High-technology equipment is available for clients who have more impairments in function. A client with quadriplegia, <u>Cerebral palsy (CP)</u>, <u>Multiple sclerosis (MS)</u>, and other neurological disabilities can benefit from an electric self-feeder that is operated through the use of a head or chin switch.

- For those with sensory sensitivities, it is important to pay attention to food texture. In addition, if swallowing is an issue, it is highly important to cut the food into small pieces.

Transfers/Mobility

A self-care activity that includes the ability to move throughout the living area, relocate from one piece of furniture to another, or position oneself within a piece of furniture (such as the bed).

- **Bed Mobility**
  - A client should use the bedside rail to help assist the client with rolling.
  - A client with hemiplegia usually demonstrates difficulty with rolling onto the unaffected side. The client may be able to hook the unaffected leg under the affected leg to help bring it across the body. The client should also use the unaffected

hand to grasp the affected hand and bring it across the body. These motions should assist the client with rolling toward the unaffected side, as well as lowering the lower extremities when attempting to sit at the edge of the bed.

- ○ A trapeze can be installed above the client's bed to assist the client with pulling him- or herself up in bed.
- ○ Additional condition-specific adaptations should be implemented for mobility.

- **Wheelchair Mobility**
  - ○ Proper fitting, seating, and utility should be considered in selection of a wheelchair.
  - ○ Consider the type of wheelchair cushion to prevent skin breakdown.
  - ○ A client with hemiplegia can learn to propel the wheelchair with the unaffected arm and leg. Clients who demonstrate incoordination can use both feet to propel the wheelchair.
  - ○ A client with quadriplegia, spastic CP, or degenerative disease will likely benefit from an electric wheelchair. Training and practice will be important to the client's progress in maneuvering the wheelchair.
  - ○ Some clients may need to wear hand protectors to prevent skin breakdown when manipulating the wheelchair.
  - ○ A client may require assistance when going up onto curbs, unless the client is able to safely complete a "wheelie" while correctly distributing his or her weight to prevent a fall. There are also newer wheelchair technologies available for curbs and uneven surfaces.

- **Transfers**
  - ○ It is very important that the wheelchair be locked during all transfers. Leg rests should be moved out of the way.
  - ○ The client should wear a transfer or gait belt during *all* transfers. This allows the therapist to hold onto the client securely without pulling on a weak extremity. Staff should be taught this principle also, as clients with hemiplegia are at risk of injury of the affected extremities.
  - ○ If the client is unable to assist with the transfer, a lift should be used. If a lift is not available, the therapist may need to ask for assistance to perform a *two-person carry transfer*. Once a

client is in a sitting position, one person stands near the client's head while the other stands nears the client's feet. While using good <u>Body mechanics</u>, the lifter nearest the client's head places the arms around the client's chest from behind the client and grasps one wrist with the opposite hand. The lifter nearest the client's feet places his or her arms behind the client's knees and grasps one wrist with the opposite hand. The lifters then lift the client and move him or her to the desired target surface. If transferring the client to a wheelchair, the lifter who is supporting the client's upper body should carefully walk behind the back of the wheelchair to lower the client nearest the back of the wheelchair.

o   If the client is unable to bear weight on the lower extremities but demonstrates fair upper extremity strength, a *sliding board transfer* can be completed. The board bridges the gap between the transfer surfaces. The board should be snugly placed under the client's bottom with the opposite end of the board resting on the surface of the target chair or location. When possible, the client should transfer toward the unaffected side. This allows the client to use the strong arm to help pull him- or herself along the board toward the target surface.

o   A client who has good upper extremity strength can depress the scapulae to lift the bottom from a chair and pivot to another surface. This method is called a *depression transfer*. The transfer surfaces should be placed as close in proximity as possible during this transfer. The client should remove the armrest of the wheelchair, if the client is in a wheelchair, and place one arm on the target surface with the other arm on the surface from which the client is transferring. The client then depresses the scapulae while lifting the bottom off the chair and swings the bottom toward the target surface.

o   A client who is able to bear weight on the lower extremities can learn to *pivot transfer*, which requires very little, if any, ambulation. The client should begin by transferring toward the unaffected side. The transfer surfaces should be placed in close proximity at a 90-degree angle, which allows the client to go from one surface to another with only a one-quarter turn. The client should scoot to the edge of the chair. With verbal cues, the client should attempt to stand while the therapist helps the client to stand and pivot. The client should push up from the armrests or surface from which the client is transferring. The client will have difficulty standing if the center of gravity is not brought over the client's feet. The therapist should instruct the client to bring the nose over the knees to help with this component. After turning, the client should reach back for the armrests of the chair to which the client is transferring. The client should not sit down until the knees are resting against the seat. Once the client has demonstrated knowledge of the transfer method, the client should also learn to pivot-transfer toward the affected side.

o   A client will complete a transfer easier if the surface he or she is transferring to is lower or the same height as the surface being transferred from.

o   The therapist should be careful to observe good body mechanics while assisting a client with a transfer to prevent injury of the therapist's back.

Bathing

A self-care activity that includes retrieving items that will be used during the activity; transferring to and from the tub or shower; and soaping, rinsing, and drying oneself.

- The client should never bathe if he or she is home alone until the client has demonstrated consistent independence with all activities included in bathing.

- After bathing, the tub should be completely drained before the client transfers out of the tub.

- If the client demonstrates poor balance or safety, the therapist should encourage the client to sponge-bathe after returning home.

- Sliding glass doors should be removed and replaced with a shower curtain. This provides the client with a larger area for transferring him- or herself to and from the tub.

- If a client has a bathtub only, a handheld shower can be purchased and easily attached to the faucet. This removes the need for the client to get all of the way down into the tub.

- A client may prefer baths and want to get into the tub after returning home. The therapist should then have the client practice this transfer a few times before returning home to make sure the client is able to do this. The therapist should also recommend grab bars.

- Liquid soap or soap on a rope may be used to facilitate handling of soap.
- Use adaptive equipment to assist with activities according to the client's needs. See <u>Assistive technology</u> and specific diagnoses/conditions for treatment ideas.

Toileting

A self-care activity that includes retrieving items that will be used during the activity; transferring to and from the toilet; managing the clothing when sitting or standing; cleaning him- or herself after voiding; and caring for other needs, such as menstruation or incontinence.

- Stool softeners can be used to make bowel movements easier for a client with poor endurance. Softeners may also be necessary to counteract the constipating side effects of some medications. (Note: Talk with the physician prior to advising use of any over-the-counter stool softeners.)
- A client with poor safety judgment should not be left alone while on the toilet. The therapist should remain with the client or stand right outside the door during toileting.
- For clients with continence issues, a toileting program and schedule may be helpful.
- Ensure secure footing and entry to the toilet (e.g., so that the client does not slip on a throw rug).
- Use adaptive equipment such as a raised toilet seat to assist with activities according to the client's needs. See <u>Assistive technology</u> and specific diagnoses/conditions for treatment ideas.

Self-Concept or Self-Image. An individual's perceptions, feelings, and attitudes about his or her own identity, values, capabilities, and weaknesses. It is an individual's assessment of self in regard to environmental mastery, ability to cope with stress, confidence in social situations, and ability to perform a job. Self-concept is determined by feedback from others, self-evaluations, and competence in performing tasks. Activities that ensure success for clients reinforce a positive self-concept and increase <u>Self-esteem</u>.

Self-Control. Modifying one's behavior in response to environmental needs, demands, constraints, personal aspirations, and feedback from others. Occupational therapists enable clients to self-regulate behaviors such as coping with stress, <u>Time management</u>, <u>Pain management</u>, behavior modification, and <u>Social skills</u> training.

Self-Efficacy. An individual's perception of being able to perform a functional task or occupation.

Self-Esteem. An individual's appraisal of his or her competencies and abilities to succeed or master tasks with which he or she is confronted on a daily basis. An individual's self-esteem can be assessed as low or high depending on his or her self-confidence in performing a task.

Self-Evaluation Method. Subjects assess their own progress. Self-evaluation is an important factor in assessing treatment effectiveness. Other factors used in assessing treatment effectiveness include objective tests, psycho-physiological measures, and mechanical procedures.

Self-Expression. A social component where an individual is able to use a variety of styles and skills to express thoughts, feelings, and needs such as pleasure, anger, distrust, agreement, and disagreement. Creative media such as art, music, Psychodrama, Role playing, and poetry can be used to help individuals to express their feelings.

Self-Fulfilling Prophecy. The expectation by a therapist, teacher, or parent that a child or adult will perform at a certain level based on expectation, prejudice, or bias toward the group to which the individual belongs, such as in stereotyping.

Sensorimotor Performance Components. The sensory components were included in the historical *Uniform Terminology* of the American Occupational Therapy Association (1994) and referred to an individual's ability to receive sensory perceptual organization and transmit neuromusculoskeletal and motor information. The sensory domain includes Sensory awareness and Sensory processing of tactile, proprioceptive, vestibular, visual, auditory, gustatory, and olfactory information. The perceptual domain includes organizing Stereognosis, Kinesthesia, Pain response, Body scheme, Right/left discrimination, Form constancy, Position in space, Visual closure, Figure/ground perception, Depth perception, Spatial relations, and Topographical orientation. The neuromusculoskeletal domain includes movements related to Reflexes and reactions, Range of motion (ROM), Muscle tone, strength, Endurance, Postural control, Postural alignment, and Soft tissue integrity. The motor domain includes gross (motor) coordination, Crossing the midline, Laterality, Bilateral integration, Motor control, Praxis, Fine motor coordination/dexterity, visual motor integration, and Oral-motor control.

Sensory Awareness. Awareness of and differentiation of stimuli that are received through the sensory channels such as auditory, visual, tactile, olfactory, gustatory, vestibular, and proprioceptive.

Sensory Defensiveness. An alternative term for *hypersensitivity*. Persons with this condition find touch uncomfortable or irritating. Treatment that may help increase the client's tolerance to touch is called <u>Desensitization</u>. See <u>Sensory deficits</u> and <u>Hypersensitivity</u> for further discussion and treatment.

Sensory Deficits. An impairment in a client's sensory system can hinder function, even though the client may have normal motor or cognitive ability. Sensory deficits may be congenital, caused by a condition, or occur during the aging process. A client may demonstrate difficulty with sensing where the extremities are or telling that the hand is holding onto an object. A client with decreased sensation is especially at risk for injury to the affected body part since the client will not be able to tell if the part has been placed on a dangerously sharp or hot object. Deficits may be displayed in the following sensory areas: <u>Touch awareness</u>, <u>Tactile attention</u>, <u>Touch localization</u>, <u>Touch/pressure threshold</u>, <u>Sharp/dull awareness</u>, <u>Temperature discrimination</u>, <u>Vibration awareness</u>, <u>Proprioception</u>, <u>Stereognosis</u>, and <u>Two-point discrimination</u>.

Specific Interventions

- **Sensory Reeducation.** Used with clients who demonstrate impaired, rather than absent, sensation. Clients are instructed to reinterpret stimuli within a new framework to decipher what the new stimuli mean. For example, following a stroke, a client may state that warm water feels different than it did previous to the stroke. The client learns what the new sensation in warm water feels like opposed to the new sensation in cold water. The client can then learn to use these new signals or stimuli to tell the difference between the temperatures of water, even though the temperature does not feel the same as it did previously.

- **Desensitization.** May be used with clients who demonstrate <u>Hypersensitivity</u> to sensory stimuli. A client who is hypersensitive may find certain sensations uncomfortable following an injury. For example, a client who has <u>Cubital tunnel syndrome</u> may find massage to the affected elbow very uncomfortable, while the same client has no discomfort when the unaffected elbow is massaged. Likewise, a client who has had a crushing injury may find a shirt sleeve to be very irritating to the affected area, even though the wound is completely healed. Desensitization is the process of presenting increasingly noxious stimuli to a client's affected area to help increase the client's tolerance to sensory stimulation.

- **Compensation.** Should be taught to clients who demonstrate absent sensation. A client who is unable to feel when an affected extremity is in danger may further damage the extremity. To avoid further injury, the client should be educated on the following principles. Sustained pressure on bony prominences will result in decreased circulation to the area. An area of low circulation is at risk of tissue damage or a sore. A sore that results from static positions is called a <u>Decubitus ulcer</u>, and clients should be taught to reposition themselves in bed or a wheelchair, as well as to protect vulnerable areas such as the elbows or heels. Pressure may also result from splint straps that do not displace pressure over a large enough surface area. A therapist should be cautious when fabricating a splint for a client with no sensation in the affected upper extremity. Splints may also cause pressure areas that the client is not able to feel. The client should be instructed to remove the splint for 15 minutes every 1 to 2 hours after first receiving the splint to check for red areas that persist longer than 15 minutes. The therapist should be notified of problem areas and make adjustments as needed. Temperature can also present danger to the affected extremity. The client should use good oven mitts/potholders and wooden or plastic utensils when cooking, good mittens if the temperature is cold outside, and thermometers to test the temperature of water, depending on the activity, if more than one extremity is affected. A client with absent sensation will also not be able to tell if repetitive motions are causing pain to the extremity. Instruction should be provided on repetitive motion injuries and methods to reduce repetitive motion if necessary. A final danger includes the use of an infected extremity, which may cause spread of the infection. The client should be instructed to allow an infected extremity to rest until sufficient healing has occurred. Finally, the client should learn to use other senses to compensate for the extremity such as vision, smell, or tactile.

General Treatment Considerations

- If sensory reeducation is going to be taught, it is essential that a client has normal cognitive ability to understand new concepts and the motivation to follow through with the training.
- Treatment should be graded so a client can demonstrate success. If activities are too difficult, the client will become frustrated and may want to discontinue therapy.

- The therapist should monitor treatment to prevent a client from accidentally injuring him- or herself on sharp objects.

- Treatment usually begins with a specific activity, but it should be generalized to situations that the client normally encounters. For example, when working on stereognosis, a client may place the hands in a sheltered area to identify objects through tactile input from a list provided by the therapist. A client does not usually have the convenience of a list to choose from in situations outside of the clinic. The client should eventually work toward identifying items in a purse without looking and with no cues provided because this more accurately resembles a real-life situation when stereognosis is used.

- The treatment environment should be free from distractions since these tasks require concentration.

- Tasks should be only 10 to 15 minutes in length, but the client should participate in two to four sessions per day for optimal benefit.

- Most specific deficits stem from a client's inability to sense tactile input; therefore, treatment should begin with the techniques listed under touch (or tactile) awareness. After the client is able to perceive tactile input, more specific input such as tactile attention, touch localization, touch/pressure threshold, temperature, etc., may be practiced. The therapist should take careful note of correct and incorrect responses to document progress.

Treatment of Specific Deficits

- **Touch Awareness**

  ○ The therapist should provide tactile input during treatment when possible. While the client completes range of motion or strengthening tasks, the therapist can lightly stroke the affected extremity.

  ○ Lotion may be applied to the affected area or extremity.

  ○ Different textures may be rubbed against the affected area. Some textures that can be used include a terrycloth towel, cotton ball, sandpaper, moleskin, foam, leather, eraser, clay, or feather.

  ○ A client can trace shapes with the finger on carpeting.

  ○ Clay can be made into shapes.

  ○ The client can wash clothes by hand.

  ○ <u>Vibration</u> or electric stimulation can be applied to the affected area.

- o Special textures can be applied to grooming or feeding equipment to increase input.
- o The client can press out pizza dough or knead bread dough.

- **Touch Localization**
  - o A client must be able to sense tactile input before localization of the input is possible. See <u>Touch awareness</u> for methods to improve tactile awareness. Treatment can then proceed with the client practicing localization of tactile input. The therapist should record the client's correct and incorrect responses (measurement from touched point to identified point) to document progress.

- **Proprioception**
  - o Weightbearing may help increase a client's awareness of the position of extremities.
  - o For clients with <u>Sensory processing</u> deficits, specific proprioceptive activities using joint compression, heavy muscle movement, or use of weighted blanket or weighted vests may be advised.

- **Stereognosis**
  - o Treatment begins while allowing the client to use other senses such as sight or hearing to compensate for tactile impairment, but the client should progress toward identification of objects through tactile input only. The client can first learn to identify if objects are similar or different. The client then learns to describe the ways in which the objects are different, such as in size or shape.
  - o Treatment should progress from larger traits and differences to finer details.
  - o A client can learn to identify objects that are placed in the hand, but the client should progress to locating the object among various objects on the table.
  - o Objects that are three-dimensional are easier to identify than those that are two-dimensional, so treatment should also proceed according to this rule.
  - o The client can practice locating small objects in a bowl of rice, sand, macaroni, and popcorn.
  - o Many small objects can be placed in a container, and the client then removes the objects and counts them.

- **Hypersensitivity**
    - ◦ A protective device may be placed over the affected extremity, but use of the device should be gradually discontinued as treatment proceeds.
    - ◦ A client should progress through the Downey Hand Center's hierarchy of textures (Yerxa, Barber, Diaz, Black, & Azen, 1983). The client should then choose a texture that is tolerable and apply the texture to the affected extremity or area for 10 minutes three to four times per day. The hierarchy is listed in order of least noxious to most noxious. For each level, a texture is first listed, which can be applied to a dowel and stroked over the affected area, and then a texture is listed that a client can place in a container for immersion of the affected area.
        - ▪ Moleskin/cotton
        - ▪ Felt/terrycloth pieces
        - ▪ Closed cell foam (Quickstick, AliMed)/dry rice
        - ▪ Velvet/popcorn
        - ▪ Semi-rough cloth/pinto beans
        - ▪ Velcro loop/macaroni
        - ▪ Hard T-foam/plastic wire insulation pieces
        - ▪ Burlap/small BBs or buckshot
        - ▪ Rug back/large BBs or buckshot
        - ▪ Velcro hook/plastic squares
    - ◦ Other mediums or activities that can be used with a hypersensitive area include the following: weightbearing, massage, an isotoner glove, <u>Transcutaneous electrical nerve stimulation (TENS)</u>, <u>Fluidotherapy</u>, or any activity that requires use of the affected extremity or area.

Sensory Integration (SI)/Sensory Processing Therapy. An occupational therapy theory and <u>Frame of reference</u> that is based on developmental, neurological, and perceptual concepts. SI theory refers to how the brain processes incoming sensation for resultant emotional, behavioral, motor, and attentional responses (Miller, Anzalone, Lane, Cermak, & Osten, 2007). Treatment includes various types of sensory input to help the brain learn to organize this input for accomplishing functional activities such as <u>Self-care</u> and academic learning. SI has been successfully applied to individuals with <u>Cerebral palsy (CP)</u>, <u>Autism</u>, <u>Learning disability/specific learning disorder</u>, <u>Intellectual disability</u> and <u>Developmental disability</u>,

Traumatic brain injury, Developmental delay, and Schizophrenia. An important component of treatment is to allow the client to collaborate with the therapist in selecting activities. Vestibular stimulation, balance exercises, visual spatial awareness, motor planning, tactile exercises, and bilateral motor coordination activities are specific techniques used in treatment (Ayres, 1972). Some of the equipment used with children include swings, bolsters, slides, large balls, mattresses filled with water and foam, scooter boards, inner tubes, flash cards, and sand. During treatment sessions, the therapist integrates various media to stimulate the client and induce positive movements in a supportive environment. The family plays an important role in reinforcing the activities in the home.

Sensory Modulation. An automatic neurological function that organizes sensory input and stimuli. Ayres (1979) defined modulation as the "brain's regulation of its own activity" (p. 182). Efficient sensory modulation facilitates one's ability to regulate incoming sensory information.

Sensory Processing. The operation of interpreting sensory stimuli so that it is meaningful to an individual (e.g., interpreting visual stimuli that are words on a sensory level without reading or understanding the words). Giving meaning to the words is a perceptual and cognitive process.

Sensory Reeducation. A method used with clients who demonstrate impaired, rather than absent, sensation. Clients are instructed to reinterpret stimuli within a new framework to decipher what the new stimuli mean. See Sensory deficits for further discussion and treatment.

Sequencing. The cognitive skill that involves placing information, concepts, and actions in a logical order. It is a critical skill that is related to motor planning tasks such as in dressing, in language (e.g., in telling a story), or in nonverbal communication when listening (e.g., using eye contact).

Serial Casting. A process of casting a spastic limb in its full available range of motion for a prolonged period to provide the spastic muscles with prolonged stretch. Some research has shown that a prolonged stretch may decrease spasticity and increase range of motion. The therapist fabricates a cast at full stretch of the spastic muscles. The cast is then applied for up to 3 months with removal twice daily for exercises/movement and cleansing of the skin on the affected arm. At that point, the therapist fabricates a new cast at a greater degree of stretch than the previous cast. Precautions include increased pain or skin breakdown, and the therapist should carefully monitor the condition of the client's extremity during serial casting.

Serotonin. A neurotransmitter that occurs naturally in the brain. It plays an important role in mood behavior and the sleep–wake cycle. The regulation of serotonin is important in treating Depression.

Sexuality. An individual's personal sexual expression, as well as one's gender identity, such as heterosexual, homosexual, or transsexual, that is influenced by genetic, physical, psychological, or sociological factors. Occupational therapists address sexuality and sexual expression with a number of populations. See Hattjar (2012) for a comprehensive approach to sexuality.

Sharp/Dull Awareness. The ability to discriminate between sharp and dull stimuli. This is one of many components included in a sensory evaluation to test for deficits. See Sensory deficits for further discussion and treatment.

Sheltered Workshop. A supportive employment environment where individuals with disabilities produce a saleable product such as in assembly work or provide a service such as lawn maintenance. Individuals are usually paid on the basis of their productivity, which can be below or at comparable wages for the job performed. The work can be transitional to competitive employment or it can be long term. Work adjustment training is usually incorporated into the program.

Side Effects of Medications. Adverse effects in an individual that accompany the actions of a drug, such as nausea, headaches, dizziness, hypertension, dryness of mouth, blurred vision, insomnia, and Tardive dyskinesia. Side effects occur because most medications have multiple effects on the body. It is important to educate the client on potential side effects and to notify the physician in the case of any serious side effects.

Signs. Objective findings of a disease or disorder that are observed by the clinician or measured objectively through a test. Psychiatric signs can be gathered through laboratory findings indicating brain lesions, through electroencephalograms indicating epilepsy, or through objective tests.

Sleep. A period of suspended or altered consciousness that most individuals engage in within the normal Circadian rhythm. Sleep occurs in rhythms known as *rapid eye movement (REM)* and *non-REM states* in which an individual moves in and out of dream states. Healthy sleep patterns often include 7 to 9 hours; however, individual differences affect the number of hours depending on age, lifestyle patterns, and medical status.

Sleep Disorders. Conditions that interfere with normal sleep patterns such as apnea (breathing interruptions), narcolepsy (uncontrollable desire to sleep), and insomnia (e.g., difficulty sleeping because of Anxiety).

Sleep Hygiene. Refers to routines and habits related to maintaining healthy sleep patterns. Interventions may be used to facilitate sleep such as guided Imagery, meditation, sleep log, environmental setup, built-in routines, use of transitions, and elimination of caffeine.

Sling. A fabric orthosis that fits around the upper extremity to help resist the downward pull of gravity on the head of the humerus when the supporting scapula muscles are weak. Slings have often been used with clients who have <u>Hemiplegia</u> to presumably help maintain the position of the head of the humerus in the glenoid fossa when the client is at risk for <u>Subluxation</u>. They are most often applied for treatment when the client is standing upright to resist the pull of gravity and help prevent further subluxation. The use of slings has been controversial. The <u>Universal hemiplegic sling</u> does relieve the shoulder from carrying the full weight of the affected arm; however, this sling does not help approximate the head of the humerus. A special sling for clients with hemiplegia has a cuff that attaches around the proximal humerus. This type of sling may assist with <u>Approximation</u> while allowing the forearm and hand to remain free to complete movement. Slings do not cure a subluxation, nor do they completely prevent further dislocation. When a sling passively positions the upper extremity, the muscles that need to position the humerus are not being asked to work. This may cause the supporting muscles to weaken and contribute to further subluxation. Slings are often used to help prevent pain; however, subluxation itself may not be painful. A sling can sometimes increase the risk of pain because immobilization may lead to shoulder–hand syndrome. Finally, some slings (including the universal hemiplegic sling) position the affected upper extremity in the <u>Typical upper extremity posture</u> seen in clients with hemiplegia, rather than attempting to disrupt the components of synergy that are acting on the extremity. Slings should be used cautiously and intermittently, while treatment should focus on the reactivation of the shoulder musculature that supports the head of the humerus in the glenoid fossa. See <u>Orthosis</u>.

SOAP Note. An organized method of recording a client's progress. SOAP is an acronym for:

- **S**ubjective findings, which are the reported symptoms of the client
- **O**bjective findings of the therapist
- **A**ssessment, which is the documented analysis and summary of the findings
- **P**lan, which includes the recommended treatments, therapeutic interventions, and further diagnostic tests, if necessary

A related form of note, the DAP note, combines the S and O as Data. Thus, the DAP note is **D**ata, **A**ssessment, and **P**lan.

Social Conduct. Refers to eye contact, social interaction, nonverbal communication, social skills, manners, and <u>Self-expression</u>. <u>Social skills</u> training is used by occupational therapists in psychosocial rehabilitation programs to improve or develop social conduct.

Social Skills. Skills in attending/listening, conversational behaviors, supportive behaviors, problem solving, and self-control. These skills include both verbal and nonverbal behaviors. There are usually four steps in teaching any social skill:

1. <u>Psychoeducational</u> instruction, where the therapist presents information to the client regarding coping strategies and information in preventing recurrence of symptoms. Films, handouts, and homework reinforce what is learned.

2. Demonstration and modeling of social skills through <u>Role playing</u> and <u>Behavior rehearsal</u> where the therapist performs the skill. Videotaping is frequently used.

3. Guided practice, where the therapist observes the client as he or she performs a social skill in a supportive <u>Group therapy</u> format and provides feedback and constructive criticism.

4. Independent activities, where the client begins to practice a social skill in the community and reports back to the therapist and group what difficulties he or she encountered.

Social Stories. A technique originally developed by Carol Gray (n.d.) to facilitate social skills for persons with <u>Autism</u>.

Soft Tissue Integrity. Prevention of breakdowns in skin and to maintain health of interstitial tissues. Damage to soft tissue occurs in industry when workers handle sharp or abrasive objects during repetitive motions. <u>Decubitus ulcers</u> occur in clients who have prolonged pressure on skin during confinement in bed or sitting in a wheelchair. Strategies to prevent skin abrasions include protective barriers such as gloves, padding, and seat covers; changing positions; and job rotation.

Souques' Phenomenon. Flexion of the client's affected shoulder may result in extension of the affected fingers. This phenomenon is not present in all clients with hemiplegia, but Brunnstrom (1970, 1996) discovered that shoulder flexion presented the optimal position if the therapist is trying to facilitate finger extension. See <u>Motor control</u> problems.

Spasms. Involuntary contractions of large muscle groups in the body. Spasms may result from lesions in the corticospinal or extrapyramidal tracts.

Spasticity. An increase in <u>Muscle tone</u>, also referred to as <u>Hypertonicity</u>, in the affected extremity of a person who has <u>Hemiplegia</u>. High muscle tone most often follows after a client has had a stroke and experienced <u>Flaccidity</u>, or low muscle tone. The client will have difficulty completing <u>Active range of motion (AROM)</u> in the opposite direction of the spastic muscles (i.e., difficulty with finger extension if the finger flexors are spastic). Complaints of pain during <u>Passive range of motion (PROM)</u> are also common, and caution should be taken when stretching tight muscles. See <u>Motor control</u> problems and <u>Cerebrovascular accident (CVA)</u> for treatment methods.

Spatial Dyscalculia. Inability to arrange numbers spatially when performing math problems (e.g., when completing subtraction, the columns are not straight, which can cause subtraction of the wrong numbers). Use of graph paper or lined paper turned sideways will help alleviate this difficulty.

Spatial Operations. Cognitive ability to mentally manipulate the position of objects in various relationships. This ability entails being able to conceptualize distance between objects, as in driving a car, throwing a ball, turning an object upside down, or visualizing the movements of the planets around the sun. Using hand tools and constructing objects stimulate spatial operations.

Spatial Relations. Perceptual process or ability to determine the position of objects in relation to each other such as hitting a ball in baseball, playing tennis, or assembling parts in a factory. See <u>Cognitive-perceptual deficits</u> for further discussion and treatment.

Spherical Grasp. Ability to grasp a ball or cylindrical object. See <u>Grasp</u>.

Spina Bifida. A condition that results in malformation of the vertebrae and can be accompanied by protrusion of the meninges, spinal cord, or both. Deficits will vary depending on the location and severity of the malformation.

Spinal Cord Injury. A condition that occurs as a result of a lesion in the spinal cord. The level and location of the lesion directly affect the client's function. Paraplegia or quadriplegia may occur, as well as sensory loss to the affected areas. The cause may be from a traumatic experience or from tumors or infectious diseases.

Specific Interventions

- Maintain both <u>Active range of motion (AROM)</u> and <u>Passive range of motion (PROM)</u>.
- Increase muscle strength and endurance of the upper extremities.

- Improve coordination and dexterity.
- Manage spasticity.
- Increase client's awareness of <u>Sensory deficits</u>.
- Increase endurance.
- Improve mobility.
- Educate client on the condition/disease process.
- Increase independence with <u>Activities of daily living (ADLs)</u>.
- Explore vocational and leisure opportunities as needed.
- Assist client with psychological adjustment to condition.
- Increase client's accessibility and safety within home and community.
- Increase independence with driving.

Contraindications/Precautions

- Monitor skin carefully as the client is at great risk for pressure sores.
- Observe the client for changes in respiration, especially if the client is taking morphine.
- Do not overstretch joints, which can cause permanent joint damage.
- Monitor the client for <u>Autonomic dysreflexia</u> and know the proper method for treating this condition.

Spirituality. An individual's focus on meaning in life and connectedness to the universe. It is the higher purposes that gives meaning to life and is evident through faith and beliefs.

Splints/Orthoses. (Note: The current term for a fabricated splint is *orthosis*). An orthosis attached to the client's body, often with the purpose of immobilization or support to facilitate client healing and restoration of function. Splints may be used to decrease the effect of abnormal tone, support a weak extremity, support a part of the body after an injury or fracture, or correct a deformity (such as in the hand). Proper construction of a splint requires knowledge of rehabilitation, biomechanics, and anatomy (Quick & Bejarano, 2014). See the next page for illustrations of seven types of splints.

Types of Splints/Orthoses

- **Static Splint/Orthosis.** These splints have no moving parts, so they are used for support and stability. The therapist fabricates a static splint to immobilize a joint or prevent contractures and/or deformity. Examples include:

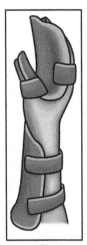

Resting hand splint.

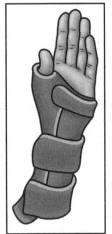

Radial gutter thumb spica splint.

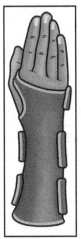

Dorsal wrist cock-up splint.

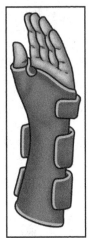

Volar thumb spica splint.

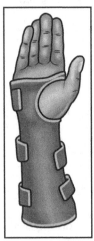

Volar wrist cock-up splint.

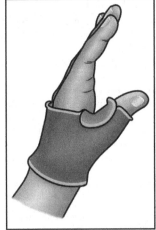

Hand-based thumb spica splint.

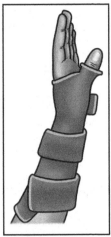

Top dorsal thumb spica splint.

- ○ Resting hand splint/orthosis
- ○ Wrist cock-up splint/orthosis
- ○ Ulnar deviation correction splint/orthosis
- ○ Thumb spica splint/orthosis
- ○ Thumb web spacer or C-bar splint/orthosis

- **Dynamic Splint/Orthosis.** These splints have moving parts that are used to assist with proper alignment of fractures, substitute for muscles that have undergone surgical repair, increase range of motion and decrease contractures, or control movement. The therapist fabricates a dynamic splint to increase mobility at a joint. Examples include:
  - ○ Flexor <u>Tendon repair</u> orthosis
  - ○ Extensor tendon repair orthosis
  - ○ Radial palsy orthosis
  - ○ Extension orthosis for an ulnar nerve injury

- **Volar Splint/Orthosis.** An orthosis applied to the volar of the forearm, hand, and/or fingers. This type of splint may be used as a static application to immobilize the wrist, or as a base for hardware, which will produce a dynamic application to increase range of motion in the fingers.

- **Dorsal Splint/Orthosis.** An orthosis applied to the dorsal surface of the forearm, hand, and/or fingers. This type of splint may be used as a static application to immobilize the wrist without compressing the carpal tunnel or as a base for hardware, which will produce a dynamic application to substitute for extensor muscles in the case of extensor tendon repair.

Standardized Tests. Assessments that have acceptable reliability and validity and are commonly used in evaluating client abilities, cognitive function, and everyday tasks.

Stereognosis. Ability to identify familiar objects through touch without visual cues. This is one of many components included in a sensory evaluation to test for deficits. Loss of tactile function will diminish stereognosis. See <u>Sensory deficits</u> for further discussion and treatment.

Stigma. Devaluation of an individual because of a disability (e.g., the stigma attached to having a psychiatric disability is marked by a prejudiced attitude by a person who devalues an individual with mental illness).

Stimulation Techniques. The term originally used by Bobath (1978) to refer to sensory techniques used to help magnify the effect of facilitation techniques. Bobath defines facilitation techniques as <u>Handling</u> patterns used by the therapist to promote normal movement, thus defining <u>Tapping</u> or <u>Brushing</u> as stimulation techniques, which are added to the handling patterns. Bobath's stimulation techniques are equal to Rood's facilitation techniques. See <u>Motor control</u> problems for further explanation of Bobath's approach versus the <u>Rood approach</u>. Additional sensory stimulation may be used in interventions for sensory integration/sensory processing disorders, sensory stimulation in coma/brain injury, and sensory stimulation as used with geriatric clients (e.g., Golden Carers, 2018).

STNR. Acronym for <u>Symmetrical tonic neck reflex (STNR)</u>. See <u>Reflexes and reactions</u>.

Storytelling. Reminiscing about events in a person's life and recapturing visual scenes. It can also be a life review of an individual. It is used with individuals with cognitive deficits, such as <u>Alzheimer's disease</u>.

Stress. A term that can mean the amount of pressure on an individual (stressor) or the end result (<u>Stress reactions</u>). Stress can either be a motivating force in a person's life (eustress) or a disabling reaction (distress). While short-term stress is often adaptive, chronic stress can lead to a number of health conditions. <u>Diathesis</u> stress models assert that persons with a predisposition for a mental illness may be more likely to develop a psychiatric condition (Dangelmaier, Docherty, & Akamatsu, 2006; Haertl, 2019).

Stress Management. The use of techniques and interventions to reduce the distress caused by life pressures, difficulties, or <u>Anxiety</u>. Chronic stress in an individual can precipitate symptoms such as anxiety, depression, hypertension, and gastrointestinal disorders. Interventions in a comprehensive stress management program include <u>Biofeedback</u>, <u>Progressive relaxation</u>, <u>Relaxation response</u>, <u>Meditation</u>, <u>Yoga</u>, <u>Tai chi</u>, <u>Music therapy</u>, <u>Prescriptive exercise</u>, and <u>Cognitive behavioral therapy</u> (Stein & Associates, 2003; Stein, Grueschow, Hoffman, Taylor, & Tronbak, 2003).

In designing a stress management group program, the therapist should consider the following questions:

- What is the target population? Examples: individuals with depression, arthritis, <u>Schizophrenia</u>, substance abuse, or <u>Stroke</u>.
- What are the specific goals for the group? Examples: reduce anxiety, increase the number of copers, learn relaxation methods, incorporate exercise into everyday life, or gain insight into stressors and symptoms.

- What are the specific techniques that the client will learn? Examples: relaxation response, progressive relaxation, biofeedback, prescriptive exercise, nutrition, creative expression, or visualization exercises.

- What will be the context for stress management? Examples: individual or <u>Group therapy</u>. How many sessions? How long will each session be? If a group, how many clients will be in the group and where will the therapy take place?

- What modalities and therapeutic strategies will be applied? Examples: <u>Psychoeducational</u> with lectures and discussion, <u>Role playing</u>, music for relaxation, demonstrations of relaxation techniques, practice in learning techniques, learning arts and crafts, or engaging in exercises such as tai chi.

- How will the occupational therapist evaluate the effectiveness of the stress management program? Examples: <u>Self-evaluation method</u>, standardized tests, physiological measures (biofeedback), and clinical observation.

- What are the potential problems that reduce the effectiveness of the program? Examples: lack of client motivation, lack of compliance to stress management recommendations, and noisy or distracting environment.

Stress Reactions. The psychophysiological reactions in an individual that are the end results of <u>Stressors</u> minus personal resources.

Stressors. The specific factors that precipitate a <u>Stress reaction</u>, such as death in the family, loss of job, or loss of income.

Stretch. Application of force elongating muscles and tendons, often used to prepare a muscle for exercise, recover from exercise, or act on <u>Muscle tone</u>. Types of stretch may include dynamic stretching, which involves stretching the muscle through movement, whereas static stretching involves holding a muscle in an elongated position. Current research suggests that dynamic stretching should be used to warm up the muscle prior to physical exercise. The use of stretch is also a technique that can be used to facilitate low muscle tone or inhibit high muscle tone.

- **Quick Stretch.** Facilitates muscle tone, but the effects are temporary. The therapist stabilizes the proximal joint while quickly moving the distal joint (i.e., stabilizing the shoulder while quickly flexing the elbow to facilitate the triceps). This type of facilitation is usually applied to flexors and adductors.

- **Maintained Stretch.** Inhibits muscle tone, according to Rood (1962); however, Rood did not suggest passive stretching. Rood's theory stated that a muscle should be positioned in its elongated state while the <u>Antagonist</u> is facilitated. This type of stretch on the <u>Agonist</u> would help lengthen the muscle's spindles and decrease the tone. A final definition of stretch is the act of applying outside forces to lengthen a muscle, as occurs during passive range of motion activities. See <u>Motor control</u> problems, <u>Rood approach</u>, and <u>Passive range of motion (PROM)</u>.

Stretch Reflex. A protective reflex that serves to limit a joint's range of motion and, therefore, protect the muscles around the joint from being stretched too far. When a muscle is quickly stretched, the muscle spindle sends a signal to the central nervous system, which returns a signal that asks the muscle to contract. The strength of the contraction is often in proportion to the speed of the stretch to the muscle; however, overprotective stretch reflexes may be present in persons who demonstrate hypertonicity. See <u>Hypertonicity</u>.

Stroke. See <u>Cerebrovascular accident (CVA)</u> for discussion and treatment.

Stroking. A technique that can either facilitate or inhibit <u>Muscle tone</u>. If facilitation is the desired outcome, then light stroking of three to five repetitions with 30-second rest breaks between repetitions is the technique of choice. If inhibition is the desired outcome, then slow stroking with a firm and constant pressure is applied. See <u>Motor control</u> problems and <u>Rood approach</u> for more discussion of <u>Facilitation and inhibition techniques</u>.

Subluxation. The process of the head of the humerus partially dislocating from the glenoid fossa as a result of abnormal tone of the supporting muscles. When the scapular muscles (specifically, the <u>Rotator cuff muscles</u>) demonstrate low tone, the head of the humerus cannot resist the downward pull of gravity. Also, the fossa may orient backward, downward, and/or medially rather than its usual forward, upward, lateral direction, which can facilitate subluxation. If the muscles that attach to the head of the humerus become spastic, subluxation can also occur. This is demonstrated in a client who shows spasticity of the pectoral muscles accompanied by an anterior subluxation of the humerus. Treatment should focus on facilitation or inhibition of the appropriate muscles to restore orientation of the fossa and pull of the humerus into the fossa. Slings have often been used to help position the humerus into the fossa, especially while a client with <u>Hemiplegia</u> stands upright and the downward pull of gravity is stronger; however, the effectiveness of slings has been questioned. See <u>Sling</u>.

Substance Abuse. A psychiatric disorder in which an individual becomes dependent on a chemical substance such as alcohol, sedatives, hypnotics, anxiolytics, amphetamines, cocaine, opium, or heroin. Effects of substance abuse include <u>Delirium</u>, <u>Psychosis</u>, and cognitive mood disorders; sleep and eating disturbances; <u>Anxiety</u>; and a general interference with functional <u>Activities of daily living (ADLs)</u>. Occupational therapy treatment goals for individuals with substance abuse include <u>Social skills</u> training, vocational readiness, anger and <u>Stress management</u>, development of <u>Leisure</u> activities, self-regulation of addictive behavior, and effective time management. Specific media can include woodworking, <u>Horticulture</u>, daily diaries, use of creative and expressive activities, <u>Role playing</u>, and <u>Values clarification</u>. Group treatment using a <u>Psychoeducational</u> approach with <u>Cognitive behavioral therapy</u> has been shown to be effective in treating individuals with substance abuse. See also <u>Addiction</u>.

Substitution. This method may be used by a client during a <u>Manual muscle test (MMT)</u> to help improve the client's results even though the client has a weakness/deficit in the motion being tested. When testing the <u>Prime movers</u> responsible for a motion, the client may use other, stronger muscles to execute a movement if the prime movers are weak. A client may also substitute body movements such as trunk rotation or lateral flexion to assist with movement such as shoulder abduction or horizontal adduction. Finally, the client may consciously substitute for movement by inching the arm along a supportive surface. See <u>Appendix H</u> for a list of common substitutions used during MMT.

Suicide. The intentional act of taking one's own life. Suicide is an unfortunate leading cause of death, particularly for those with ages in their teens through thirties. According to the Centers for Disease Control (2014), in 2014 suicide was the second leading cause of death for the age groups of 10 to 14 years, 15 to 24 years, and 25 to 34 years. Warning signs of suicide include expressing intent to commit suicide, progressive social withdrawal or isolation, increase in alcohol and drug abuse, extreme <u>Depression</u> or mood swings (may or may not be accompanied by anger), giving away one's things, and expression of feelings of helplessness and/or hopelessness. In the event of someone expressing suicidal behavior, it is important to stay with him or her and seek professional help. For those with a suicidal history, often a crisis and prevention plan are developed. Interventions may include <u>Cognitive behavioral therapy</u>, <u>Dialectical behavioral therapy (DBT)</u>, and other psychosocial interventions. In addition, Calear et al. (2016) found that system-wide interventions (such as those in schools) may be effective for preventing youth suicide.

Superficial. On the surface or shallow, as in near the skin. See <u>Anatomical position</u>.

Superior. Above a specific part of the body. See <u>Anatomical position</u>.

Supination. Rotating the palm so the hand faces up, or outward rotation of the foot. See <u>Anatomical position</u>.

Supine. A term that refers to the position of a client while the client lies on a horizontal surface with the back and bottom touching the supporting surface.

Support Groups. Community groups that meet regularly and provide opportunities for individuals and their families and friends to discuss their problems openly. There are hundreds of support groups for almost every disability. Meeting times and places are often listed in local newspapers. Examples include:

- Alliance for the Mentally Ill
- Recovery Incorporated
- Alcoholics Anonymous
- Alzheimer's support groups
- <u>Multiple sclerosis (MS)</u> groups
- <u>Stroke</u> groups
- Brain Injury Association
- Learning Disabilities of America
- <u>Autism</u> groups
- <u>Post-traumatic stress disorder (PTSD)</u> groups

Lectures, educational films, and literature are also available at support group meetings.

Supported Employment. A concept first used with individuals with developmental disabilities. It includes job placement, work adjustment, advocacy, job coaching, and follow-up. The concept has been expanded to individuals with mental illness and other disabilities to include transitional employment and access to career development and training.

Supported Housing. Refers to enabling individuals to live in affordable housing by improving access to existing housing through federal subsidies or cooperative ventures. Rental units, single-family homes, or public housing can be supported housing.

Suspension Sling. An assistive device similar to the mobile arm support, the sling attaches to the edge of the seat back on the client's affected side. A client can use this device to help complete functional activities; however, the client will need to have stronger and more controlled movement of the upper extremity to use the sling successfully. See <u>Assistive technology</u> for further discussion of adaptive equipment.

Swan Neck Deformity. A digit that demonstrates hyperextension of the proximal interphalangeal (PIP) joint with flexion of the distal interphalangeal (DIP) joint. This condition can result from the rupture of distal extensor tendons, dorsal migration of the extensor mechanism, dislocation, and volar plate laxity.

Symmetrical Tonic Neck Reflex (STNR). Response by infants by extending arms and bending knees. See <u>Reflexes and reactions</u>.

Symptoms. Reported changes in an individual that are subjective sensations such as pain, hearing voices, <u>Anxiety</u>, or seeing double images.

Syncope. Dizziness caused by a temporary decrease in blood pressure or blood flow to the brain.

Syndrome. Refers to a group of symptoms or signs of an impairment or dysfunction. For example, Korsakoff syndrome is characterized by <u>Delirium</u>, <u>Hallucinations</u>, memory disturbances, disorientation of time and space, confusion, and personality deterioration. Persian Gulf syndrome is characterized by respiratory and gastrointestinal disturbances, fatigue, muscle and joint pain, and memory impairment.

Synergist. A muscle that assists the <u>Prime mover</u> in completing an action by preventing other muscles from interrupting the motion.

Systematic Desensitization. A technique developed by Wolpe (1991) and used in <u>Behavior therapy</u> for eliminating phobias in which the client is exposed to <u>Anxiety</u>-producing stimuli in gradual increments until the <u>Phobia</u> is eliminated.

T

Tactile Attention. General ability to tell that the body is being touched in two different places/areas simultaneously (e.g., the client can tell that the arm and the leg are both being touched at the same time). This is one of many components included in a sensory evaluation to test for deficits. See <u>Sensory deficits</u> for further discussion and treatment.

Tactile Defensiveness. Syndrome conceptualized by Jean Ayres (1972) and identified in the sensory integration literature in which an individual has an aversive reaction to being handled or touched. See <u>Sensory defensiveness</u>.

Tactile Sensation. Receiving and interpreting stimuli through nerve endings for touch as light pressure on the skin, temperature awareness, pain, and <u>Vibration</u>.

Tai Chi. Ancient Chinese exercise designed to develop *chi* within the body. It can be used to rejuvenate, to heal and prevent illness and injuries, and to lead to spiritual enlightenment. It is based on principles of rhythmic movements, equilibrium of body, effective breathing, and development of life forces in the body through a series of slow-moving, circular movements.

Tapping. The act of lightly tapping or touching the belly of a muscle with the fingertips to facilitate low <u>Muscle tone</u>. The suggested frequency in the literature is three to five taps, which may be completed prior to or during the client's attempt to voluntarily contract the muscle. See <u>Motor control</u> problems and <u>Rood approach</u> for further discussion of facilitation techniques.

Tardive Dyskinesia. A motor disorder that can be a chronic symptom. It is similar to symptoms occurring in <u>Parkinson's disease</u> such as slow, rhythmic involuntary movements; tremors; and muscular weakness. It can occur as a side effect of long-term dosage of phenothiazines or

Stein, F., & Haertl, K.
Pocket Guide to Intervention in Occupational Therapy, Second Edition (pp 287-297).
© 2019 Taylor & Francis Group.

neuroleptics (particularly the traditional neuroleptics), which are major antipsychotics used in the treatment of <u>Schizophrenia</u>.

Task Analysis. The component-based breakdown and analysis of a given task. See <u>Activity analysis</u>.

Telemedicine. The use of computer equipment to send lab results, video images, x-rays, and client records to remote sites.

Temperature Discrimination. Ability to discriminate between hot and cold stimuli. This is one of many components included in a sensory evaluation to test for deficits. See <u>Sensory deficits</u> for further discussion and treatment.

Tendon Repairs. These injuries result in treatment that is very specialized according to the location of the laceration. Other references should be consulted for treatment as well, depending on the type of treatment preferred by the physician and surgical repair technique. To help clarify treatment approaches, the zones of the hand have been listed here.

Flexor Zones of the Hand

- Zone I: The distal part of the middle phalanx, distal interphalangeal (DIP) joint, and fingertip
- Zone II: The metacarpal bones, metacarpophalangeal (MCP) joint, proximal phalanx, proximal interphalangeal (PIP) joint, and proximal half of the middle phalanx
- Zone III: The area proximal to the metacarpal heads and the proximal palm of the hand to the carpal tunnel
- Zone IV: The carpal tunnel area
- Zone V: The crease at the wrist and up toward the forearm

Extensor Zones of the Hand

- Zone I: The DIP joint
- Zone II: The middle phalanx
- Zone III: The PIP joint
- Zone IV: The proximal phalanx
- Zone V: The MCP joint
- Zone VI: The metacarpal
- Zone VII: The carpal bones
- Zone VII: The wrist and forearm

Zones of the Thumb

- Zone I: The interphalangeal joint

- Zone II: The proximal phalanx
- Zone III: The MCP joint
- Zone IV: The metacarpal
- Zone V: The carpal bones on the radial side of the hand

Repairs

- **Flexor Tendon Repairs**
    - The therapist should fabricate a dorsal blocking splint to prevent overextension of the affected finger, which may rupture the repair.
    - A dynamic outrigger should be placed on the strap on the volar side of the wrist to allow rubber bands to substitute for the action of the flexor tendons while allowing the client to actively extend the fingers within the protected range of extension in the dorsal blocking splint.
    - The wrist is usually positioned in 20 to 40 degrees of flexion, and the MCP joints are positioned in 35 to 40 degrees of flexion with the interphalangeal joints at 0 degrees flexion to prevent contractures. Initiation of active motion is dependent upon surgical repair technique. Protocols range from protected early motion protocols, <u>Tenodesis</u> wrist movement, and <u>Place-and-hold</u> exercises to no active flexion or passive extension until 6 weeks postsurgery. Protocols are customized to client healing based on scar formation and tendon glide.
    - Typically, 6 to 8 weeks postsurgery the day splint is discontinued and light functional use, <u>Active range of motion (AROM)</u>, and tendon gliding exercises are initiated. Graded strengthening is initiated around 8 weeks postinjury.
    - Generally, the client may begin normal activity with the affected hand at or near 12 weeks after surgery.
    - Please refer to specific protocols for more detailed treatment of tendon laceration injuries, including specific zones where those tendons have been lacerated.

- **Extensor Tendon Repairs**
    - Injuries to Zones I and II usually result in immobilization for 6 to 8 weeks. Following immobilization, initiation of AROM is gradually progressed weekly, monitoring closely for joint drop. Nighttime splinting is continued until full extension is maintained.

- Protocols for Zones III and IV vary according to physician and surgical repair technique, from immobilization to weekly progressed graded movement through template or dynamic extension assist splinting. Tendon glide is closely monitored as AROM is progressed.

- Injuries to Zones IV and VII usually result in immobilization for 3 to 4 weeks.

- For injuries to Zones V and VII, the therapist will need to fabricate a dorsal-based splint, which places the wrist in 40 to 45 degrees of extension.

- Early protected AROM is initiated via either a dynamic splint or a template to assist movement. If a dynamic splint is ordered, the outrigger should hold the MCP and interphalangeal joints in 0 degrees extension. A stop may be placed on the outrigger to allow the client to actively flex the fingers within a safe range to avoid rupture of the repaired tendons. Movement is gradually increased as the tendon repair heals. Again, the client allows the outrigger or rubber bands to extend the fingers rather than actively using the extensor tendons.

- At around 6 to 8 weeks, the daytime dynamic splint may be discontinued, and light functional use is initiated along with progressive strengthening graded to tendon healing.

- Normal activity is resumed at 10 to 12 weeks after surgery.

- Please refer to specific protocols for more detailed treatment of specific tendons and zones where those tendons have been lacerated.

Tendon Transfers. This is not an injury, but a surgery that is completed following an injury. Once the physician knows that nerve or muscle damage is permanent, the physician may choose to transfer a tendon from a working muscle to a bone or joint that is not able to move due to an injury. This allows the working muscle to now move the affected joint. Once surgery has been completed, the affected part should be immobilized for 3 to 4 weeks if the transferred tendon is a flexor tendon. Immobilization may be necessary for 4 to 6 weeks if the transferred tendon is a weaker extensor tendon. The therapist should fabricate a splint to help protect the tendon for 2 to 3 more weeks, but the splint may be removed for exercise. Gentle Active range of motion (AROM) may be started while using Icing, compression, or elevation to help decrease Edema. The therapist should gradually increase the exercise program while adding resistance to strengthen the transferred tendon.

Tenodesis. A natural action of the hand that results from the length of the extrinsic flexor and extensor muscles of the forearm or hand. When a person flexes the wrist, the fingers naturally extend through partial range of motion. When a person extends the wrist, the fingers naturally flex through partial range of motion. A client with <u>Spinal cord injury</u> can learn to use this motion to help compensate for weak finger flexors/extensors. By voluntarily extending the wrist, the client can learn to flex the fingers to help grasp items. Likewise, by voluntarily flexing the wrist, the client can learn to extend the fingers to release items.

Tenolysis. Surgery that helps free a tendon from adhesion to improve tendon gliding, which will, in turn, improve movement at the affected joints. This procedure may be necessary if a client has not achieved sufficient tendon gliding following a <u>Tendon repair</u>. The physician may need to perform surgery to free the tendon from scar tissue. Therapy should begin as soon as possible following the surgery, with the client completing <u>Active range of motion (AROM)</u> to achieve good tendon gliding. The client should not complete resistive activities until 6 to 8 weeks following surgery because surgery usually decreases blood flow to the tendon and results in a weaker tendon that could rupture.

TENS. See <u>Transcutaneous electrical nerve stimulation</u>.

Terminal Behavior. Refers to the target goal in <u>Behavior therapy</u>, such as the cessation of smoking, reduction of temper tantrums, or elimination of <u>Phobias</u>.

Termination or Stopping a Physical or Mental Activity. Cognitive task that requires the individual to understand the sequence of an activity. Individuals with brain damage or severe intellectual deficit may have difficulty in terminating an activity and may perseverate on the same aspects of the activity. The therapist can structure the sequence of activity to eliminate perseveration.

Tertiary Prevention. Prevention of secondary problems that can result from a disability, such as preventing decubiti in individuals with <u>Spinal cord injury</u>.

Test Battery. A group of tests selected to comprehensively measure an individual's capacity. In occupational therapy, typical areas assessed include behavior, vocational and <u>Leisure</u> interests, aptitudes, <u>Self-care</u>, and <u>Work</u> capacity.

Theory. A comprehensive conceptual framework that attempts to explain, for example, how individuals contract and resist disease, learn motor tasks, and develop cognitive and language functions. Theory is used to develop a <u>Frame of reference</u>.

Therapeutic Community. A term first coined by Maxwell Jones (1953) to describe a treatment environment created in psychiatric hospitals or Community mental health centers (CMHC) where community meetings of staff, clients, and family are held; client government is encouraged; and each individual takes responsibility for housekeeping tasks.

Therapeutic Milieu. An environment of support where clients feel comfortable in learning and developing social, cognitive, employment, Leisure, and Self-care skills while feeling empowered to change behavior.

Therapeutic Social Clubs. Client-centered groups where individuals can socialize and engage in recreational activities. They can be incorporated in hospitals or in the community as drop-in centers. Beard at Fountain House in New York City was an innovator in developing therapeutic social clubs (Fountain House, n.d.).

Therapeutic Use of Self. Within occupational therapy literature, this term was conceptualized by Jerome Frank (1958), a psychotherapist. It refers to a therapist using his or her personal behavior and feelings in providing feedback to the client.

Three-Jaw Chuck Pinch. A prehension pattern involving the thumb and first two digits. See Palmar prehension.

Time Management. Involves planning and participating in a balance of daily activities such as Self-care, education, Work, Leisure, and rest to promote satisfaction and health. Healthy time management is related to wellness and a balance in a person's life. Individuals balance time to meet a desired healthy lifestyle such as 8 hours work, 8 hours sleep, and 8 hours of self-care and leisure. The amount of time spent in each area is dependent on client and environmental factors. Occupational therapists can help clients to establish priorities and to schedule activities that reduce Stressors in their everyday life.

Tip Prehension. A pattern that combines opposition and flexion of the interphalangeal (IP) joint of the thumb with proximal interphalangeal (PIP) and distal interphalangeal (DIP) flexion of the index finger so that the tips of the distal phalanxes are touching. This pattern is used when picking up a very small object such as a hairpin or penny.

Toileting. An Activity of daily living (ADL) essential to an individual's self-care. See Self-care for specific adaptive techniques, Assistive technology for adaptive equipment, and specific diagnoses/conditions for further discussion and treatment.

Token Economy. A technique of Behavior therapy in which clients earn tokens for specific positive behaviors or mastery of skills. Token economies have been used in psychiatric hospitals and residential schools. Tokens can be exchanged for desired foods or privileges.

Tonic Labyrinthine Reflex. Infantile reflex that is opposite of <u>Symmetrical tonic neck reflex (STNR)</u>. See <u>Reflexes and reactions</u>.

Tonic Lumbar Reflex. A prone lying position that initiates flexion. See <u>Reflexes and reactions</u>.

Topographical Orientation. The perceptual ability to move from one location to another without assistance. This ability is enhanced by our awareness of directionality, memory of places, and spatial relations (e.g., moving from one department to another within a hospital, or from one geographical location to another within a city or state). See <u>Cognitive-perceptual deficits</u> for further discussion and treatment.

Total Active Motion (TAM). A measurement used to help record the motion of the metacarpophalangeal joints (MCPs), proximal interphalangeal joints (PIPs), and distal interphalangeal joints (DIPs) due to tendon excursion. To find this number, the therapist measures active flexion and extension at each joint of a digit. The number of degrees of flexion available at each joint is added together, and the number of degrees that each joint lacks from 0 degrees is subtracted from that sum. For example, the therapist measures the client's joints as follows: MCP = 90 degrees flexion and lacking 5 degrees extension (-5 degrees); PIP = 105 degrees flexion and lacking 15 degrees extension (-15 degrees); DIP = 40 degrees flexion and full extension. To find the TAM of the digit, the therapist should add $90 + 105 + 40 - 5 - 15 = 215$ degrees. The digit should be measured while the client makes a fist; the client should not attempt to flex only the digit being measured. The TAM is then compared to the TAM of the corresponding finger on the opposite hand.

Total Passive Motion (TPM). A measurement used to help record the motion of the metacarpophalangeal joints (MCPs), proximal interphalangeal joints (PIPs), and distal interphalangeal joints (DIPs), which is due to joint mobility. The method for measurement and comparison is similar to total active motion; the only difference is that passive motion, rather than active motion, is measured. See <u>Total active motion (TAM)</u> for method, comparison, and computation instructions.

Touch Awareness. The ability to tell that someone or something is touching the body. This is one of many components included in a sensory evaluation to test for deficits. See <u>Sensory deficits</u> for further discussion and treatment.

Touch Localization. The ability to identify the approximate area where the body is touched without visual cues. This is one of many components included in a sensory evaluation to test for deficits. See <u>Sensory deficits</u> for further discussion and treatment.

Touch/Pressure Threshold. The amount of touch or pressure needed so that a client is able to sense the stimuli. This is one of many components included in a sensory evaluation to test for deficits. See <u>Sensory deficits</u> for further discussion and treatment.

Traction. A separation of joint surfaces that facilitates joint receptors and promotes movement, historically used by Voss (1967) within the framework of proprioceptive neuromuscular facilitation. This technique may decrease pain or increase range of motion during treatment. Currently, traction is used by a number of health professionals, including rehabilitation therapists, chiropractors, and others. See <u>Motor control</u> problems and <u>Proprioceptive neuromuscular facilitation (PNF)</u> for more techniques.

Transactional Analysis (TA). A <u>Psychotherapy</u> technique developed by Berne (1961) that analyzes the roles individuals assume in interpersonal relationships, such as parent (superego), child (id), or adult (ego). Current versions of the original publication are still in print.

Transcutaneous Electrical Nerve Stimulation (TENS). A noninvasive physical agent modality that uses electrical current to help decrease pain, based on the endorphin release principle and on the gate-control theory principle. It consists of a small battery-operated unit that sends mild electrical current through the skin that interferes with transmission of painful stimuli. It is usually placed near the site of the pain, such as in the lower back. Precautions noted in using TENS include skin irritations and interfering with pacemakers. See <u>Physical agent modalities (PAMs)</u> for further discussion and treatment.

Transdisciplinary Team. Professionals from various disciplines who share their roles with one another (e.g., an occupational therapist may use <u>Family therapy</u> or behavior management techniques in treatment sessions after consulting with the social worker or behavioral psychologist about the procedures). Additional similar terms include interprofessional and <u>Multidisciplinary teams</u>.

Transfers/Mobility. An <u>Activity of daily living (ADL)</u> that is essential to an individual's self-care. See <u>Self-care</u> for specific adaptive techniques, <u>Assistive technology</u> for adaptive equipment, and specific diagnoses/conditions for further discussion and treatment.

Traumatic Brain Injury. An insult to the brain resulting from an injury occurred in a car accident, sports, combat, or fall. The movement of the brain within the skull damages brain tissue. Injury occurs at the point of impact and the counter-coup.

Specific Interventions

- Increase response to stimuli and environment.
- Improve client's positioning.
- Maintain <u>Passive range of motion (PROM)</u>.
- Improve swallowing.
- Increase independence with <u>Activities of daily living (ADLs)</u>.
- Improve cognitive functions.
- Improve perceptual functions.
- Improve visual tracking and scanning.
- Improve <u>Tactile sensation</u> and teach safety with regard to sensory loss.
- Teach <u>Pain management</u>.
- Teach <u>Stress management</u>.
- Increase voluntary movement of the affected upper extremity.
- Increase muscle strength.
- Improve coordination.
- Increase endurance.
- Assist client with psychological adjustment to condition.
- Educate client on condition/disease process.
- Increase client's accessibility and safety within the home and community.
- Explore vocational opportunities as needed.
- Assist client in finding leisure activities.

Contraindications/Precautions

- Monitor the skin for breakdown if splints are used.
- Expect plateaus during treatment as the client's progression can vary from one day to another.
- Be aware of the client's medications and their side effects. Also be prepared for seizures.
- When a client is going through an agitated stage, do not overly frustrate the client.

Treatment Protocol. A standardized intervention procedure that is detailed and can be replicated. In many instances, it may be adapted to meet the specific needs of a client, such as in hand therapy, stroke rehabilitation, or sensory-based interventions.

Tremor. A rhythmic contraction of opposing muscles that results in small involuntary movements at a joint.

Types of Tremors

- **Resting Tremor.** Small, involuntary rhythmic movements at one or more joints that occur while the client rests. When the client completes voluntary movement, the movement is smooth and the small, involuntary rhythmic movements disappear. Once the voluntary movement is complete, the involuntary oscillations reappear. A lesion in the basal ganglia may result in this deficit. Clients who have Parkinson's disease often display resting tremors, which occur in a pill-rolling motion. See <u>Parkinson's disease</u> for treatment and further discussion.

- **Intention Tremor.** A client with this deficit demonstrates small involuntary rhythmic movements at one or more joints when attempting voluntary movement. While the client is at rest, tremors will decrease or may disappear. Once the client attempts movement, tremors will reappear and may hinder the client's ability to complete the desired tasks. This deficit results from a cerebellar lesion, and clients who have multiple sclerosis often demonstrate intention tremors. See <u>Multiple sclerosis (MS)</u> for treatment and further discussion.

Turner Syndrome. A congenital condition that results from only 45 chromosomes with only a single X sex chromosome. Symptoms include dwarfism, <u>Valgus</u> of elbows, webbed neck, amenorrhea, and immature sexual development.

Two-Point Discrimination. The ability to sense two different stimuli touching the client on the same body part and the threshold (or farthest distance apart) at which the two separate stimuli feel like only one stimulus (e.g., the therapist may test the client's hand to see how far apart two pin points must be before the client can feel that he or she is receiving two separate stimuli simultaneously). This is one of many components included in a sensory evaluation to test for deficits. See <u>Sensory deficits</u> for further discussion and treatment.

Typical Upper Extremity Posturing. A position mainly observed in a client with hemiplegia who is beginning to develop <u>Spasticity</u>. Often, the client will begin developing both the <u>Flexor</u> and <u>Extensor synergies</u> simultaneously; however, only one motion can be demonstrated at a time. The strongest components from each of the synergies "wins" so the client demonstrates a pattern that includes both flexor and extensor motions. The typical motions observed are shoulder adduction and internal rotation, elbow flexion, forearm pronation, and wrist and finger flexion. See <u>Motor control</u> problems for further discussion of synergies and treatment.

U

Ultrasound. A physical agent modality that uses conversion of sound waves to heat deeper physiological tissue. Ultrasound can also be used in a nonthermal way to help drive topical medication into deeper tissue; this is called <u>Phonophoresis</u>. See <u>Physical agent modalities (PAMs)</u> for further discussion and treatment.

Uniform Terminology. A historical document of the American Occupational Therapy Association (AOTA) first published in 1979. The third edition was approved in 1994 (AOTA, 1994). The purpose of the document was to create a common terminology that can be used by occupational therapists in education, treatment, and documentation of practice. The document includes <u>Performance areas</u>, <u>Performance components</u>, and <u>Performance contexts</u>. It has now been replaced by the *Occupational Therapy Practice Framework* (AOTA, 2014).

Unilateral Neglect. The inability to sense or perceive stimuli presented on the side of the client's body that is contralateral to the site of the brain lesion. This perceptual deficit may be demonstrated by the client who has had a right <u>Cerebrovascular accident (CVA)</u> and does not dress the hemiplegic left arm or turn toward the left to look for food on the left side of the plate. This deficit differs from homonymous <u>Hemianopsia</u>. A client with neglect does not understand that the affected side exists, while the client with homonymous hemianopsia simply cannot see the affected side. See <u>Cognitive-perceptual deficits</u> for further discussion and treatment.

Universal Design. Refers to design concepts in architecture, environments, classrooms, and products in order to make them accessible for persons with and without disabilities. Examples include wheelchair ramps, first-floor elevators, accessible homes, and kitchen devices.

Stein, F., & Haertl, K.
Pocket Guide to Intervention in Occupational Therapy, Second Edition (pp 299-301).
© 2019 Taylor & Francis Group.

Universal Hemiplegic Sling. A sling often used by a client with <u>Hemiplegia</u> who has a flaccid or weak upper extremity for the purpose of preventing subluxation. The sling usually has a fabric piece that fits around the affected arm from the elbow to the hand. This fabric is attached to a strap, which is fastened from the fabric near the elbow, around the client's back and/or neck, to the fabric near the client's wrist/hand. The strap may need to be padded with a wider, thicker pad to provide more surface area and help displace pressure from the weight of the arm in the sling. The use of slings is very controversial. If <u>Subluxation</u> has already occurred, this type of sling does not help approximate the head of the humerus into the glenoid fossa; however, the sling could benefit the client by relieving stress on the shoulder from the weight of the entire arm. Also, a client who is beginning to demonstrate return of muscle tone and movement in the affected extremity will not be able to use the arm while it is positioned in the sling. <u>Neurodevelopmental treatment (NDT)</u> views the use of slings as a risk as immobilization that may lead to shoulder–hand syndrome. This treatment theory also dislikes slings (including the universal hemiplegic sling), as they position the affected upper extremity in the <u>Typical upper extremity posture</u> seen in clients with hemiplegia, rather than attempting to disrupt the components of synergy that are acting on the extremity. Slings should be used cautiously and intermittently, while treatment should focus on the reactivation of the shoulder musculature that supports the head of the humerus in the glenoid fossa. See <u>Sling</u>.

Universal Precautions. Written guidelines established by the Occupational Safety and Health Administration to protect health care workers who are exposed to contagious diseases that produce bloodborne pathogens, such as HIV and hepatitis. Methods of control include protective clothing, puncture-resistant containers, and washing of hands after contact with infectious materials.

Upper Motor Neuron Disorders. Lesions of the central nervous system may cause a disruption of the cell bodies or axons in the tracts of the brain and spinal cord that run to the lower motor neurons. These are referred to as *upper motor neuron lesions*, and they result in increased muscle tone or spasticity, hyperreflexia or increased <u>Deep tendon reflexes</u>, <u>Clonus</u>, and pathological reflexes. Disorders and diseases that may result in an upper motor lesion include stroke, <u>Cerebral palsy (CP)</u>, <u>Multiple sclerosis (MS)</u>, meningitis, AIDS, syringomyelia, <u>Traumatic brain injury</u>, <u>Spinal cord injury</u>, <u>Amyotrophic lateral sclerosis (ALS)</u>, and <u>Spina bifida</u>.

Urinary Incontinence/Urinary Infections (and Use of Catheters). Infections pertaining to the urinary tract, including the kidneys, bladder, urethra, and ureter. Infections may be caused by a number of conditions, including catheters. Occupational therapists may use intervention techniques for incontinence, such as coping strategies, toileting programs, pelvic floor exercises, <u>Biofeedback</u>, and client education. Therapists must also be apprised of precautions and signs of a urinary tract infection. Client and caregiver education on proper use of catheters is imperative.

V

Valgus. An orthopedic term that refers to the outward bending or twisting of a body part away from the midline of the body; usually referring to the lower extremities. A similar, more common term that is often used is *bowlegged*.

Values. Psychological components that include an individual's belief systems regarding ethics, moral behavior, standards of conduct, tolerance for others, occupational choices, and cultural mores. Values are formed by family, cultural influences, peers, and religious beliefs. Group activities such as Values clarification exercises can be helpful in clarifying and shaping an individual's values and beliefs.

Values Clarification. "An intervention approach that utilizes a form of questioning and a set of activities or strategies to help individuals learn the valuing process" (Franklin, 1986, p. 41). This process helps an individual to choose, affirm, and act on one's beliefs.

Varus. An orthopedic term that refers to the inward bending or twisting of a body part toward the midline of the body; usually refers to the lower extremities. A similar, more common term which is often used is *knock-kneed*.

Verbal Cues. Directions given prior to movement or feedback from the therapist during movement to assist the client in completing a desired motion, behavior, or activity. Verbal cues are also heavily used in communication and coincide with nonverbal gestures such as eye contact and body language.

Vestibular Rehabilitation. Rehabilitation techniques for those with vestibular dysfunction. Often, therapists require advanced training and use individualized approaches and exercises designed to improve occupational performance.

Stein, F., & Haertl, K.
Pocket Guide to Intervention in Occupational Therapy, Second Edition (pp 303-306).
© 2019 Taylor & Francis Group.

Vestibular Sensation. Receiving and interpreting stimuli from the receptors of the inner ear in regard to the position and movement of the head. It is influenced by gravitational factors and affects balance while moving (e.g., an individual with a vestibular dysfunction could experience dizziness and have a staggered walk).

Vestibular Stimulation. Stimulation of the vestibular system, which controls equilibrium and reactions to gravity. Sensory integrative therapists use vestibular stimulation in treatment by using swings, hassocks, therapy balls, and scooter boards.

Vertigo. An unpleasant sensation of moving around in space. It may be caused by visual disorders or disturbances to the inner or middle ear, or to the areas of the brain governing the vestibular system. It may be confused with dizziness. In recent years occupational therapists have been increasingly involved with specialty interventions for vertigo.

Vibration. A facilitation technique that helps increase low <u>Muscle tone</u>. An electrical vibrator, which has a high speed of vibration per second, is the most effective tool for this technique. The vibration should be applied to the muscle belly, which is slightly stretched, and it should be applied parallel to the muscle fibers for 1 to 2 minutes. The effects of this method are present only while the vibration is being applied. Vibration is also sometimes used in therapy for persons with sensory integration/sensory processing difficulties. See <u>Motor control</u> problems and <u>Rood approach</u> for further discussion of facilitation techniques.

Vibration Awareness. The ability to sense <u>Vibration</u>. This is one of many components included in a sensory evaluation to test for deficits. See <u>Sensory deficits</u> for further discussion and treatment.

Vision. The ability to take in sensory information through the eyes and process it in the nervous system in order to see. Vision involves both sensation and perception.

Vision Therapy. Therapy that includes both remedial and adaptive techniques to strengthen vision or adapt for vision loss (see <u>Low vision</u>). Remedial techniques may include specific eye interventions, often under the direction of an ophthalmologist or optometrist. Adaptive techniques use magnification, adaptive equipment, sensory replacement (e.g., audiobooks), and other techniques to compensate for the vision loss.

Visual Acuity. The ability to focus on objects both at near and far distances. Visual acuity, <u>Visual fields</u>, and <u>Oculomotor function</u> comprise the <u>Visual foundation skills</u>, which may decrease perception or negatively affect a test of perception. See <u>Cognitive-perceptual deficits</u> for further discussion and treatment of perceptual problems.

Visual Closure. The perceptual process of identifying a form or word from an incomplete presentation. Reading is an example of visual closure when individuals scan words quickly.

Visual Cues. Cues that assist a client in understanding the desired movement or action. Demonstration of the desired movement by the therapist or positioning of an activity or the therapist in the place where movement is supposed to end. Visual cues are increasingly used as a teaching technique for a number of populations, such as those with <u>Autism</u>. See also <u>Motor control</u> problems and <u>Proprioceptive neuromuscular facilitation (PNF)</u> for more techniques.

Visual Fields. A person with intact visual fields must be able to see objects in each of the four quadrants of vision with each eye. Visual fields, <u>Visual acuity</u>, and <u>Oculomotor function</u> comprise the <u>Visual foundation skills</u> that may decrease perception or negatively affect a test of perception. See <u>Cognitive-perceptual deficits</u> for further discussion and treatment of perceptual problems.

Visual Foundation Skills. These skills are composed of <u>Visual acuity</u>, <u>Visual fields</u>, and <u>Oculomotor function</u>. A person with impaired visual foundation skills may demonstrate either decreased perception or a poor score on a test of perception (even though some perceptual skills can be functional without vision, such as <u>Right/left discrimination</u>). See <u>Cognitive-perceptual deficits</u> for further discussion and treatment of perceptual problems.

Visual Sensation. Receiving and interpreting stimuli through the eyes, such as form, color, and pattern. Damage to visual sensation includes *myopia* (nearsightedness), *presbyopia* (farsightedness), *strabismus* (crossed eyes), *stigmatism* (inability to focus clearly), *hemianopia* (<u>Blindness</u> in one-half of the visual field), and <u>Nystagmus</u> (involuntary movements of the eyeball).

Visualization. Imagining one's own body or inner experiences to encourage healing and well-being. Visualization exercises are used in conjunction with relaxation and meditation in comprising a <u>Stress</u> or <u>Pain management</u> program. The steps in a visualization exercise are:

- Have the client sit in a comfortable chair with his or her feet on the floor and hands in the lap.
- With the client's eyes closed, have the client create a relaxed state through meditation or the <u>Relaxation response</u>.

- The therapist should explain to the client the purpose of the visualization exercise, such as to reduce <u>Anxiety</u>, decrease <u>Stress reactions</u>, or facilitate sleep.
- The therapist uses a visualization tape or guides the client through the exercise such as building a dream house.

Vocational Rehabilitation. The restoration of <u>Work</u> functions in individuals with mental or physical disabilities.

Volar. A term referring to the surface of the palm or sole of the foot.

Volar Splint. See <u>Splints/orthoses.</u>

Weakness. Lack of the muscle tension necessary for maintaining posture or moving body parts through controlled and purposeful patterns to complete a task. Various conditions can lead to weakness, which may be generalized to the entire body or specifically located in one area of the body. Weakness should be treated to increase a client's independence with functional activities, as well as to prevent deformities. To increase a client's strength, the muscle needs to recruit more motor units to fire during contraction of the muscle. This may be accomplished by applying stress to the muscle to the point of fatigue. Stress may be in the form of increased resistance to movement, velocity of movement, type of contraction, duration of exercise, or the frequency of exercise. The therapist includes this in the client's plan of treatment as an adjunctive treatment to help enable the client to have sufficient strength in order to complete functional activities. Some examples of strengthening activities are listed next. See <u>Manual muscle test (MMT)</u> for the method of testing the client's strength to monitor progress during treatment.

Specific Interventions

- Theraband exercises: For the upper extremity, the client should hold a stretchy piece of rubber to give resistance while completing all shoulder and elbow motions, including shoulder flexion/extension, abduction/adduction, internal/external rotation, horizontal abduction/adduction, and elbow flexion/extension
- Bilateral sander
- Beanbag activities: The client slides the bags off a large table, to either the side or forward, or tosses the bags into a bucket placed at a distance

Stein, F., & Haertl, K.
Pocket Guide to Intervention in Occupational Therapy, Second Edition (pp 307-314).
© 2019 Taylor & Francis Group.

- Skateboard with or without weights applied: The client places the affected upper extremity on a skateboard and moves it across the surface of a table from side to side and forward/back

- Ring tree: The client may use one or both extremities to retrieve one ring at a time from a horizontal rod on one side of the "tree" and move it to a horizontal rod on the other side of the "tree"

- Removing items from cupboards/shelves

- Wheelchair pushups

- Dressing

- Pulleys

- Clothespins: The client can place or remove clothespins from various heights and widths of horizontal and vertical bars

- Any activity that requires lifting the upper extremity against gravity

- Upper extremity bicycle: Most bicycles allow the therapist to adjust the tension to provide greater resistance to movement when needed

- Theraputty exercises: The client should squeeze the putty and complete exercises to help strengthen gross grasp, wrist flexion/extension, finger flexion/extension, abduction/adduction, thumb flexion/extension, abduction/adduction, and opposition

- Resistive pegboards: The client can place pegs into a pegboard that provides resistance to insertion and removal of the pegs

- Stirring mixtures

- Opening containers

- Drying dishes

- Lifting pans

- Sliding an object up and down an inclined surface will produce a dynamic application to increase range of motion in the fingers

Weightbearing. A term used in a variety of contexts, including the amount of weight an individual places on a limb following injury or surgery. Weightbearing is also used in rehabilitation and was a technique used by Bobath (1978) to help normalize abnormal muscle tone and increase the client's voluntary control of movement with the involved extremity. See Motor control problems and Neurodevelopmental treatment (NDT) for further explanation of weightbearing

Wernicke's Aphasia. Receptive aphasia causing difficulty understanding speech and the written word. See <u>Aphasia</u>.

Wheelchair Positioning. A client should be positioned in a wheelchair to decrease the risk of falling, provide safety in swallowing, prevent contractures, maintain skin integrity, reduce the use of restraints (when possible), and decrease abnormal tone or abnormal postures. See <u>Positioning</u> for treatment.

Whirlpool. A physical agent modality that can be classified as <u>Hydrotherapy</u>. This modality is used for many purposes during treatment, including the heating of superficial tissue, <u>Debridement</u> of wounds, and providing assistance or resistance to active motion. See <u>Physical agent modalities (PAMs)</u> for further discussion and treatment.

Williams Syndrome. A congenital condition that results in cognitive disability, a mild stunt in growth, cardiovascular problems, and high blood calcium levels in some cases.

Work. Paid or unpaid activity that contributes to subsistence, produces a service or product, and is culturally meaningful to the worker. Work can be driven by internal motivation if the individual engages in work purely for the inherent job satisfaction, pleasure, or self-accomplishment that results. For example, a creative artist or composer may be working to express a feeling or create a new composition without concern for material reward. The creative individual may spend many hours on work without pay as <u>Intrinsic motivation</u>. On the other extreme is the individual who dislikes his or her job, such as a factory worker who works for subsistence only. This is an example of extrinsic motivation. Probably the highest level of job satisfaction is to work at a job that one enjoys and to be paid a high salary. This may be true for some professional athletes or successful artists. Most individuals work to support their standard of living while selecting a job that they enjoy. Some individuals engage in full-time volunteer work in activities that they find rewarding. Housewives or house husbands work at home for no monetary compensation while performing full-time work in child care, household tasks, and cooking. All of these activities are work. For the occupational therapist, evaluating the client's work and role as a worker are important aspects of treatment.

Work Hardening/Work Conditioning. An interdisciplinary team approach that applies a highly structured environment with supervised, goal-oriented activities, designed to maximize the injured worker's return to work (Demers, 1992). The components of a work conditioning program include the following activities:

- Increase muscle strengthening, range of motion, and coordination by using purposeful and graded activities to improve function in biomechanical, neuromuscular, and cardiovascular areas
- Intervene with psychosocial and <u>Stress management</u> programs
- Employ functional goal-directed activities
- On-the-job work tasks using functional work capacity evaluations such as the Baltimore Therapeutic Equipment or Isenhagen
- Simulated <u>Work samples</u>
- <u>Self-care</u> activities
- <u>Body mechanic</u> exercises
- Transition from acute treatment to return to work considering these factors:
    - What are the results of an ergonomic job assessment?
    - Would modifying the job or altering the work environment reduce risks for on-the-job injury?
    - Is the worker able to regain the before-injury level of productivity?
    - Does the worker adhere to safety rules of industry?
    - Can the worker tolerate the physical demands of the job?
    - Is the worker's behavior consistent with employee expectations?

Work Samples. Well-defined activities that are similar to an actual job. They can be used to assess an individual's vocational aptitude, worker characteristics, and vocational interests. Examples of work samples include Valpar (http://valparint.com) and McCarron-Dial (http://mccarrondial.com).

Work Simplification. A treatment technique that divides tasks into smaller steps or uses simple methods to make activities easier. A client who has low endurance may require this technique to help preserve energy. A client who has arthritis may benefit from work simplification to reduce stress on the joints. Any person with decreased strength will improve his or her ability to complete activities independently if the person uses the easiest method possible. See <u>Energy conservation</u>, a related topic, for techniques to preserve a client's energy during tasks.

Self-Care Tasks

- Gather the necessary items before beginning each task.
- Choose light, loose-fitting clothing or clothing with elastic waistbands and cuffs. Make sure the elastic is loose enough to slip over the hips or hands.

- Use Velcro closures instead of buttons, hooks, or shoelaces.
- Sit in a firm, straight-backed chair for good support when dressing.
- Fasten a brassiere at the front of the body and then turn it around to the back.
- Wear slip-on shoes. Elastic shoelaces may be used to convert tie shoes into slip-on shoes. A long-handled shoehorn can help a person avoid bending.
- Use belts with magnetic fasteners that require little force to fasten.
- Carry lightweight wallets or purses and eliminate all unnecessary articles from them.
- Sit while grooming whenever possible.
- Use built-up handles on grooming items to provide an easier grip.
- Shave with an electric razor rather than a handheld razor.
- Have hair done by a professional or family member. Consider a short, easy style to maintain good appearance.
- Use a shower caddy to hold necessary items in the shower.
- Sit while undressing, showering, drying, and dressing.
- Keep baking soda in the bathroom and sprinkle some into bathwater to prevent a ring from forming around the tub. This will prevent scrubbing later.
- Use a long-handled sponge to reach feet and back.
- A terrycloth robe will help absorb water after bathing and prevent the need for thorough drying.

Kitchen/Meal Preparation Tasks

- Plan menus before shopping.
- Plan the shopping list according to the layout of the store to eliminate extra trips.
- Shop when the store is not busy.
- Shop at a store where employees will unload the cart, bag the groceries, and carry the groceries to the car.
- Ask an employee to help lift heavy items.
- Ask an employee to bag your groceries lightly to make lifting and carrying from the car easier.
- If possible, have a family member sort and store groceries.
- Use a wheeled cart to transport groceries or take rest breaks between trips to the car for the groceries.

- Store canned goods so that the same items are lined up behind one another. This eliminates the need to remove many cans when looking for ingredients.
- Plan menus that require short preparation time and little effort. Use frozen foods, mixes, and convenience foods.
- Sit on a stool or at the table when preparing a meal.
- Use convenient appliances such as an electric can opener, food processor, or electric mixer, when possible.
- Slide items to transport them to the sink, refrigerator, or stove.
- Use a wheeled cart to carry items to the table for the meal and remove dirty dishes after the meal.
- Serve directly from the baking dish or pan used to cook the food to prevent extra dirty dishes.
- If entertaining, arrange a buffet where guests serve themselves.
- Use disposable dishes, napkins, and silverware.

Household/Cleaning Tasks

- Ask a family member to make the bed for you.
- Allow space on both sides of the bed to enable the person to walk around it easily.
- Make only one trip around the bed. Begin by smoothing the sheets and blankets at the head of the bed on one side. Walk to the foot of the bed and smooth covers there. Then, walk around to the other side of the bed and smooth toward the head of the bed on that side.
- Use a ping-pong paddle or yardstick to tuck in sheets.
- Eliminate knickknacks to decrease the amount of dusting.
- Use a feather duster. Sit while dusting when possible.
- Use a lightweight broom, mop, or vacuum. A self-propelled vacuum will further reduce work.
- Use a long-handled dust pan.
- Place a wastebasket in every room to eliminate trips.
- Place a pail of water for mopping on a dolly with wheels.
- Use a mop with a squeeze control on the handle.
- Store all cleaning supplies together in a bucket that can be placed on a dolly with wheels.
- Purchase duplicate sets of cleaning supplies for each story of the house.
- Ask family members for assistance with heavier cleaning tasks.

Laundry

- Use paper towels to reduce the amount of laundry.
- Have frequent wash days to avoid large loads.
- Position the laundry facilities on the main floor of the home if possible.
- Use a wheeled cart to transport dirty clothes to the laundry area.
- If the laundry facilities are in the basement, use a laundry chute.
- Sit while sorting clothes at a table.
- Place brassieres, aprons, or other fine clothing in plastic bags with holes in them or special laundry bags to avoid tangling.
- When transferring wet clothes from the washer, remove a small amount at a time.
- Purchase a laundry basket on wheels.
- Use tongs to remove articles that cannot be easily reached from the washer or dryer.
- Consider taking heavy items such as blankets or bedspreads to the laundromat for the attendants to launder.
- Sit while removing items from the dryer. Position a table on the other side of the chair so the person can fold and sort clean laundry on the table while remaining seated.
- Avoid line drying if possible. If this is not possible, have the line within easy reach. Use push-type rather than the spring-type clothespins. Keep pins within easy reach also. Ask for assistance to transport clothing to the line or use a wheeled cart.
- Purchase permanent-press or wrinkle-free articles of clothing.
- Do not press items that can "pass" like sleepwear, sheets, T-shirts, etc.
- Consider using a handheld steamer unit like department stores use to get rid of wrinkles.
- Select a lightweight iron and pad the handle if needed.
- Sit while ironing. Use an adjustable ironing board.
- Slide the iron rather than lifting it on and off the garment.
- Use a rack on wheels for hanger items.
- Iron in several short sessions rather than completing all the clothes at once.

Yard Work

- Take frequent rest breaks.
- Sit on a stool when working in the garden.
- Use long-handled equipment for gardening.
- Store tools together in a container and store the tools near the garden if possible.
- Consider using raised boxes for gardening.
- Ask for help from a family member or friend if the activity causes pain.
- Take advantage of power tools and labor-saving devices such as a riding or self-propelled lawn mower.

Recreation

- Use <u>Assistive technology</u>, such as a cardholder, during activities. A clean, upturned hairbrush can also hold cards.
- Use an automatic card shuffler.
- Substitute weaving for knitting and crocheting.
- Avoid prolonged flexion of the fingers. Let a hoop hold needlework.
- Take frequent rest breaks.
- Use elastic scissors that remain open and require little pressure to close and cut items.
- Prop a book in a bookstand, or place it on a pillow on the lap.
- Lay a newspaper flat across a table.
- Use good posture while reading, playing cards, sewing, or completing other recreational activities.
- When fishing, use a rod holder to free hands during long waits.
- Use a golf cart to conserve energy for the game itself.

Y

Yoga. As used in the Western world, an Eastern meditative discipline that has been associated almost exclusively with exercises, physical postures, and regulation of breathing. The aim is to achieve the harmony of body, mind, and spirit.

Stein, F., & Haertl, K.
Pocket Guide to Intervention in Occupational Therapy, Second Edition (p 315).
© 2019 Taylor & Francis Group.

References

Aebischer, B., Elsig, S., & Taeymans, J. (2016). Effectiveness of physical and occupational therapy on pain, function and quality of life in patients with trapeziometacarpal osteoarthritis: A systematic review and meta-analysis. *Hand Therapy, 21,* 5-15. doi:10.1177/1758998315614037

Allen, C. K. (1985). *Occupational therapy for psychiatric diseases: Measurement and management of cognitive disabilities.* Boston, MA: Little Brown and Co.

Almhdawi, K. A., Mathiowetz, V. G., White, M., & delMas, R. C. (2016). Efficacy of occupational therapy task-oriented approach in upper extremity post-stroke rehabilitation. *Occupational Therapy International, 23,* 444-456. doi: 10.1002/oti.1447

Altizer, L. (2005). Hip fractures. *Orthopaedic Nursing, 24,* 283-292.

American Occupational Therapy Association. (1994). *Uniform terminology for occupational therapy: Application to practice* (3rd ed.). Rockville, MD: Author.

American Occupational Therapy Association. (2007). Obesity and occupational therapy [position paper]. *American Journal of Occupational Therapy, 61,* 701-703. doi:10.5014/ajot.61.6.701

American Occupational Therapy Association. (2014). Occupational therapy practice framework. Domain and process (3rd ed.). *American Journal of Occupational Therapy, 68*(Supp 1), S1-S48. http://dx.doi.org/10.5014/ajot.2014.682006

American Psychiatric Association. (1952). *Diagnostic and statistical manual of mental disorders.* Washington, DC: Author.

American Psychiatric Association. (1994). *Diagnostic and statistical manual of psychiatric disorders* (4th ed.). Washington, DC: Author.

American Psychiatric Association. (2013). *Diagnostic and statistical manual of mental disorders* (5th ed.). Arlington, VA: Author.

American Society of Addiction Medicine. (2017). *Definition of addiction.* Retrieved from https://www.asam.org/quality-practice/definition-of-addiction

Americans with Disabilities Act of 1990, Pub.L. No. 101-336 42 U.S.C. § 12101.

Anthony, W. A. (1979). *The principles of psychiatric rehabilitation.* Amherst, MA: Human Resources Press.

Stein, F., & Haertl, K.
Pocket Guide to Intervention in Occupational Therapy, Second Edition (pp 317-326).
© 2019 Taylor & Francis Group.

Asher, E. (2014). *Asher's occupational therapy assessment tools* (4th ed.). Bethesda, MD: AOTA Press.

Avery, W. (2011). *American Occupational Therapy Association fact sheet: Occupational therapy: A vital role in dysphagia care.* Bethesda, MD: American Occupational Therapy Association.

Ayres, A. J. (1972). *Sensory integration and learning disorders.* Los Angeles, CA: Western Psychological Services.

Ayres, A. J. (1979). *Sensory integration and the child.* Los Angeles, CA: Western Psychological Services.

Ayres, A. J. (2005). *Sensory integration and the child: 25th anniversary edition.* Los Angeles, CA: Western Psychological Services.

Bandura, A. (1977). *Social learning theory.* Englewood Cliffs, NJ: Prentice-Hall.

Bebbington, P., & Kuipers, L. (1994). The predictive utility of expressed emotion in schizophrenia: An aggregate analysis. *Psychological Medicine, 24,* 707-718.

Beck, A. T. (1976). *Cognitive therapy and the emotional disorders.* New York, NY: Meridian.

Benson, H. (1975). *The relaxation response.* New York, NY: Harper Collins.

Berne, E. (1961). *Transactional analysis in psychotherapy.* New York, NY: Grove.

Bobath, B. (1978). *Adult hemiplegia: Evaluation and treatment* (2nd ed.). London, England: Butterworth-Heinemann LTD.

Bobath, B. (1990). *Adult hemiplegia: Evaluation and treatment* (3rd ed.). London, England: William Heinemann Medical Books.

Bonsaksen, T., & Kvarsnes, H. (2016). Role performance and role valuation among occupational therapy student in Norway. *Open Journal of Occupational Therapy, 4,* 1-12.

Bracciano, A. (2008). *Physical agent modalities: Theory and application for the occupational therapist* (2nd ed.). Thorofare, NJ: SLACK Incorporated.

Brazier, M. (1968). *The electrical activity of the nervous system: A textbook for students* (3rd ed.). London, England: Pitman Medical Publishing Co., Ltd.

Bridle, C., Spanjers, K., Patel, S., Atherton, N., & Lamb, S. E. (2012). Effect of exercise on depression severity in older people: Systematic review and meta-analysis of randomised controlled trials. *The British Journal of Psychiatry, 201,* 180-185. DOI: 10.1192/bjp.bp.111.095174

Brunnstrom, S. (1970). *Movement therapy in hemiplegia.* New York, NY: Harper & Row.

Brunnstrom, S. (1996). *Clinical kinesiology* (5th ed.). Philadelphia, PA: F. A. Davis.

Burke, R. E. (2007). Sir Charles Sherrington's the integrative action of the nervous system: A centenary appreciation. *Brain, 130*(4), 887-894.

Burns, T. (2018). *Cognitive Performance Test Revised Manual 2018.* Pequannock, NJ: Maddak.

Buron, K. D., & Curtis, M. (2003). *The incredible 5-point scale.* Shawnee, KS: Autism Asperger Publishing Co.

Calear, C., Christensen, H., Freeman, A., Fenton, K., Busby, G. J., van Spiker, B., & Donker, T. (2016). A systematic review of psychosocial suicide prevention interventions for youth. *European Child & Adolescent Psychiatry, 5,* 467-482.

California Board of Occupational Therapy. (n.d.). *Occupational Therapy Practice Act, Sections 2570.2, 2570.3.* Retrieved from www.bot.ca.gov/board_activity/laws_regs/occupational_act.shtml

Cannon, N. M. (2001). *Diagnosis and treatment manual for physicians and therapists* (4th ed). Indianapolis, ID: Hand Rehabilitation Center of Indiana.

Cannon, W. B. (1932). *The wisdom of the body.* New York, NY: Norton.

Carol Gray Social Stories. (n.d.). About. Retrieved from https://carolgraysocialstories.com/about-2/carol-gray

Case-Smith, J., & Arbesman, M. (2008). Evidenced-based review of interventions for autism used in or of relevance to occupational therapy. *American Journal of Occupational Therapy, 62,* 416-425. doi:10.5014/ajot.62.4.416

Case-Smith, J., Frolek Clark, G. J., & Schlabach, T. L. (2013). Systematic review of interventions used in occupational therapy to promote motor performance for children birth-5 years. *American Journal of Occupational Therapy, 67,* 413-424. doi: 10.5014/ajot.2013.005959

Centers for Disease Control and Prevention. (2014). *Ten leading causes of death by age group—United States—2014.* Retrieved from https://www.cdc.gov/injury/images/lc-charts/leading_causes_of_death_age_group_2014_1050w760h.gif

Centers for Disease Control and Prevention. (2015). *Vision health initiative.* Retrieved from https://www.cdc.gov/visionhealth/basics/ced/index.html

Centers for Disease Control and Prevention. (2016). *HRQOL concepts.* Retrieved from https://www.cdc.gov/hrqol/concept.htm

Centers for Disease Control and Prevention. (2017a). *Cerebral palsy.* Retrieved from https://www.cdc.gov/ncbddd/cp/index.html

Centers for Disease Control and Prevention. (2017b). *Stroke.* Retrieved from https://www.cdc.gov/stroke/facts.htm

Centers for Medicare and Medicaid Services. (2014). *Community mental health centers.* Retrieved from https://www.cms.gov/Medicare/Provider-Enrollment-and-Certification/CertificationandComplianc/CommunityHealthCenters.html

Chang, M., Chen, C., & Huang, K. (2008). Effects of music therapy on psychological health of women during pregnancy. *Journal of Clinical Nursing, 17,* 2580-2587. DOI: 10.1111/j.1365-2702.2007.02064.x

Cook, A. M., & Polgar, S. M. (2008). *Cook and Hussey's assistive technologies principles and practices* (3rd ed.) St. Louis, MO: Mosby.

Coppard, B. M., & Lohman, H. (Eds.). (2015). *Introduction to orthotics: A clinical reasoning and problem-solving approach* (4th ed.). Toronto, Ontario: Elsevier.

Corbetta D., Sirtori V., Castellini G., Moja L., & Gatti, R. (2015). Constraint-induced movement therapy for upper extremities in people with stroke. *Cochrane Database Systematic Reviews,* (10), CD004433. doi: 10.1002/14651858.CD004433.pub3

Couturier, J., Kimber, M., & Szatmari, P. (2013). Efficacy of family based treatment for adolescents with eating disorders: A systematic review and meta-analysis. *International Journal of Eating Disorders, 46*, 3-11. doi: 10.1002/eat.22042

Dangelmaier, R. E., Docherty, N. M., & Akamatsu, T. J. (2006). Psychosis proneness, coping, and perceptions of social support. *American Journal of Orthopsychiatry, 76*, 13-17. http://dx.doi.org/10.1037/0002-9432.76.1.13

De Baets, S., Calders, P., Schalley, N., Vermeulen, K., Vertriest, S., Van Peteghem, L., … Van de Velde, D. (2018). Updating the evidence on functional capacity evaluation methods: A systematic review. *Journal of Occupational Rehabilitation, 28*(3), 418-428.

Demers, L. (1992). *Work hardening: A practical guide.* Stoneham, MA: Andover.

DeVahl, J. (1992). Neuromuscular electrical stimulation (NMES) in rehabilitation. In M. R. Gersh (Ed.), *Electrotherapy in rehabilitation* (pp. 218-268). Philadelphia, PA: F. A. Davis.

Dugosh, K., Abraham, A., Seymour, B., McLoyd, K., Chalk, M., & Festinger, D. (2016). A systematic review on the use of psychosocial interventions in conjunction with medications for the treatment of opioid addiction. *Journal of Addiction Medicine, 10*, 91-101. doi: 10.1097/ADM.0000000000000193

Ekelman, B. A., Hooker, L., Davis, A., Newburn, D., & Ricchino, N. (2014). Occupational therapy interventions for adults with rheumatoid arthritis: An appraisal of the evidence. *Occupational Therapy in Health Care, 28*, 347-361. doi: 10.3109/07380577.2014.919687

Ellis, A., & Whiteley, J. M. (Eds.). (1979). *Theoretical and empirical foundations of rational-emotive therapy.* Pacific Grove: CA: Brooks/Cole.

Farbu, E., Gilhus, N. E., Barnes, M. P., Borg, K., De Vissor, M., Driessen, A. … Stalburg, E. (2006). EFNS guideline on diagnosis and management of post polio syndrome. Report of an EFNS task force. *European Journal of Neurology, 13*, 795-801. doi: 10.1111/j.1468-1331.2006.01385.x

Feix, T., Romero, J., Schmiedmayer, H., Dollar, A. M., & Kragic, D. (2015). The GRASP taxonomy of human grasp types. *IEEE Transactions on Human-Machine Systems, 46*, 1-12.

Foster, E. R., Bedeker, M., & Tickle-Degnen, L. (2014). Systematic review of the effectiveness of occupational therapy related interventions for people with Parkinson's disease. *American Journal of Occupational Therapy, 68*, 39-49. doi: 10.5014/ajot.2014.008706

Fountain House. (n.d.). Retrieved from https://www.fountainhouse.org

Frank, J. (1958). The therapeutic use of self. *American Journal of Occupational Therapy, 12*, 215-225.

Frankl, V. (1967). *Psychotherapy and existentialism.* New York, NY: Simon and Shuster.

Franklin, D. (1986). A comparison of the effectiveness of values clarification presented as a personal computer program versus a traditional therapy group: A pilot study. *Occupational Therapy in Mental Health, 6*(3), 39-52.

Freud, S. (1937). *The ego and the mechanisms of defense.* London, England: Hogarth Press.

Frick, P. J. (2001). Effective interventions for children and adolescents with conduct disorder. *Canadian Journal of Psychiatry, 46,* 597-608.

Garcia, B. M., Arratibel, A., & Azpiroz, M. E. (2015). The Bobath concept in walking activity in chronic stroke measured through the International Classification of Functioning, Disability and Health. *Physiotherapy Research International, 20*(4), 242-250. Epub 2014 Dec 4.

Gillespie, L. D., Robertson, M., Gillespie, W. J., Sherrington, C., Gates, S., Clemson, L. M., & Lamb, S. E. (2012). *Interventions for preventing falls in older people living in the community.* London, England: Cochrane Library, Wiley and Sons.

Glasser, W. (1965). *Reality therapy; A new approach to psychiatry.* New York, NY: Harper & Row.

Gold, C., Voracek, M., & Wigram, T. (2004). Effects of music therapy for children and adolescents with psychopathology: A meta-analysis. *The Journal of Child Psychology and Psychiatry, 45,* 1054-1063. doi: 10.1111/j.1469-7610.2004. t01-1-00298.x

Golden Carers. (2018). *30+ sensory activities for people living with dementia.* Retrieved from https://www.goldencarers.com/sensory-stimulation-for-dementia-care/4184

Grob, G. N. (1991). *From asylum to community mental health policy in modern America.* Princeton, NJ: Princeton University Press.

Haehl, R. (1922). *Hahnemann: His life and work* [trans.]. Warwick, England: Homeopathic Publishing Company.

Haertl, K. (2014). Introduction to intellectual and developmental disabilities. In K. Haertl (Ed.), *Adults with intellectual and developmental disabilities: Strategies for occupational therapy* (pp. 3-17). Bethesda, MD: AOTA Press.

Haertl, K. (2019). Coping and resilience. In C. Brown, V. Stoffel, & J. Munoz (Eds.), *Occupational therapy in mental health: A vision for participation* (2nd ed., pp. 342-365). Philadelphia, PA: F.A. Davis.

Hattjar, B. (2012). *Sexuality and occupational therapy: Strategies for persons with disabilities.* Bethesda, MD: AOTA Press.

Hindle, K. B., Whitcomb, T. J., Briggs, W. O., & Hong, J. (2012). Proprioceptive neuromuscular facilitation (PNF): Its mechanisms and effects on range of motion and muscular function. *Journal of Human Kinetics, 31,* 105-113. doi: 10.2478/v10078-012-0011-y

Houglum, P. A., & Bertoti, D. B. (2012). *Brunnstrom's clinical kinesiology* (6th ed.). Philadelphia, PA: FA Davis.

Hoy, D., March, L., Brooks, P., Blyth, F., Woolf, A., Bain, C. ... Buchbinder, R. (2014). The global burden of low back pain: Estimates from the Global Burden of Disease 2010 study. *Annals of Rheumatic Diseases, 73,* 968-974. doi:10.1136/annrheumdis-2013-204428

Jacobson, E. (1929). *Progressive relaxation*. Chicago, IL: University of Chicago.

Jacobson, E. (1978). *You must relax* (4th ed.). New York, NY: McGraw-Hill.

Jones, M. (1953). *The therapeutic community*. New York, NY: Basic Books.

Kabat, H. (1961). Proprioceptive facilitation in therapeutic exercise. In S. Licht (Ed.), *Therapeutic exercise* (2nd ed., pp. 327-343). New Haven, CT: Elizabeth Licht.

Kaczkurkin, A. N., & Foa, E. B. (2015). Cognitive-behavioral therapy for anxiety disorders: An update on the empirical evidence. *Dialogues in Clinical Neuroscience, 17*, 337-346.

Katusić, A., Alimovic, S., & Mejaski-Bosnjak, V. (2013). The effect of vibration therapy on spasticity and motor function in children with cerebral palsy: A randomized controlled trial. *NeuroRehabilitation, 32*(1), 1-8. doi: 10.3233/NRE-130817

Kielhofner, G. (Ed.). (1985). *A model of human occupation*. Baltimore, MD: Williams & Wilkins.

Kielhofner, G. (2008). *Conceptual foundations of occupational therapy* (4th ed.). Philadelphia, PA: F. A. Davis.

Knott, M., & Voss, D. E. (1968). *Proprioceptive neuromuscular facilitation patterns and techniques*. New York, NY: Harper and Row.

Knutson, J. S., Fu, M. J., Sheffler, L. R., & Chae, J. (2015). Neuromuscular electric stimulation for motor restoration in hemiplegia. *Physical Medicine & Rehabilitation in Clinics of North America, 26*, 729-745. doi: 10.1016/j.pmr.2015.06.002

Krause-Parello, C. A., Sarni, S., & Padden, E. (2016). Military veterans and canine assistance for post-traumatic stress disorder: A narrative review of the literature. *Nurse Education Today, 47*, 43-50. doi: 10.1016/j.nedt.2016.04.020

Kuypers, L. (2011). *The zones of regulation: A curriculum designed to foster self-regulation and emotional control*. Santa Clara, CA: Social Thinking Publishing.

LaGasse, A. B. (2014). Effects of a music therapy group intervention on enhancing social skills in children with autism. *Journal of Music Therapy, 51*, 250-275. doi:10.1093/jmt/thu012

Lareau, C., & Sawyer, G. (2010). Hip fracture surgical treatment and rehabilitation. *Medicine & Health/Rhode Island, 93*, 108-111.

Lee, J., Park, S., & Na, S. (2013). The effect of proprioceptive neuromuscular facilitation on pain and function. *Journal of Physical Therapy Science, 25*, 713-716. doi: 10.1589/jpts.25.713

Linehan, M. M. (1993). *Cognitive behavioral treatment for borderline personality disorder*. New York, NY: Guilford Press.

Lubahn, J., Wolfe, T. L., & Feldscher, S. B. (2011). Joint replacement in the hand and wrist: Surgery and therapy. In T. M. Skirvin, A. L. Osterman, J. M. Fedorczyk, & P. C. Amadio (Eds.), *Rehabilitation of the hand and upper extremity* (6th ed., pp. 1376-1398). Philadelphia, PA: Elsevier.

Maher, C. (2014). Orthopaedic conditions. In C. Trombly, & M. Vining Radomski (Eds.), *Occupational therapy for physical dysfunction* (7th ed., pp. 1103-1128). Philadelphia, PA: Lippincott.

Mathiowetz, V., & Bass-Haugen, J. (1994). Motor behavior research: Implications for therapeutic approaches for central nervous system dysfunction. *American Journal of Occupational Therapy, 48*, 733-745. doi: 10.5014/ajot.48.8.733

McGraw-Hill Global Education. (2018). *Principles of manual muscle testing.* Retrieved from http://highered.mheducation.com/sites/0071474013/student_view0/chapter8/manuaul_muscle_testing.html

McGurk, S. R., Twamley, E. W., McHugo, G. J., & Mueser, K. T. (2007). A meta-analysis of cognitive remediation in schizophrenia. *American Journal of Psychiatry, 164*, 1791-1802. doi:10.1176/appi.ajp.2007.07060906

Meibeyer, E. (2015). Visual impairments. In B. Boyt Schell, G. Gillen, & M. Scaffa (Eds.), *Willard & Spackman's occupational therapy* (12th ed., pp. 1187-1189). Philadelphia, PA: Lippincott Williams & Wilkins.

Mental Retardation Facilities Construction Act of 1963, P.L. 88-164 Stat 77 (1963).

Miller, L. J., Anzalone, M. E., Lane, S. J., Cermak, S. A., & Osten, E. T. (2007). Concept evolution in sensory integration: A proposed nosology for diagnosis. *American Journal of Occupational Therapy, 61*, 135-140. doi:10.5014/ajot.61.2.135

Mosey, A. C. (1970). *Three frames of reference for mental health.* Thorofare, NJ: SLACK Incorporated.

Mosey, A. C. (1973). *Activities therapy.* New York, NY: Raven Press.

Mosey, A. C. (1986). *Psychosocial components of occupational therapy.* Philadelphia, PA: Lippincott-Raven.

Mukherjee, R. A., Hollins, S., & Turk, J. (2006). Fetal alcohol spectrum disorder: An overview. *Journal of the Royal Society of Medicine, 99*, 298-302. doi: 10.1258/jrsm.99.6.298

National Collaborating Centre for Mental Health. (2010). *Antisocial personality disorder: The NICE guideline on treatment, management and prevention.* London, England: British Psychological Society and the Royal College of Psychiatrists.

National Eye Institute. (n.d.). *Low vision.* Retrieved from https://nei.nih.gov/eyedata/lowvision

National Stroke Association. (2017). *Act FAST.* Retrieved from http://www.stroke.org/understand-stroke/recognizing-stroke/act-fast

Norkin, C. C., & Levangie, P. K. (1992). *Joint structure and function: A comprehensive analysis* (2nd ed.). Philadelphia, PA: F. A. Davis.

Occupational Performance Model (Australia). (2014). *Definitions.* Retrieved from http://www.occupationalperformance.com/definitions

Pagnin, D., de Queiroz, V., Pini, S., & Cassano, G. B. (2008). Efficacy of ECT in depression: A meta-analytic review. *The Journal of Lifelong Learning in Psychiatry, 6*, 155-162. https://doi.org/10.1176/foc.6.1.foc155

Pendleton, H. M., & Schultz-Krohn, W. (2012). *Pedretti's occupational therapy practice skills for physical dysfunction* (7th ed.). St Louis, MO: Mosby.

Perls, F. (1969). *Gestalt therapy verbatim.* Moab, UT: Real People Press.

Perneros, G., & Tropp, H. (2009). Development, validity and reliability of the Assessment of Pain and Occupational Performance (POP): A new instrument using two dimensions in the investigation of disability in the investigation of disability in back pain. *The Spine Journal, 6*, 486-498. doi: 10.1016/j.spinee.2009.03.001

Quick, C. D., & Bejarano, P. D. (2014). Construction of hand splints. In M. Vining Radomski & C. A. Trombly Latham (Eds.), *Occupational therapy for physical dysfunction* (7th ed., pp. 472-494). Philadelphia, PA: Lippincott Williams & Wilkins.

Rao, A. K., Chou, A., Bursley, B., Smulofsky, J., & Jezequel, J. (2014). Systematic review of the effects of exercise on activities of daily living in people with Alzheimer's disease. *American Journal of Occupational Therapy, 68*, 50-56. doi:10.5014/ajot.2014.009035

Reilly, M. (Ed.). (1974). *Play as exploratory learning.* Beverly Hills, CA: Sage Publications.

Reips, U., & Funke, F. (2008). Interval-level measurement with visual analogue scales in Internet-based research: VAS Generator. *Behavior Research Methods, 40*, 699-704. doi: 10.3758/BRM.40.3.699

Rogers, C. (1951). *Client-centered therapy: Its current practice, implications and theory.* Boston, MA: Houghton Mifflin.

Rolf, I. (1977). *Rolfing: The integration of human structures.* Santa Monica, CA: Dennis-Landman.

Rood, M. (1962). The use of sensory receptors to activate, facilitate and inhibit motor response, autonomic and somatic in developmental sequence. In C. Stately (Ed.), *Approaches to treatment of clients with neuromuscular dysfunction* (pp. 36-37). Dubuque, IA: William Brown Group.

Satu, H., & Maruyama, H. (2009). The effects of indirect treatment of proprioceptive neuromuscular facilitation. *Journal of Physical Therapy Science, 21*, 189-193. doi: https://doi.org/10.1589/jpts.21.189

Scott, S. (2007). An update on interventions for conduct disorder. *Advances in Psychiatric Treatment, 14*, 61-70. doi: 10.1192/apt.bp.106.002626

Selye, H. (1993). History of the stress concept. In L. Goldberger & S. Breznitz (Eds.), *Handbook of stress: Theoretical and clinical aspects* (pp. 7-17). New York, NY: Free Press.

Skinner, B. F. (1938). *The behavior of organisms: An experimental analysis.* Englewood Cliffs, NJ: Prentice-Hall.

Skirven, T. M., Osterman, A. L., Fedorczyk, J. M., & Amadio, P. C. (Eds.). (2011a). *Rehabilitation of the hand and upper extremity* (6th ed., Vol. 1). Philadelphia, PA: Elsevier-Mosby.

Skirven, T. M., Osterman, A. L., Fedorczyk, J. M., & Amadio, P. C. (Eds.). (2011b). *Rehabilitation of the hand and upper extremity* (6th ed., Vol. 2). Philadelphia, PA: Elsevier-Mosby.

Slavson, S. R. (1943). *An introduction to group therapy.* New York, NY: The Commonwealth Fund.

Smallfield, S., Clem, K., & Myers, A. (2013). Occupational therapy interventions to improve the reading ability of older adults with low vision: A systematic review. *American Journal of Occupational Therapy, 67,* 288-295. doi:10.5014/ajot.2013.004929

Snead, C. C. (2005). *A meta-analysis of attention deficit/hyperactivity disorder interventions: An empirical road to practical solutions* [doctoral dissertation]. Blacksburg, VA: Virginia Polytechnic Institute and State University.

Speck, R. M., Courneya, K. S., Masse, L. C., Duval, S., & Schmitz, K. H. (2010). An update of controlled physical activity trials in cancer survivors: A systematic review and meta-analysis. *Journal of Cancer Survivorship, 4,* 87-100. doi: 10.1007/s11764-009-0110-5

Stein, F., & Associates. (2003). *Stress Management Questionnaire: An instrument for self-regulating stress.* Albany, NY: Thomson Delmar Learning.

Stein, F., & Cutler, S. K. (2002). *Psychosocial occupational therapy: A holistic approach* (2nd ed.). Albany, NY: Delmar Publishers.

Stein, F., Grueschow, D., Hoffman, M., Taylor, S., & Tronbak, R. (2003). The Sorting Out Stress Cards—A version of the SMQ: A reliability study. *Occupational Therapy in Mental Health, 19,* 41-59.

Stein, F., Soderback, I., Cutler, S., & Larson B. (2006). *Occupational therapy and ergonomics: Applying ergonomic principles to everyday occupation in the home and work.* London, England: Whurr Publishers

Sullivan, H. S. (1963). *The fusion of psychiatry and social science.* New York, NY: W. W. Norton.

Taylor, P., Pezzullo, L., Grant, S. J., & Bensoussan, A. (2014). Cost-effectiveness of acupuncture for chronic nonspecific low back pain. *Pain Practice, 14, 7,* 599-606. doi: 10.1111/papr.12116

Taylor, R. (2017). *Kielhofner's model of human occupation: Theory and application.* Philadelphia, PA: Wolters Kluwer.

Taylor, R. S., Brown, A., Ebrahim, S., Jolliff, J., Noorani, H., Rees, K. ... Oldridge, N. (2004). Exercise-based rehabilitation for patients with coronary heart disease: Systematic review and meta-analysis of randomized controlled trials. *American Journal of Medicine, 116,* 682-692. doi: 10.1016/j.amjmed.2004.01.009

Teasdale, G., Maas, A., Lecky, F., Manly, G., Stocchetti, N., & Murray, G. (2014). The Glasgow Coma Scale at 40 years: Standing the test of time. *Lancet Neurology, 8,* 844-854. doi: 10.1016/S1474-4422(14)70120-6

Thieme, H., Mehrholz, J., Pohl, M., Behrens, J., & Dohle, C. (2013). Mirror therapy for improving motor function after stroke. *Stroke, 44,* e1-e2.

Thrane, G., Friborg, O., Anke, A., & Indredavik, B. (2014). A meta-analysis of constraint induced movement therapy after stroke. *Journal of Rehabilitation Medicine, 46,* 833-842. doi: 10.2340/16501977-1859

Turner-Stokes, L. (n.d.). *Goal attainment scaling in rehabilitation: A practical guide.* London, England: Kings College, University of London.

U.S. Department of Health and Human Services. (2017). *About the epidemic*. Retrieved from https://www.hhs.gov/opioids/about-the-epidemic/index.html

Van Deusen, J., & Harlowe, D. (1987). The efficacy of the ROM dance program for adults with rheumatoid arthritis. *American Journal of Occupational Therapy, 41,* 90-95. doi:10.5014/ajot.41.2.90

Vaughan-Graham, J., Cott, C., & Wright, F. V. (2015). The Bobath (NDT) concept in neurological rehabilitation: What is the state of the knowledge? A scoping review: Part I: Conceptual practices. *Disability and Rehabilitation, 37,* 1793-1807. doi: 10.3109/09638288.2014.985802

von Bertalanffy, L. (1950). The theory of open systems in physics and biology. *Science, 111,* 23-29.

Voss, D. E. (1967). Proprioceptive neuromuscular facilitation. *American Journal of Physical Medicine, 46,* 838-898.

Voss, D. E., Ionta, M. K., & Myers, B. J. (1985). *Proprioceptive neuromuscular facilitation: Patterns and techniques* (3rd ed.). Philadelphia, PA: Lippincott Williams & Wilkins.

Watson, J. B. (1913). Psychology as the behaviorist views it. *Psychological Review, 20*(2), 158-177. http://dx.doi.org/10.1037/h0074428

Wilbarger, P. (1995). The sensory diet: Activity programs based on sensory processing theory. *Sensory Integration Special Interest Section Newsletter, 18,* 1-4.

Williams, M. S., & Shellenberger, S. (1996). *How does your engine run? A leader's guide to The Alert Program for self-regulation.* Albuquerque, NM: Therapyworks Inc.

Wolpe, J. (1991). *The practice of behavior therapy* (4th ed.). Elmsford, NY: Persimmon.

World Health Organization. (2017). *Health topics: Disabilities.* Retrieved from http://www.who.int/topics/disabilities/en

Wykoff, W. (1993). The psychological effects of exercise on nonclinical and clinical populations of adult woman: A critical review of the literature. *Occupational Therapy in Mental Health, 12*(3), 69-106.

Yang, J. L., Jan, M. H., Chang, C. W., & Lin, J. J. (2012). Effectiveness of the end-range scapular mobilization approach in a subgroup of subjects with frozen shoulder syndrome: A random controlled trial. *Manual Therapy, 17,* 47-52. doi: 10.1016/j.math.2011.08.006

Yerxa, E. J., Barber, L. M., Diaz, O., Black, W., & Azen, S. P. (1983). Development of a hand sensitivity test for the hypersensitive hand. *American Journal of Occupational Therapy, 37*(3), 176-181.

Yu, C. H., & Mathiowetz, V. (2014). Systematic review of occupational therapy-related interventions for people with multiple sclerosis: Part 2. Impairment. *American Journal of Occupational Therapy, 68,* 33-38. doi: 10.5014/ajot.2014.008680

Zeng, C., Li, H., Yang, T., Deng, Z. H., Yang, Y., & Zhang, Y. (2015). Electrical stimulation for pain relief in knee osteoarthritis: Systematic review and network meta-analysis. *Osteoarthritis Cartilage, 23*(2), 189-202. doi: 10.1016/j.joca.2014.11.014. Epub 2014 Nov 26.

Appendix A

Ten Essential Clinical Skills for Occupational Therapists

1. Listening and being responsive to a client expressing his or her feelings
2. Ability to establish rapport and a positive relationship with a client
3. Ability to communicate with a client in a clear, understandable manner in explaining the purposes and aims of occupational therapy
4. Being curious and a lifelong learner in relation to understanding a client's strengths, needs, disability, validated interventions, and quality-of-life issues
5. Established writing skills, especially in evaluation, progress notes, and case studies
6. Positive social skills necessary to work with others such as client groups, colleagues, families, and within interprofessional meetings
7. Problem-solving and critical thinking skills in planning interventions and working with clients in a therapeutic alliance to motivate a client to put forth his or her best efforts
8. Ability to apply evidence-based practice by keeping current with published research and attending educational seminars

Stein, F., & Haertl, K.
Pocket Guide to Intervention in Occupational Therapy, Second Edition (pp 327-328).
© 2019 Taylor & Francis Group.

9. Respecting diversity among clients such as gender, sexual orientation, age, ethnic backgrounds, and class distinctions

10. Maintaining ethical standards without compromising integrity or financial gain

Appendix B

Commonly Used Medical Abbreviations

/d	per day
a	of each
a.c.	before a meal
ACTH	adrenocorticotropic hormone
ad lib.	freely
ADA	Americans with Disabilities Act
ADD	attention deficit disorder
ADHD	attention deficit hyperactivity disorder
admov.	apply
AIDS	acquired immunodeficiency syndrome
ALS	amyotrophic lateral sclerosis
alt.dieb	every other day
ap	before dinner
b.i.d.	twice a day
bib.	drink
bol.	pill
BP	blood pressure
c	with

Stein, F., & Haertl, K.
Pocket Guide to Intervention in Occupational Therapy, Second Edition (pp 329-331).
© 2019 Taylor & Francis Group.

CBC	complete blood count
CMC	carpometacarpal joint
CNS	central nervous system
CP	cerebral palsy
CSF	cerebrospinal fluid
CVA	cerebrovascular accident
D and C	dilatation and curettage
DIP	distal interphalangeal
Dx	diagnosis
ECG	electrocardiogram
ECT	electroconvulsive therapy
ED	emergency departure
EEG	electroencephalogram
EMG	electromyogram
ER	emergency room
FAS	fetal alcohol syndrome
GBS	Guillain-Barré syndrome
GI	gastrointestinal
HIV	human immunodeficiency virus
IDEA	Individuals with Disabilities Education Act of 1990
IEP	Individualized Education Plan
IFSP	Individualized Family Service Plan
IM	intramuscular
in d.	daily
IQ	intelligence quotient
ITP	Individualized Transition Plan
IV	intravenous
kg	kilogram
lb	pound
MCP	metacarpophalangeal
MD	muscular dystrophy
MED	minimum effective dose
MMR	measles-mumps-rubella vaccine
MR	mental retardation
MS	multiple sclerosis
p	after
p.c.	after meals

PIP	proximal interphalangeal
p.r.n.	as needed
q.h.	every hour
q.i.d.	four times a day
quotid	every day (comes from the French)
RBC	red blood cell
REM	rapid eye movement
RESNA	Rehabilitation Engineering and Assistive Technology Society of North America
s (sans)	without
SCI	spinal cord injury
SES	socioeconomic status
STD	sexually transmitted disease
t.i.d.	three times a day
TBI	traumatic brain injury

Appendix C

Developmental Milestones
Birth to 5 Years

Stein, F., & Haertl, K.
Pocket Guide to Intervention in Occupational
Therapy, Second Edition (pp 333-337).
© 2019 Taylor & Francis Group.

AGE	GROSS MOTOR	FINE MOTOR	SOCIAL/EMOTIONAL	COGNITIVE/VISUAL	COMMUNICATION
1 to 3 Months	• Demonstrates primarily asymmetric postures • Begins to develop head/midline control in supine, prone, and supported sitting • Pushes up on forearms	• Fisted hands gradually open • Sustains grasp if object is placed in hand • Adapts hands to shape of objects without visual attention (tactile accommodation)	• Imitates facial expressions • Smiles reciprocally • Indicates anger, happiness, joy, sadness, pleasure, and displeasure with facial and body reactions	• Turns toward sources of light • Localizes faces, sounds, and moving objects in near space • Eyes follow hand/object/person, jerky movements, eyes/head together	• Coos, chuckles, and makes single-vowel sounds (e.g., ah, eh, uh) • Discriminates cries to express discomfort (e.g., hunger or pain) • Echoes another's vocalizations
4 to 6 Months	• Achieves mature and symmetrical head control on forearms and supported sitting • Hands reach and grasp knees/feet, may bring foot to mouth • Rolls from prone/supine/prone	• Primitive grasps develop into efficient power grasps, involving thumb • Engages hands in midline • Eats finger food without biting fingers (tactile discrimination)	• Smiles, reaches, and vocalizes to initiate social interactions • Smiles at self in mirror • Anticipates food by sight and smell • Indicates fear and stranger anxiety with crying and facial expressions	• Visually attends to object within 1 inch • Eyes gradually separate from head to track objects • Searches for missing object, but distracted by new stimulus (begins object permanence)	• Vocalizes polysyllabic vowel sounds • Begins consonant sounds (e.g., m-m-m) • Excites to stimuli, breathing heavily • Listens to speaker, vocalizes when speaker stops

(continued)

Chart compiled by Rhoda Erhardt, MS, OTR/L, FAOTA.

Age	Gross Motor	Fine Motor	Social/Emotional	Cognitive/Visual	Communication
7 to 9 Months	• Sits alone • Pushes up to hands and knees • Pushes up to sitting • Crawls on hands and knees • Rotates from hands and knees, to sitting, to hand to knees	• Explores objects with mouth more than hands • Achieves more precise grasping of large objects • Begins primitive grasp of pellet • Transfers object from one hand to the other	• Waves bye • Extends object to person without release. • Reacts appropriately to other person's emotions (e.g., frowns when spoken to angrily) • Comforts self (e.g, with blanket)	• Searches for lost object, ignoring new stimulus (achieves object permanence) • Intentionally manipulates objects only with visual monitoring • Begins reciprocal assimilation	• Babbles randomly, with increased meaning through adult reinforcement • Responds to own name • Imitates sounds • Says ma-ma, da-da • Plays peek-a-boo
10 to 12 Months	• Pulls to stand • Stands alone • Bends over to pick up object without falling • Walks by cruising along furniture • Walks with one hand held • Tries to walk without support	• Replaces oral exploration with tactile, except for novel objects • Isolates index finger to poke and refine pincer grasp of pellet • Releases objects into another's hand or container	• Shows sense of humor by smiling and laughing • Amuses self with toys • Plays with other children • May show tantrum behavior when frustrated (e.g., crying, throwing food)	• Learns cause and effect (e.g., inverts container to reach contents) • Finds hidden object (object permanence) • Explores objects by shaking, banging, pushing, pulling, dropping	• Babbles with conversational tones • Imitates gestures • Points to desired object (means-end) • Responds to simple one-step verbal command with gestures

(continued)

Chart compiled by Rhoda Erhardt, MS, OTR/L, FAOTA.

Age	Gross Motor	Fine Motor	Social/Emotional	Cognitive/Visual	Communication
1 to 2 Years	• Walks alone • Squats in play • Carries one or more toys while walking • Begins to run • Kicks large ball • Crawls up steps, then learns to walk up and down stairs, holding rail • Climbs up on furniture	• Manipulates object with one hand, other stabilizes or assists • Uses palmar-supinate grasp of utensils (e.g., spoon and crayon) • Scribbles spontaneously, draws vertical, horizontal, and circular strokes	• Imitates behaviors of adults and older children • Shows excitement about being with other children • Gradually releases separation anxiety • Begins to show defiant behavior • Helps with undressing	• Manipulates objects intentionally without visual monitoring (reciprocal assimilation) • Inverts container to reach contents • Engages in solitary play, then parallel play	• Begins speaking several single words, then simple two- to four-word phrases • Points to body parts • Responds to one-step verbal command, without gestures • Follows a two-step command
3 to 4 Years	• Runs easily • Throws and catches ball • Hops on one foot • Begins to skip • Goes up stairs without support, alternating feet	• Uses more mature digital-pronate and static tripod grasps (e.g., pencil and paint brush) • Draws circle and cross • Uses scissors	• Imitates adults and playmates • Shows affection for playmates • Dresses and undresses • Separates easily from parents	• Names three to four colors • Counts to four • Knows own gender and age • Participates in associative and cooperative play • Begins turn-taking	• Uses four- to five-word sentences • Uses plurals • Tells stories • Comprehends prepositions and follows directions (e.g., put toy in or under object.)

(continued)

Chart compiled by Rhoda Erhardt, MS, OTR/L, FAOTA.

Age	Gross Motor	Fine Motor	Social/Emotional	Cognitive/Visual	Communication
5 Years	• Stands on one foot for 8 to 10 seconds • Walks backward • Hops (one foot) • Jumps (both feet) • Skips • Walks downstairs without rail, alternating feet	• Achieves mature dynamic tripod grasp of utensils • Draws square and triangle • Cuts on line consistently • Prints own first name	• Verbalizes feelings to others • Pours liquid from one container to another • Ties shoelaces • Cares for own toileting needs	• Names five to six colors • Counts 10 objects, pointing correctly • Identifies at least three coins • Joins in dramatic play • Plays games, following rules	• Discusses both past and future experiences • Says name, address, and phone number • Names categories of sorted objects

Chart compiled by Rhoda Erhardt, MS, OTR/L, FAOTA.

Appendix D

Orthotics and Orthoses
Exoskeletal or External
Devices to Limit or Assist
Motion in Joints of Body

Stein, F., & Haertl, K.
*Pocket Guide to Intervention in Occupational
Therapy, Second Edition* (pp 339-341).
© 2019 Taylor & Francis Group.

CATEGORY OF DEVICE	TYPES	MATERIALS	PURPOSE	DISABILITY EXAMPLES
Crutch	Straight canes, forearm crutches, underarm crutches, quad canes, walkers	Wood, metal, plastic	Support or replace limb	Amputee, fracture, sprain
Orthosis	Static: no moving parts • Wrist cock-up splint • Resting hand splint • Ulnar deviation correction splint • Thumb web spacer Dynamic: moving parts • Flexor tendon repair splint • Extensor tendon repair splint • Radial palsy splint Volar splint Dorsal splint	Aluminum, metal, and plastic	Immobilization: prevent movement Correction: correct deformity Preventive: contractures in muscles Functional position Therapeutic: strengthen weak muscle	Fracture Burns Arthritis Peripheral nerve injury Spinal cord injury
Brace	Foot attachments, leg braces, knee joint, pelvic band, Milwaukee brace, cervical collar, trunk, hip, knee, ankle, foot	Surgical steel, aluminum, leather, plastic	Support the body, prevent and correct deformity; control involuntary movements	Scoliosis Spinal cord injury Orthopedic deformities Cerebral palsy

(continued)

Category of Device	Types	Materials	Purpose	Disability Examples
Wheelchair, client vehicles, tricycles, and scooters	Manual Battery powered Scooter: battery Folding	Light chromium plated, plastic, fabric, battery	Transport • Indoor • Outdoor • Transfer to car	Spinal cord injury Amputee Muscular dystrophy Multiple sclerosis Cerebral palsy
Automobile controls	Upper extremity: hand controls Lower extremity controls	Metal, leather, plastic	Enable individuals with disabilities to drive Controls gas, brake, signals, dimmer switch, steering, and transmission	Amputee Spinal cord injury Traumatic brain injury Cerebral palsy
Slings	Overhead (wheelchair) Universal hemiplegic sling	Cotton webbing	Back support, flail shoulder, support subluxated shoulder joint	Quadriplegia Hemiplegia
Traction	Cervical, lumbar, pelvic	Cotton	Reduce pain by relieving pressure on joint	Dislocation, arthritis, herniated disc
Foot and shoe orthoses	Inserts, heel, cushions, sole vamps, pads	Leather, plastic, metal, cotton, sponge	Assist gait, reduce pain, correct deformity	Back pain, arthritis, hammer toes, leg shortening, cerebral palsy

Appendix E

Table of Muscles

Muscles	Origin	Insertion	Innervation	Action
MUSCLES OF THE BACK				
Superficial Muscles				
Trapezius	External occipital protuberance, superior nuchal line, ligamentum nuchae, spines of C7–T12	Spine of scapula, acromion, and lateral third of clavicle	Spinal accessory n., C3–C4	Adducts, rotates, elevates, and depresses scapula
Levator scapulae	Transverse processes of C1–C4	Medial border of scapula	Nerves to levator scapulae, C3–C4; dorsal scapular n.	Elevates scapula
Rhomboid minor	Spines of C7–T1	Root of spine of scapula	Dorsal scapular n., C5	Adducts scapula
Rhomboid major	Spines of T2–T5	Medial border of scapula	Dorsal scapular n.	Adducts scapula
Latissimus dorsi	Spines of T5–T12, thoracodorsal fascia, iliac crest, ribs 9–12	Floor of bicipital groove of humerus	Thoracodorsal n.	Adducts, extends, and rotates arm medially
Intermediate Muscles				
Serratus posterior–superior	Ligamentum nuchae, supraspinal ligament, and spines of C7–T3	Upper border of ribs 2–5	Intercostal n., T1–T4	Elevates ribs
Serratus posterior–inferior	Supraspinous ligament and spines of T11–L3	Lower border of ribs 9–12	Intercostal n., T9–T12	Depresses ribs

(continued)

MUSCLES	ORIGIN	INSERTION	INNERVATION	ACTION
Deep Muscles (Intrinsics)				
Superficial Layer of Deep Muscles (Spinotransverse Group)				
Splenius capitis	Inferior half of ligamentum nuchae, spinous processes of T1–T6	Lateral aspect of mastoid process, lateral third of superior nuchal line	Dorsal rami of inferior cervical n.	Alone, it laterally flexes and rotates head and neck to same side; it works with the other splenius muscle to extend the head and neck
Splenius cervicis	Inferior half of ligamentum nuchae, spinous processes of T1–T6	Posterior tubercles of transverse processes of C1–C4	Dorsal rami of inferior cervical n.	Alone, it laterally flexes and rotates head and neck to same side; it works with the other splenius muscle to extend the head and neck
Intermediate Layer of Deep Muscles (Sacrospinalis or Erector Spinae Group)				
Iliocostalis (lateral column)	Posterior part of iliac crest, posterior aspect of sacrum, sacroiliac ligaments, and sacral and inferior lumbar spinous processes	Angles of the ribs, cervical transverse processes	Dorsal rami of spinal n.	Bilaterally, they extend the head and vertebral column; unilaterally, they laterally flex the head or vertebral column

(continued)

MUSCLES	ORIGIN	INSERTION	INNERVATION	ACTION
Longissimus (intermediate column)	Posterior part of iliac crest, posterior aspect of sacrum, sacroiliac ligaments, and sacral and inferior lumbar spinous processes	Transverse processes of thoracic and cervical vertebrae, mastoid process	Dorsal rami of spinal n.	Same as previous; also, the longissimus capitis rotates the head to the same side
Spinalis (medial column)	Posterior part of iliac crest, posterior aspect of sacrum, sacroiliac ligaments, and sacral and inferior lumbar spinous processes	Spinous processes from lumbar to thoracic region	Dorsal rami of spinal n.	Bilaterally, they extend the head and vertebral column; unilaterally, they laterally flex the head or vertebral column
Deep Layer of Deep Muscles (Transversospinalis Group)				
Semispinalis thoracis	Transverse processes	Thoracic and cervical spinous processes	Dorsal rami of cervical spinal n.	Bilaterally, extends the cervical and thoracic regions of vertebral column; unilaterally, rotates toward the opposite side
Semispinalis cervicis	Transverse processes	Thoracic and cervical spinous processes	Dorsal rami of cervical spinal n.	Bilaterally, extends the cervical and thoracic regions of vertebral column; unilaterally, rotates toward the opposite side

(continued)

Muscles	Origin	Insertion	Innervation	Action
Semispinalis capitis	Transverse processes of T1–T6	Medial half of area between superior and inferior nuchal line on occipital bone	Dorsal rami of cervical spinal n.	Bilaterally, extends the head; unilaterally, rotates toward the opposite side
Multifidus	Laminae of S4–C2	Span one to three vertebrae before inserting in spinous processes	Dorsal rami of cervical spinal n.	Bilaterally, extend the trunk and stabilize the vertebral column; unilaterally, flex the trunk laterally and rotate it to the opposite side
Rotators	Transverse processes	Base of the spinous process superior to vertebra of origin	Dorsal rami of cervical spinal n.	Rotate the superior vertebra to the opposite side and stabilize it
SEGMENTAL MUSCLES				
Interspinales	Spinous processes	Adjacent spinous processes	Dorsal rami of cervical spinal n.	Extend the vertebral column
Intertransversarii	Transverse processes	Adjacent transverse processes	Ventral and dorsal rami of cervical spinal n.	Bilaterally, extend the vertebral column; unilaterally, laterally flex the superior vertebra
Levator costarum	Transverse processes	Rib just inferior to vertebra of origin	Dorsal rami of spinal n.	Elevate the ribs during inspiration
				(continued)

Muscles	Origin	Insertion	Innervation	Action
SUBOCCIPITAL MUSCLES				
Rectus capitis posterior major	Spine of axis	Lateral portion of inferior nuchal line	Suboccipital n.	Extends, rotates, and flexes head laterally
Rectus capitis posterior minor	Posterior tubercle of atlas	Occipital bone below inferior nuchal line	Suboccipital n.	Extends and flexes head laterally
Obliquus capitis superior	Transverse process of atlas	Occipital bone above inferior nuchal line	Suboccipital n.	Extends, rotates, and flexes head laterally
Obliquus capitis inferior	Spine of axis	Transverse process of atlas	Suboccipital n.	Extends head and rotates it laterally
MUSCLES OF THE NECK				
Platysma	Superficial fascia over upper part of deltoid and pectoralis major	Mandible; skin and muscles over mandible and angle of mouth	Facial n.	Depresses lower jaw and lip and angle of mouth; wrinkle skin of neck
Sternocleidomastoid	Manubrium sterni and medial one-third of clavicle	Mastoid process and lateral one-half of superior nuchal line	Spinal accessory n.; C2–C3 (sensory)	Unilaterally, turns face toward opposite side; bilaterally, flexes head, raises thorax
SUPRAHYOID MUSCLES				
Digastric	Anterior belly from digastric fossa of mandible; posterior belly from mastoid notch	Intermediate tendon attached to body of hyoid	Anterior belly by mylohyoid n. of trigeminal n.; posterior belly by facial n.	Elevates hyoid and tongue; depresses mandible
				(continued)

MUSCLES	ORIGIN	INSERTION	INNERVATION	ACTION
Mylohyoid	Mylohyoid line of mandible	Median raphe and body of hyoid bone	Mylohyoid n. of trigeminal n.	Elevates hyoid and tongue; depresses mandible
Stylohyoid	Styloid process	Body of hyoid	Facial n.	Elevates hyoid
Geniohyoid	Genial tubercle of mandible	Body of hyoid	C1 via hypoglossal n.	Elevates hyoid and tongue
INFRAHYOID MUSCLES				
Sternohyoid	Manubrium sterni and medial end of clavicle	Body of hyoid	Ansa cervicalis	Depresses hyoid and larynx
Sternothyroid	Manubrium sterni; first costal cartilage	Oblique line of thyroid cartilage	Ansa cervicalis	Depresses thyroid cartilage and larynx
Thyrohyoid	Oblique line of thyroid cartilage	Body and greater horn of hyoid	C1 via hypoglossal n.	Depresses and retracts hyoid and larynx
Omohyoid	Inferior belly from medial lip of suprascapular notch and suprascapular ligament; superior belly from intermediate tendon	Inferior belly to intermediate tendon; superior belly to body of hyoid	Ansa cervicalis	Depresses and retracts hyoid and larynx

(continued)

Muscles	Origin	Insertion	Innervation	Action
		PREVERTEBRAL MUSCLES		
Anterior scalene	Transverse processes of C3–C6	Scalene tubercle on first rib	Ventral rami of cervical spinal n. (C3–C8)	Elevates first rib, bends neck
Middle scalene	Transverse processes of C2–C7	Upper surface of first rib	Ventral rami of cervical spinal n. (C3–C8)	Flexes neck laterally, elevates first rib during forced inspiration
Posterior scalene	Transverse processes of C4–C6	Outer surface of second rib	Ventral rami of cervical spinal n. (C7–C8)	Flexes neck laterally, elevates second rib during forced inspiration
Longus capitis	Transverse processes of C3–C6	Basilar part of occipital bone	Ventral rami of cervical spinal n. (C1–C4)	Flexes and rotates head
Longus colli	Transverse processes and bodies of C3–T3	Anterior tubercle of atlas; bodies of C2–C4; transverse process of C5–C6	Ventral rami of cervical spinal n. (C2–C6)	Flexes and rotates head
Rectus capitis anterior	Lateral mass of atlas	Basilar part of occipital bone	Ventral rami of cervical spinal n. (C1–C2)	Flexes and rotates head
Rectus capitis lateralis	Transverse process of atlas	Jugular process of occipital bone	Ventral rami of cervical spinal n. (C1–C2)	Flexes head laterally

(continued)

MUSCLES	ORIGIN	INSERTION	INNERVATION	ACTION
MUSCLES OF FACIAL EXPRESSION				
Occipitofrontalis	Superior nuchal line; upper orbital margin	Epicranial aponeurosis	Facial n.	Elevates eyebrows, wrinkles forehead
Corrugator supercilii	Medial supraorbital margin	Skin of medial eyebrow	Facial n.	Draws eyebrows downward medially
Orbicularis oculi	Medial orbital margin; medial palpebral ligament; lacrimal bone	Skin and rim of orbit; tarsal plate; lateral palpebral raphe	Facial n.	Closes eyelids
Procerus	Nasal bone and cartilage	Skin between eyebrows	Facial n.	Wrinkles skin over bones
Nasalis	Maxilla lateral to incisive fossa	Ala of nose	Facial n.	Draws ala of nose toward septum
Depressor septi	Incisive fossa of maxilla	Ala and nasal septum	Facial n.	Constricts nares
Orbicularis oris	Maxilla above incisor teeth	Skin of lip	Facial n.	Closes lips
Levator anguli oris	Canine fossa of maxilla	Angle of mouth	Facial n.	Elevates angle of mouth medially
Levator labii superioris	Maxilla above infraorbital foramen	Skin of upper lip	Facial n.	Elevates upper lip, dilates nares

(continued)

Muscles	Origin	Insertion	Innervation	Action
Levator labii superioris alaeque nasi	Frontal process of maxilla	Skin of upper lip	Facial n.	Elevates ala of nose and upper lip
Zygomaticus major	Zygomatic arch	Angle of mouth	Facial n.	Draws angle of mouth backward and upward
Zygomaticus minor	Zygomatic arch	Angle of mouth	Facial n.	Elevates upper lip
Depressor labii inferioris	Mandible below mental foramen	Orbicularis oris and skin of lower lip	Facial n.	Depresses lower lip
Depressor anguli oris	Oblique line of mandible	Angle of mouth	Facial n.	Depresses angle of mouth
Risorius	Fascia over masseter	Angle of mouth	Facial n.	Retracts angle of mouth
Buccinator	Mandible; pterygomandibular raphe; alveolar processes	Angle of mouth	Facial n.	Presses cheek to keep it taut
Mentalis	Incisive fossa of mandible	Skin of chin	Facial n.	Elevates and protrudes lower tip
Auricularis anterior, superior, and posterior	Temporal fascia; epicranial aponeurosis; mastoid process	Anterior, superior, and posterior sides of auricle	Facial n.	Retract and elevate ear
				(continued)

Muscles	Origin	Insertion	Innervation	Action
MUSCLES OF MASTICATION				
Temporalis	Temporal fossa	Coronoid process and ramus of mandible	Trigeminal n.	Elevates and retracts mandible
Masseter	Lower border and medial surface of zygomatic arch	Lateral surface of coronoid process, ramus and angle of mandible	Trigeminal n.	Elevates mandible
Lateral pterygoid	Superior head from infratemporal surface of sphenoid; inferior head from lateral surface of lateral pterygoid plate	Neck of mandible; articular disk and capsule of temporomandibular joint	Trigeminal n.	Protracts (protrudes) and depresses mandible
Medial pterygoid	Tuber of maxilla; medial surface of lateral pterygoid plate; pyramidal process of palatine bone	Medial surface of angle and ramus of mandible	Trigeminal n.	Protracts (protrudes) and elevates mandible
MUSCLES OF EYE MOVEMENT				
Superior rectus	Common tendinous ring	Sclera just behind cornea	Oculomotor n.	Elevates eyeball
Inferior rectus	Common tendinous ring	Sclera just behind cornea	Oculomotor n.	Depresses eyeball

(continued)

Muscles	Origin	Insertion	Innervation	Action
Medial rectus	Common tendinous ring	Sclera just behind cornea	Oculomotor n.	Adducts eyeball
Lateral rectus	Common tendinous ring	Sclera just behind cornea	Abducens n.	Adducts eyeball
Levator palpebrae superioris	Lesser wing of sphenoid above and anterior to optic canal	Tarsal plate and skin of upper eyelid	Oculomotor n.	Elevates upper eyelid
Superior oblique	Body of sphenoid bone above optic canal	Sclera beneath superior rectus	Trochlear n.	Rotates downward and medially, depresses adducted eye
Inferior oblique	Floor of orbit lateral to lacrimal groove	Sclera beneath lateral rectus	Oculomotor n.	Rotates upward and laterally, elevates adducted eye
MUSCLES OF THE PALATE				
Tensor veli palatini	Scaphoid fossa; spine of sphenoid; cartilage of auditory tube	Tendon hooks around hamulus of medial pterygoid plate to insert into aponeurosis of soft palate	Mandibular branch of trigeminal n.	Tenses soft palate

(continued)

MUSCLES	ORIGIN	INSERTION	INNERVATION	ACTION
Levator veli palatini	Petrous part of temporal bone; cartilage of auditory tube	Aponeurosis of soft palate	Vagus n. via pharyngeal plexus	Elevates soft palate
Palatoglossus	Aponeurosis of soft palate	Dorsolateral side of tongue	Vagus n. via pharyngeal plexus	Elevates tongue
Palatopharyngeus	Aponeurosis of soft palate; hard palate	Thyroid cartilage and side of pharynx; muscles of pharynx	Vagus n. via pharyngeal plexus	Elevates pharynx; closes nasopharynx
Musculus uvulae	Posterior nasal spine of palatine bone; palatine aponeurosis	Mucous membrane of uvula	Vagus n. via pharyngeal plexus	Elevates uvula
MUSCLES OF THE TONGUE				
Styloglossus	Styloid process	Side and inferior aspect of tongue	Hypoglossal n.	Retracts and elevates tongue
Hyoglossus	Body and greater horn of hyoid bone	Side and inferior aspect of tongue	Hypoglossal n.	Depresses and retracts tongue
Genioglossus	Genial tubercle of mandible	Inferior aspect of tongue; body of hyoid bone	Hypoglossal n.	Protrudes and depresses tongue
See Palatoglossus				

(continued)

MUSCLES	ORIGIN	INSERTION	INNERVATION	ACTION
MUSCLES OF THE PHARYNX				
Superior constrictor	Medial pterygoid plate; pterygoid hamulus; pterygomandibular raphe; mylohyoid line of mandible; side of tongue	Median raphe and pharyngeal tubercle of skull	Vagus n. via pharyngeal plexus	Constricts upper pharynx
Middle constrictor	Greater and lesser horns of hyoid; stylohyoid ligament	Median raphe	Vagus n. via pharyngeal plexus	Constricts lower pharynx
Inferior constrictor	Arch of cricoid and oblique line of thyroid cartilages	Median raphe of pharynx	Vagus n. via pharyngeal plexus, recurrent and external laryngeal n.	Constricts lower pharynx
Stylopharyngeus	Styloid process	Thyroid cartilage and muscles of pharynx	Glossopharyngeal n.	Elevates pharynx and larynx
Salpingopharyngeus	Cartilage of auditory tube	Muscles of pharynx	Vagus n. via pharyngeal plexus	Elevates nasopharynx, opens auditory tube
See Palatopharyngeus				

(continued)

MUSCLES	ORIGIN	INSERTION	INNERVATION	ACTION
MUSCLES OF THE LARYNX				
Cricothyroid	Arch of cricoid cartilage	Inferior horn and lower lamina of thyroid cartilage	External laryngeal n.	Tenses vocal folds
Posterior cricoarytenoid	Posterior surface of lamina of cricoid cartilage	Muscular process of arytenoid cartilage	Recurrent laryngeal n.	Abducts vocal folds
Lateral cricoarytenoid	Arch of cricoid cartilage	Muscular process of arytenoid cartilage	Recurrent laryngeal n.	Abducts vocal folds
Transverse arytenoid	Posterior surface of arytenoid cartilage	Opposite arytenoid cartilage	Recurrent laryngeal n.	Abducts vocal folds
Oblique arytenoid	Muscular process of arytenoid cartilage	Apex of opposite arytenoid	Recurrent laryngeal n.	Abducts vocal folds
Aryepiglottic	Apex of arytenoid cartilage	Side of epiglottic cartilage	Recurrent laryngeal n.	Abducts vocal folds
Thyroarytenoid	Inner surface of thyroid lamina	Lateral margin of epiglottic cartilage	Recurrent laryngeal n.	Adducts vocal folds
Thyroepiglottic	Anteromedial surface of lamina of thyroid cartilage	Vocal process	Recurrent laryngeal n.	Adducts and tenses vocal folds
Vocalis	Anteromedial surface of lamina of thyroid cartilage	Anterolateral surface of arytenoid thyroid cartilage	Laryngeal n.	Adducts vocal folds

(continued)

MUSCLES	ORIGIN	INSERTION	INNERVATION	ACTION
MUSCLES OF THE MIDDLE EAR				
Stapedius	Pyramidal eminence	Neck of the stapes	Branch of the facial n.	Pulls the head of the stapes posteriorly, thereby tilting the base of the stapes, and protects the inner ear from injury during a loud noise
Tensor tympani	Cartilaginous portion of the auditory tube	Handle of the malleus	Mandibular branch of trigeminal n.	Draws the manubrium medially, pulling the tympanic membrane taut
MUSCLES OF THE UPPER LIMB				
Muscles of the Shoulder Region				
Deltoid	Lateral third of clavicle, acromion, and spine of scapula	Deltoid tuberosity of humerus	Axillary n.	Anterior part: flexes and medially rotates arm; Middle part: abducts arm; Posterior part: extends and laterally rotates arm
Supraspinatus	Supraspinous fossa of scapula	Superior facet of greater tubercle of humerus	Suprascapular n.	Abducts arm
				(continued)

Muscles	Origin	Insertion	Innervation	Action
Infraspinatus	Infraspinous fossa	Middle facet of greater tubercle of humerus	Suprascapular n.	Rotates arm laterally
Subscapularis	Subscapular fossa	Lesser tubercle of humerus	Upper and lower subscapular n.	Rotates arm medially
Teres major	Dorsal surface of inferior angle of scapula	Medial lip of intertubercular groove of humerus	Lower subscapular n.	Adducts and rotates arm medially
Teres minor	Upper portion of lateral border of scapula	Lower facet of greater tubercle of humerus	Axillary n.	Rotates arm laterally
Latissimus dorsi	Spines of T7–T12 thoracolumbar fascia, iliac crest, ribs 9–12	Floor of bicipital groove of humerus	Thoracodorsal n.	Adducts, extends, and rotates arm medially
Muscles of the Arm				
Coracobrachialis	Coracoid process	Middle third of medial surface of humerus	Musculocutaneous n.	Flexes and adducts arm
Biceps brachii	Long head: supra glenoid tubercle of scapula; short head: tip of coracoid process of scapula	Radial tuberosity of radius	Musculocutaneous n.	Flexes arm and forearm, supinates forearm when it is supine

(continued)

MUSCLES	ORIGIN	INSERTION	INNERVATION	ACTION
Brachialis	Distal half of anterior surface of humerus	Coronoid process of ulna and ulnar tuberosity	Musculocutaneous n.	Flexes forearm
Triceps brachii	Long head: infraglenoid tubercle of scapula; Lateral head: posterior surface of humerus, superior to radial groove; medial head: posterior surface of humerus, inferior radial groove	Posterior surface of olecranon process; of ulna	Radial n.	Extends forearm
Anconeus	Lateral epicondyle of humerus	Olecranon and upper posterior surface of ulna	Radial n.	Extends forearm with triceps; stabilizes elbow joint
Muscles of the Anterior Forearm				
Pronator teres	Medial epicondyle and coronoid process of ulna	Middle of lateral side of radius	Median n.	Pronates forearm
Flexor carpi radialis	Medial epicondyle of humerus	Bases of second and third metacarpals	Median n.	Flexes forearm, flexes and abducts hand
Palmaris longus	Medial epicondyle of humerus	Flexor retinaculum, palmar aponeurosis	Median n.	Flexes hand and forearm
				(continued)

Muscles	Origin	Insertion	Innervation	Action
Flexor carpi ulnaris	Medial epicondyle, medial olecranon, and posterior border of ulna	Pisiform, hook of hamate, and base of fifth metacarpal	Ulnar n.	Flexes and adducts hand, flexes forearm
Flexor digitorum superficialis	Medial epicondyle, coronoid process, oblique line of radius	Middle phalanges of finger	Median n.	Flexes proximal interphalangeal joints, flexes hand and forearm
Flexor digitorum profundus	Anteromedial surface of ulna, interosseous membrane	Bases of distal phalanges of fingers	Ulnar and median n.	Flexes distal interphalangeal joints and hand
Flexor pollicis longus	Anterior surface of radius, interosseous membrane, and coronoid process	Base of distal phalanx of thumb	Median n.	Flexes thumb
Pronator quadratus	Anterior surface of distal ulna	Anterior surface of distal radius	Median n.	Pronates forearm
Muscles of the Posterior Forearm				
Brachioradialis	Lateral supracondylar ridge of humerus	Base of radial styloid process	Radial n.	Flexes forearm
Extensor carpi radialis longus	Lateral supracondylar ridge of humerus	Dorsum of base of second metacarpal	Radial n.	Extends and abducts hand
Extensor carpi radialis brevis	Lateral epicondyle of humerus	Posterior base of third metacarpal	Radial n.	Extends fingers and abducts hands

(continued)

MUSCLES	ORIGIN	INSERTION	INNERVATION	ACTION
Extensor digitorum	Lateral epicondyle of humerus	Extensor expansion, base of middle and digital phalanges	Radial n.	Extends fingers and hand
Extensor digiti minimi	Common extensor tendon and interosseous membrane	Extensor expansion, base of middle and distal phalanges	Radial n.	Extends little finger
Extensor carpi ulnaris	Lateral epicondyle and posterior surface of ulna	Base of fifth	Radial n.	Extends and adducts hand
Supinator	Lateral epicondyle, radial collateral and annular ligaments	Lateral side of upper part of radius	Radial n.	Supinates forearm
Abductor pollicis longus	Interosseous membrane, middle third of posterior surfaces of radius and ulna	Lateral surface of base of first metacarpal	Radial n.	Abducts thumb and hand
Extensor pollicis longus	Interosseous membrane and middle third of posterior surface of ulna	Base of distal phalanx of thumb	Radial n.	Extends distal phalanx of thumb and abducts hand

(continued)

Muscles	Origin	Insertion	Innervation	Action
Extensor pollicis brevis	Interosseous membrane and posterior surface of middle third radius	Base of proximal phalanx of thumb	Radial n.	Extends proximal phalanx of thumb and abducts hand
Extensor indicis	Posterior surface of ulna and interosseous membrane	Extensor expansion of index finger	Radial n.	Extends index finger
Muscles of the Hand				
Abductor pollicis brevis	Flexor retinaculum, scaphoid, and trapezium	Lateral side of base of proximal phalanx of thumb	Median n.	Abducts thumb
Flexor pollicis brevis	Flexor retinaculum and trapezium	Base of proximal phalanx of thumb	Median n.	Flexes thumb
Opponens pollicis	Flexor retinaculum and trapezium	Lateral side of first metacarpal	Median n.	Opposes thumb to other digits
Adductor pollicis	Oblique head: capitate and bases of second and third metacarpals Transverse head: palmar surface of third metacarpal	Medial side of base of proximal phalanx of thumb	Ulnar n.	Adducts thumb
Palmaris brevis	Medial side of flexor retinaculum, palmar aponeurosis	Skin of medial side of palm	Ulnar n.	Wrinkles skin on medial side of palm

(continued)

Muscles	Origin	Insertion	Innervation	Action
Abductor digiti minimi	Pisiform and tendon of flexor carpi ulnaris	Medial side of base of proximal phalanx of little finger	Ulnar n.	Abducts little finger
Flexor digiti minimi brevis	Flexor retinaculum and hook of hamate	Medial side of base of proximal phalanx of little finger	Ulnar n.	Flexes proximal phalanx of little finger
Opponens digiti minimi	Flexor retinaculum and hook of hamate	Medial side of fifth metacarpal	Ulnar n.	Opposes little finger
Lumbricals (4)	Lateral side of tendons of flexor digitorum profundus	Lateral side of extensor expansion	Median (2 lateral) and ulnar (2 medial) n.	Flex metacarpophalangeal joints and extend interphalangeal joints
Dorsal interossei (4)	Adjacent sides of metacarpal bones	Lateral sides of bases of proximal phalanges; extensor expansion	Ulnar n.	Abduct fingers; flex metacarpophalangeal joints; extend interphalangeal joints
Palmar interossei (3)	Medial side of second metacarpal; lateral sides of fourth and fifth metacarpals	Bases of proximal phalanges in same sides as their origins; extensor expansion	Ulnar n.	Adduct fingers; flex metacarpophalangeal joints; extend interphalangeal joints

Appendix F

Average Range of Motion Measurements

Shoulder

Flexion	0 to 180°
Extension	0 to 60°
Adduction/Abduction	0 to 180°
Horizontal Abduction	0 to 90°
Horizontal Adduction	0 to 45°
Internal Rotation	0 to 70°
External Rotation	0 to 90°
Internal Rotation (alternate method)	0 to 80°
External Rotation (alternate method)	0 to 60°

Elbow and Forearm

Extension/Flexion	0 to 150°
Supination	0 to 80°
Pronation	0 to 80°

Stein, F., & Haertl, K.
*Pocket Guide to Intervention in Occupational
Therapy, Second Edition* (pp 365-366).
© 2019 Taylor & Francis Group.

Wrist

Flexion	0 to 80°
Extension	0 to 70°
Ulnar Deviation	0 to 30°
Radial Deviation	0 to 20°

Thumb

CM Flexion	0 to 15°
CM Extension/Thumb Radial Abduction	0 to 20°
MCP Extension/Flexion	0 to 50°
IP Extension/Flexion	0 to 80°
Palmar Abduction	0 to 70°/Cm
Opposition	Cm

Fingers

MCP Flexion	0 to 90°
PIP Extension/Flexion	0 to 100°
DIP Extension/Flexion	0 to 90°
Abduction	No Norm
Adduction	No Norm

Appendix G

Prime Movers for Upper and Selected Lower Extremity Motions

Scapular elevation
Upper trapezius
Levator scapulae

Scapular depression
Lower trapezius
Latissimus dorsi

Scapular adduction
Middle trapezius
Rhomboids

Scapular abduction
Serratus anterior

Shoulder flexion
Anterior deltoid
Coracobrachialis
Pectoralis major, clavicular head
Biceps, both heads

Shoulder extension
Latissimus dorsi
Teres major
Posterior deltoid
Triceps, long head

Stein, F., & Haertl, K.
Pocket Guide to Intervention in Occupational Therapy, Second Edition (pp 367-370).
© 2019 Taylor & Francis Group.

Shoulder abduction	Supraspinatus Middle deltoid
Shoulder adduction	Pectoralis major Teres major Latissimus dorsi
Shoulder horizontal abduction	Posterior deltoid
Shoulder horizontal adduction	Pectoralis major Anterior deltoid
Shoulder external rotation	Infraspinatus Teres minor Posterior deltoid
Shoulder internal rotation	Subscapularis Teres major Latissimus dorsi Pectoralis major Anterior deltoid
Elbow flexion	Biceps Brachialis Brachioradialis
Elbow extension	Triceps
Pronation	Pronator teres Pronator quadratus
Supination	Supinator Biceps
Wrist extension	Extensor carpi radialis longus (ECRL) Extensor carpi radialis brevis (ECRB) Extensor carpi ulnaris (ECU)
Wrist flexion	Flexor carpi radialis (FCR) Palmaris longus Flexor carpi ulnaris (FCU)
Finger DIP flexion	Flexor digitorum profundus (FDP)

Finger PIP flexion	Flexor digitorum superficialis (FDS) Flexor digitorum profundus (FDP)
Finger MCP flexion	Flexor digitorum profundus (FDP) Flexor digitorum superficialis (FDS) Dorsal interossei Volar (palmar) interossei Flexor digiti minimi (small finger only)
Finger adduction	Volar (palmar) interossei
Finger abduction	Dorsal interossei Abductor digiti minimi (small finger only)
Finger MCP extension	Extensor digitorum (ED) Extensor indicis proprius (index finger only) Extensor digiti minimi (small finger only)
Finger PIP/DIP extension	Lumbrical and interossei if MCP is flexed Dorsal and volar (palmar) interossei Extensor digitorum (ED) Extensor indicis proprius (index finger only) Extensor digiti minimi (small finger only)
Thumb IP extension	Extensor pollicis longus (EPL)
Thumb MCP extension	Extensor pollicis brevis (EPB) Extensor pollicis longus (EPL)
Thumb abduction	Abductor pollicis longus (APL) Abductor pollicis brevis (APB)
Thumb IP flexion	Flexor pollicis longus (FPL)
Thumb MCP flexion	Flexor pollicis brevis (FPB) Flexor pollicis longus (FPL)
Thumb adduction	Adductor pollicis
Opposition	Opponens pollicis (thumb) Opponens digiti minimi (small finger)
Hip flexion	Iliopsoas (iliacus and psoas major)
Hip extension	Gluteus maximus Biceps femoris

Knee flexion	Semimembranosus
	Semitendinosus
	Biceps femoris
Knee extension	Rectus femoris
	Vastus medialis
	Vastus intermedius
	Vastus lateralis
Ankle dorsiflexion	Tibialis anterior
	Extensor hallucis longus
	Extensor digitorum longus
Ankle plantarflexion	Gastrocnemius
	Soleus

Appendix H

Substitutions for Muscle Contraction

Scapular elevation	Pushing on the knees when sitting
Scapular depression	Gravity if sitting or using the fingers to inch the arm downward along a surface if prone
Scapular adduction	Gravity if sitting
Scapular abduction	Using the fingers to inch the arm outward along a surface if supine
Shoulder flexion	Trunk extension or substitution by shoulder abductors
Shoulder extension	Hunching the shoulders forward or shoulder abductors
Shoulder abduction	Long head of the biceps if humerus is externally rotated or trunk lateral flexion
Shoulder adduction	Gravity if sitting or using the fingers to inch the arm downward along a surface if supine

Stein, F., & Haertl, K.
Pocket Guide to Intervention in Occupational Therapy, Second Edition (pp 371-373).
© 2019 Taylor & Francis Group.

Shoulder horizontal abduction	Trunk rotation
Shoulder horizontal adduction	Trunk rotation
Shoulder external rotation	Scapula adduction + downward rotation, the triceps, or supination
Shoulder internal rotation	Scapula abduction + upward rotation, the triceps, or pronation
Elbow flexion	Wrist flexors
Elbow extension	Gravity if sitting, or external rotation to help gravity assist if in gravity-eliminated position
Pronation	Wrist and finger flexors
Supination	Wrist and finger extensors
Wrist extension	Extensor pollicis longus, extensor digitorum
Wrist flexion	Abductor pollicis longus, flexor pollicis longus, flexor digitorum superficial, and flexor digitorum profundus
Finger DIP flexion	Rebound of fingers following extension or tenodesis
Finger PIP flexion	Rebound of fingers following extension or tenodesis
Finger MCP flexion	Rebound of fingers following extension or tenodesis
Finger adduction	Extrinsic finger flexors or gravity for first palmar interosseus
Finger abduction	Extensor digitorum or gravity for dorsal interossei 3 and 4 and abductor digiti minimi
Finger MCP extension	Rebound of fingers following flexion or tenodesis
Finger PIP/DIP extension	Other muscles of extension if MCP is flexed

Thumb IP extension	Rebound of thumb following flexion, abductor pollicis brevis, adductor pollicis, and flexor pollicis brevis
Thumb MCP extension	Rebound of thumb following flexion
Thumb abduction	Extensor pollicis brevis
Thumb IP flexion	Rebound of thumb following extension
Thumb MCP flexion	Rebound of thumb following extension, abductor pollicis brevis, and adductor pollicis
Thumb adduction	Extensor pollicis longus, flexor pollicis longus, and flexor pollicis brevis
Opposition	Abductor pollicis brevis, flexor pollicis brevis, and flexor pollicis longus

Appendix I

Health Organization
Web Resources

ABLEDATA	part of NIDILRR: www.abledata.com
ACRM	American Congress of Rehabilitation Medicine: www.acrm.org
ADA	Americans with Disabilities Act: www.ada.gov
ADA-JAN	Job Accommodation Network (JAN): janweb.icdi.wvu.edu
ADAPT	American Disabled for Attendant Programs Today: www.adapt.org
AF	Arthritis Foundation: www.arthritis.org
AFB	American Foundation for the Blind: www.afb.org
AHA	American Heart Association: www.heart.org
AMA	American Medical Association: www.ama-assn.org
AOTA	American Occupational Therapy Association: www.aota.org
APA	American Psychological Association: www.apa.org

Stein, F., & Haertl, K.
*Pocket Guide to Intervention in Occupational
Therapy, Second Edition* (pp 375-377).
© 2019 Taylor & Francis Group.

APS	American Pain Society: http://americanpainsociety.org
APTA	American Physical Therapy Association: www.apta.org
ARC	The ARC (IDD): www.theArc.org
ARTSUSA	Americans for the Arts: www.artsusa.org
ASA	Autism Society of America: www.autism-society.org
ASHA	American Speech-Language Hearing Association: www.asha.org
ASHT	American Society of Hand Therapists: www.asht.org
CARF	The Rehabilitation Accreditation Commission: www.carf.org
CC	Canine Companions: www.cci.org
CDC	Centers for Disease Control: www.cdc.gov/injury
CPIR	Center for Parent Information and Resources: www.parentcenterhub.org
DHHS	Department of Health and Human Services: www.hhs.gov
DS	Down Syndrome (National Down Syndrome Society): www.ndss.org
ES	Easter Seals: www.easterseals.com
JCAHO	Joint Commission on Accreditation of Healthcare Organizations: www.jointcommission.org
MHN	Mental Health America: www.mentalhealthamerica.net
NAMI	National Alliance for the Mentally Ill: www.nami.org
NARHA	North American Riding for the Handicapped Association: http://narha.org
NARIC	National Rehabilitation Information Center: www.naric.com
NIDRR	National Institute on Disability and Rehabilitation Research: www.ed.gov/category/program/national-institute-disability-and-rehabilitation-research

NIH	National Institutes of Health: www.nih.gov
NIMH	National Institute of Mental Health: www.nimh.nih.gov
NINDS	National Institute of Neurological Disorders and Stroke: www.ninds.nih.gov
NIOSH	National Institute for Occupational Safety and Health: www.cdc.gov/niosh
NRCTBI	National Resource Center for Traumatic Brain Injury: http://www.tbinrc.com
OP	Orthotics and Prosthetics Professional Network: www.oandpnet.com
OSEP	Office of Special Education and Rehabilitation Programs: www2.ed.gov/about/offices/list/osers/index.html
OSHA	Occupational Safety and Health Administration: www.osha.gov
RESNA	Rehabilitation Engineering and Assistive Technology Society of North America: www.resna.org
RN	Rehab NET: https://rehabnet.com
SCI-USA	Spinal Cord Injury (United Spinal Association): https://unitedspinal.org
SIA	Spinal Injuries Association: www.goweb.com/sia
UCP	United Cerebral Palsy: www.ucp.org
USDE	United States Department of Education: www.ed.gov
WFOT	World Federation of Occupational Therapy: www.wfot.org
WHO	World Health Organization: www.who.int

Printed in the United States
by Baker & Taylor Publisher Services